Gastroenterology Research and Clinical Developments

nova
Medicine & Health
New York

Gastroenterology Research and Clinical Developments

Colonoscopy: Screening, Procedures and Preparation
Jihwan Ko, MD (Editor)
2023. ISBN: 979-8-89113-014-2 (Softcover)
2023. ISBN: 979-8-89113-071-5 (eBook)

Exercise and Diet as Modulators of Cognitive Function through Gut Microbiota
Natalia Arias, PhD (Editor)
Ismael Martínez-Guardado, PhD (Editor)
Francisco J. Grijota Pérez, PhD (Editor)
2022. ISBN: 979-8-88697-164-4 (Hardcover)
2022. ISBN: 979-8-88697-318-1 (eBook)

Gut Microbiome: Simplified! (For Medical, Nursing, Nutrition Students and Practitioners)
Ujjwal Sonika, MD, DM (Editor)
2022. ISBN: 979-8-88697-340-2 (Softcover)
2022. ISBN: 979-8-88697-379-2 (eBook)

Effects of Healthful Bioactive Compounds on the Gastrointestinal Tract
Amir M. Mortazavian, PhD, Nasim Khorshidian, PhD, Zahra Yari, PhD (Editors)
2022. ISBN: 978-1-68507-624-5 (Hardcover)
2022. ISBN: 978-1-68507-624-5 (eBook)

Probiotics and their Role in Health and Disease
Yusuf Olsen (Editor)
2021. ISBN: 978-1-53619-965-9 (Hardcover)
2021. ISBN: 978-1-53619-997-0 (eBook)

More information about this series can be found at
https://novapublishers.com/product-category/series/gastroenterology-research-and-clinical-developments/

Edward L. Stillman
Editor

Exploring Microbiotics in Health and Disease

Postbiotics, Probiotics, and Prebiotics

nova
Medicine & Health
New York

Library of Congress Cataloging-in-Publication Data

ISBN: 978-8-89113-410-2

Published by Nova Science Publishers, Inc. † New York

Contents

Preface

This book consists of thirteen chapters which will examine the role of microbiotics in health and disease. Chapter One encompasses the origin, selection, and identification of bifidobacteria in traditional foods, the impact of environmental factors on their presence in food, the production of bioactive compounds, as well as the immune response, antimicrobial effect, and antiparasitic effect induced by bifidobacteria found in traditional foods. Chapter Two discusses the biological role of postbiotic compounds as a promising tool for improving oral health. Chapter Three investigates the beneficial properties of honey as a natural postbiotic, including microbe metabolites, plant waste products, and bees. An overview of the concept of postbiotics and their clinical role in host health is presented in Chapter Four. Chapter Five touches upon how postbiotic compounds with safety profile and unique function in degradation of gluten peptides and promotion of the intestinal cell integrity can be considered novel and accessible approach in celiac diet-based therapy. Chapter Six gives a comprehensive overview of the latest developments in the field of drug delivery and discusses the primary in vivo pathways for the targeted delivery of postbiotics. Chapter Seven provides a clinical review of postbiotics described in the literature, including their mechanisms of action, characteristics, and potential therapeutic applications. In Chapter Eight a proteomic analysis of postbiotics in medical bacteriology is conducted. The authors of Chapter Nine provide research on how postbiotics are used in different mechanisms to treat many diseases, as well as improve the symptoms of colorectal cancer. In Chapter Ten the types, physiological functions and biosynthesis methods of HMOs are reviewed in order to make the future application of HMOs possible, such as additives for infant milk powder. The aim of Chapter Eleven is to approach the advantages of application of postbiotics as functional components in foods. In Chapter Twelve the authors discuss the therapeutic benefits of different postbiotic compounds for the therapy of food allergies in light of the numerous publications demonstrating the high biological function and safety of postbiotics. And finally, a review of the most recent applications of postbiotics for food bio-preservation and maintenance of their microbial safety status, current challenges, and future perspectives is provided in Chapter Thirteen.

Chapter 1

Bifidobacteria in Traditional Foods

Sarahí del Carmen Rangel-Ortega[1]
Rocío Guadalupe Castillo-Godina[1]
Martha Monzerrath Orozco-Sifuentes[1]
Sendar Daniel Nery-Flores[1]
Lissethe Palomo-Ligas[1]
Dora Elisa Cruz-Casas[1]
Carlos Neftali Cano-Gonzalez[2]
Lluvia de Abril Alexandra Soriano-Melgar[1]
Mariela Michel-Michel[3]
Jesús David García-Ortiz[1]
Sandra Lucía Teniente[1]
Stephany Nefertari Chávez-García[1]
Raúl Rodríguez-Herrera[1]
and Lizeth Guadalupe Campos-Muzquiz[1,*]

[1]Facultad de Ciencias Químicas, Universidad Autónoma de Coahuila, Saltillo, Coahuila, México
[2]Centro de Investigación en Química Aplicada, Saltillo, Coahuila, Mexico
[3]Tecnológico Nacional de México/ Instituto Tecnológico de Ciudad Valles, San Luis Potosí, México

[*] Corresponding Author's Email: l_campos@uadec.edu.mx.

In: Exploring Microbiotics in Health and Disease
Editor: Edward L. Stillman
ISBN: 978-8-89113-410-2

Abstract

Traditional foods play a significant role in the dietary habits of numerous cultures. These food items have been associated with nutritional benefits owing to the by-products generated through microbial starter culture fermentation. With the expanding field of functional foods, the utilization of certain bacteria, such as *Bifidobacterium* sp., as probiotics, has witnessed a notable increase. *Bifidobacterium*, a natural inhabitant of the human colon, exerts beneficial effects on the balance of the intestinal microbiota. It enhances defenses against pathogens, possesses antimicrobial and anticancer properties, and contributes to overall intestinal health. *Bifidobacterium* strains, including *B. animalis*, *B. bifidum*, *B. longum*, and *B. breve*, have been reported to exhibit biofunctional attributes and are commonly employed in traditional foods such as cheeses, beverages, sausages, and yogurts. These strains exert a positive influence on intestinal health. This chapter encompasses the origin, selection, and identification of bifidobacteria in traditional foods, the impact of environmental factors on their presence in food, the production of bioactive compounds (such as bioactive peptides, exopolysaccharides, conjugated linoleic acid, and short-chain fatty acids), as well as the immune response, antimicrobial effect, and antiparasitic effect induced by bifidobacteria found in traditional foods. Furthermore, the response of these bifidobacteria in *in vivo* models is discussed, along with the production of foods containing bifidobacteria as probiotics. Finally, future trends in the utilization of bifidobacteria derived from traditional foods to enhance intestinal health are addressed.

Keywords: traditional food, gut health, bifidobacteria

Introduction

The digestive system organs are colonized by a microbial ecosystem composed of trillions of microorganisms, including bifidobacteria (Zuo, Chen, and Marcotte 2020). Bifidobacteria are gram-positive, obligate anaerobic bacteria that do not form spores. They are related to the host's health since they participate in different metabolic processes not only related to the digestive tract but also to processes of the immune and nervous systems (Shori 2022; He et al. 2002). Therefore, they have been associated with reducing disorders such as diarrhea, hypertension, inflammation processes, cholesterol, pathogen colonization, effects of lactose intolerance, and cancer prevention (Chugh and Kamal-Eldin 2020; Zuo, Chen, and Marcotte 2020; Sharma, Wasan, and Sharma 2021). Among their multiple properties, these microorganisms' potential as a treatment against allergenic diseases, including food allergies, particularly those with high levels of immunoglobulin E (IgE), is particularly remarkable (An et al. 2022).

Probiotics are microorganisms that provide different health benefits in adequate concentrations or proportions, but they should remain alive and, therefore, must survive the components of the intestinal tract (bile and gastric fluids) (Bocchi et al. 2020). The most well-known probiotics come from the *Bifidobacterium* and *Lactobacillus* genera. The most used as commercial probiotics emphasizing *B. animalis* subsp. *lactis*, *B. bifidum*, *B. longum* subsp. *infantis*, *B. longum* subsp. *longum*, and *B. breve* (Li et al. 2023). These probiotic bacteria are widely used to produce foods, called functional because of their potential beneficial effect on human health (Chugh and Kamal-Eldin 2020).

Since time immemorial, humans have used different microorganisms directly or indirectly for food production and preservation, generating multiple applications in the food industry (Gholami-Shabani, Shams-Ghahfarokhi, and Razzaghi-Abyaneh 2023). One of the most used processes is fermentation, which modifies the flavor, texture, and nutraceutical composition of various foods, such as cheese, cream, yogurt, salami, pepperoni, bread, vinegar, wine, beer, and ice cream, among others (Gholami-Shabani, Shams-Ghahfarokhi, and Razzaghi-Abyaneh 2023; Patel et al. 2023). Foods, mainly fermented foods, are an important source of probiotics. Therefore, probiotics are usually present in traditional foods, mainly in dairy products (Bocchi et al. 2020). However, only a few bifidobacteria strains are known to be present in traditionally processed foods without a known or controlled microbiological substrate source. This chapter addresses the origin, selection, and identification of bifidobacteria in traditional foods, as well as the influence of the environment on the presence of bifidobacteria in foods, and the different responses of bifidobacteria and their effects as a source of probiotics, with a final focus on future trends.

Origin, Selection, and Identification of Bifidobacteria in Traditional Foods

Bifidobacteria Are Present in Traditional Food

Bifidobacteria are normal inhabitants of the human colon, and some strains have been isolated and used as starter cultures for milk fermentation (Chung et al. 2008). These bacteria can also be found in milk, cheeses made from raw milk, and meat (Martín et al. 2009; Yasmin et al. 2020; Bunesova et al. 2014). In fact, strains isolated from meat and raw milk serve as indicators of fecal contamination from animal sources (Gavini et al. 2006).

These microbes contained in traditional foods can improve the quality of the overall diet by providing health-related microbial metabolites. Researchers have been studying how these foodborne microbes impact the composition of gut microbes and have suggested that this could be a strategy to improve overall health through nutritional interventions (Roselli et al. 2021). Certain foods of Mexican origin have been used since pre-Hispanic times and are still commonly consumed in the present diet. According to reports, these foods contain various nutrients such as vitamins, minerals, antioxidants, and prebiotics. Many of these foods are considered functional and prebiotic since they stimulate the growth of beneficial strains of intestinal microbiota, such as *Bifidobacterium*, due to their prebiotic content (Valerino-Perea et al. 2019). For instance, cocoa (*Theobroma cacao*) has been shown to have prebiotic effects, which can promote the growth of intestinal bacteria such as *Bifidobacterium* spp. and alter bacterial diversity (Escutia-Gutiérrez, Almeida-López, and Sandoval-Rodríguez 2023). The consumption of crickets (*Acheta domesticus*) has been linked to the growth of *Bifidobacterium animalis*, which can improve intestinal health by reducing serum levels of the proinflammatory cytokine TNFα. Additionally, fiber derived from the cactus *Opuntia ficus-indica* has been reported to modify the composition of intestinal microbiota and increase bacterial diversity, including specific genera such as *Bifidobacterium* spp. The by-products of nixtamalized corn may be a source of prebiotic compounds such as ferulated arabinoxylans (Paz-Samaniego et al. 2019), which can promote the growth of probiotic bacteria of the genus *Bifidobacterium* (Martínez-López et al. 2016). Torres-Maravilla et al. (2022) mentioned that monosaccharides and oligosaccharides derived from simple cereals, including maize (*Zea mays* L.), showed antioxidant and prebiotic effects, stimulating the development of *Bifidobacterium* spp. and *Lactobacillus* spp. The fiber components of the agave (*Agave americana*) favor the growth of lactic acid bacteria, yeast communities, and *Bifidobacterium*. In nopal (*Opuntia ficus-indica*), the metabolic and prebiotic effect of the peel was analyzed by means of an *in vivo* model. They assessed an increase in cecal lactic acid bacteria and bifidobacteria (Perez-Chabela et al. 2015). The juice of the nopal fruit showed a significant increase in the growth of intestinal bacteria. The mucilage and stems were also analyzed, and prebiotic effects were found *in vitro*. Pinto beans (*Phaseolus vulgaris* L.)

increased the activity of *Lactobacillus* and *Bifidobacterium* in an *in vivo* model of *Gallus gallus* (Dias et al. 2019).

The probiotic potential of bifidobacteria allows its culture to be used in various food systems due to its safety aspects and different functional attributes. For the detection and selection of probiotics, the Food and Agriculture Organization (FAO) and the World Health Organization (WHO) have developed basic criteria (Yasmin et al. 2020), which suggest the identification of genera, species, and strains using genotypic and phenotypic methods (FAO/WHO 2006). Phenotypic methods are less reproducible and have less discriminatory power than genotypic methods because the expression of a phenotypic character results from the interaction of the genotype with the environment and is, therefore, susceptible to modification when environmental conditions vary (Pérez et al. 2012).

In general, strains used in the industry must maintain their properties during storage and survive processing conditions similar to those of the digestive tract (Moreno et al. 2018). The criteria used to select starter cultures include their ability to produce flavor and their acidification rate. The key characteristics required for lactic acid bacteria (LAB) to be used as probiotics in the manufacturing industry include recognition as safe (GRAS - generally recognized as safe), viability during processing and storage, antagonistic effects against pathogens, tolerance to bile acid challenge, adherence to the host's intestinal epithelium, and other relevant characteristics (Vélez et al. 2007).

Culture-dependent methods for isolating microbial populations have been widely studied, but the current focus is on selection and identification using molecular techniques, DNA extraction methods, and the choice of polymerase chain reaction (PCR) primers to generate amplicons for next-generation sequencing (NGS) analysis. REP-PCR is a typing technique that uses primers that hybridize with repeated (rep) DNA sequences, which are found distributed in the chromosomes of many organisms, such as Enterobacteriaceae, some gram-positive bacteria, and even fungi. With this technique, the regions that separate the repeated sequences are amplified, so that the polymorphism results from both the variability in the repetition of the sequences and the distance between contiguous copies. For the identification of *Bifidobacterium*, analysis of the 16S rRNA gene sequences is the most widely used due to its high reproducibility (Cifuentes-Orjuela 2018). For instance, Nzingula et al. (2023) identified the 16S rRNA gene of *Bifidobacterium* in breast milk. Since the genus *Bifidobacterium* inhabits a wide range of hosts, such as insects, birds, and mammals. Dyachkova,

Chekalin, and Danilenko (2019) established a host-bacteria relationship by analyzing a selection of PFNA genes (*pkb2, fn3, aaa-atp*) present in the genomes of species of the genus *Bifidobacterium* to identify codons that underwent adaptive evolution of the *Bifidobacterium* phylogenetic tree.

Traditional Food Production with Bifidobacteria as a Source of Probiotics

Bifidobacteria have been used in the production of various foods throughout history. Their main purpose in the food industry is to produce fermented products such as yogurt, cheese, milk, and juice. Recently, the effects of bifidobacteria on the production of other products with prebiotic, antioxidant, and anti-inflammatory properties have been studied. Bifidobacteria are known for their saccharolytic metabolism, which results in the production of mainly acetic and lactic acid. Although the production of ethanol and formic acid from fermentation is possible, their yield is relatively low (Bottacini, van Sinderen, and Ventura 2017).

The production of short-chain fatty acids (SCFAs) from substrates has been reported in the literature. These SCFAs serve as prebiotic sources and are used in products with thickening properties, such as starch and various gums (e.g., locust bean, guar, tragacanth, arabic, xanthan, and karaya gums). The production of these by-products depends on the species of bifidobacteria and the characteristics of the strain used. Apart from their prebiotic effects, bifidobacteria have been suggested to be used in symbiotic mixtures with other probiotics to achieve a synergistic effect. Studies have shown the beneficial effects of such mixtures, in improving gut health (Luo et al. 2018; Modrackova et al. 2019).

Some studies suggest that bifidobacteria can influence the production of functional foods with a higher content of isoflavones, which are phytoestrogens, that have been recognized for their beneficial health effects. Daidzin and genistin are the main isoflavones present in soy-containing foods (Gaya, Peirotén, and Landete 2017). By combining bifidobacteria, which have biotechnological capabilities to produce bioactive compounds, with functional foods that are rich in isoflavones, these compounds could become more bioavailable, thus providing a beneficial effect on consumer health (Huang, Cai, and Xu 2014; Delgado et al. 2019).

Fermentation with bifidobacteria not only increases the absorption of bioactive compounds such as isoflavones, but it can also reduce the content of antinutrients present in soy drinks, such as phytic acid, and increase the concentration of B complex vitamins. These beneficial properties are believed to be due to the presence of β-glucosidases (Bowey, Adlercreutz, and Rowland 2003). Similarly, the use of bifidobacteria to produce fermented flaxseed beverages has gained attention due to the presence of biologically active compounds, such as lignans and flavonoids, which are often present in non-bioavailable forms and require metabolism by these bacteria to become available (Landete et al. 2016; Peirotén, Bravo, and Landete 2020).

Therefore, research is being conducted to explore the use of cocultures of bifidobacteria strains as an alternative to improving the nutritional properties of flaxseed-based beverages. This approach could ensure the production of enterolignans and flavonoids such as herbacetin and quercetagetin. Although foods like soybeans and flaxseeds have health benefits, these effects are attributed to the metabolism of bifidobacteria present in the intestinal microbiota, which transform functional compounds into metabolites with greater availability for the consumer. Hence, adding bifidobacteria to products could help provide additional amounts of these biocompounds (Ghedini et al. 2017; Ruiz de la Bastida et al. 2021; Gaya et al. 2016).

The fermentative process with bifidobacteria has been found to produce various metabolites, including exopolysaccharides. These polysaccharides have been shown to have several beneficial effects such as antitumor, cholesterol-lowering, and immunomodulatory properties, as well as technological properties like the production of biofilms to increase the shelf life of different foods. Furthermore, exopolysaccharides have been utilized as emulsifying agents in the food industry (Llamas-Arriba et al. 2019). Bifidobacteria also possess specific enzymes for the synthesis of isomers of conjugated linoleic acid (CLA) and conjugated linolenic acid (CLNA), which exhibit anti-cancer and anti-inflammatory properties. Therefore, bifidobacteria have been used as a starter culture to produce functional foods with high levels of these specific isomers of CLA and CLNA, as well as for the preparation of dietary supplements offering the consumer additional health benefits (Gorissen et al. 2012).

Influence of the Environment on the Presence of Bifidobacteria in Food

The upward trend in the production of bifidobacteria-containing food products is predicted to persist. To achieve favorable outcomes, manufacturers must consider the impact of the food's environmental conditions during production and storage, to guarantee that the concentration of bifidobacteria at the time of consumption delivers an effective dose to consumers. Furthermore, foods that have been fortified with bifidobacteria must maintain their sensory properties that are characteristic of the respective traditional food (Boylston et al. 2004).

Effect of Traditional Food Environment on Survival of Bifidobacteria

It is assumed that the effectiveness of probiotics can be measured by their ability to remain alive and viable. The viability of probiotics is often compromised by environmental factors, including the acidity of the food, temperature, shelf conservation, and the presence of oxygen in the packaging (Mayorga-Reyes et al. 2009). To classify a food as functional due to its probiotic activity, it is important to ensure that a sufficient number of live bacteria (10^6 CFU/mL or g) reach the colon, which mainly requires the bacteria to withstand pH changes, as they will be exposed to the gastric juices of the stomach and bile salts during the digestion process in the gastrointestinal tract (GIT) (Castillo-Escandón et al. 2019; Ventura et al. 2006).

There are factors that decrease the viability of bacteria in food and modify its quality, among them are acidity, dissolved oxygen, the concentration of metabolites produced by the bacteria itself (organic acids), water activity, osmotic pressure, interaction with the food matrix, processing, and shelf life. The survival of probiotics depends to a large extent on the type of food matrix and the species of microorganism used, for which it is necessary to analyze and study in a particular way for each interaction (Castillo-Escandón et al. 2019; Allouche et al. 2018). Studies have shown that bifidobacteria that have been subjected to stress conditions during the exponential growth phase or stationary phase can develop greater resistance to stress conditions (Takahashi et al. 2004).

The tolerance to survive under acidic conditions is influenced by the species and it is very likely that this process is mediated by the increase in the expression of membrane proteins. *In vitro* gastric juice simulation tests have shown the behavior of different strains of bifidobacteria under acidic conditions. It has been observed that this resistance is dependent on the pH and the time they remain exposed to acid, their contact and exposure to bile salts (Bezkorovainy 2001; Ventura et al. 2006; Mayorga-Reyes et al. 2009).

In a study conducted by Vinderola et al. (2000), the feasibility of utilizing Argentinian Fresco cheese as a vehicle for probiotic cultures was assessed. The research indicated that nine distinct combinations of *Lactobacillus acidophilus* and bifidobacteria exhibited adequate viability levels (decrease in counts of less than one log order in 60 days) in the cheese and demonstrated good adaptation to the Fresco cheese microenvironment. Furthermore, in a simulated test under acidic conditions resembling the stomach, the probiotic cultures displayed exceptional survival rates for up to 3 hours. Notably, *Bifidobacterium bifidum* exhibited the highest level of resistance among the evaluated microorganisms. Table 1 shows some species of bifidobacteria and their tolerance to acid conditions and the use of some food matrices to increase tolerance.

Table 1. *Bifidobacterium* species and their tolerance to acidic conditions

Species	Conditions/matrices	Authors
B. bifidum	Tolerant to pH 1.8 in periods of 80 min, with a 20% decrease in active biomass.	Marteau et al. 1997
B. animalis subps. lactis	Tolerant to pH 3 for 180 min	Pochart et al. 1992
B. infantis 25962	It tolerates gastric transit in the presence of milk proteins, which act as buffering agents.	Charteris et al. 1998
B. longum BL1	Survives in fermented milk at pH 3 for 2 hours.	Takahashi et al. 2004
B. infantis	Bacteria from fermentation (24h) inoculated in pH 4 media remain stable for 4 hours.	Mayorga-Reyes et al. 2009
Bifidobacterium BB-12	Goat milk fat maintains its viability up to 94% in acidic environments	Verruck et al. 2017
B. animalis	Goat milk ice cream maintains the viability of bifidobacteria strains in in vitro digestion at pH 4.	Kowalczyk et al. 2022

Bifidobacteria are categorized as strict anaerobes. Nonetheless, the level of oxygen tolerance exhibited by bifidobacteria is reliant on the particular species and culture medium. Studies have demonstrated that selecting oxygen-resistant mutants of *Bifidobacterium bifidum* and other bifidobacteria can improve the survival of bifidobacterial strains in foods during processing and storage (Mutai et al. 1980). Goat cheese is typically considered an anaerobic environment with a low redox potential ranging from -250 to -350 mV (Gomes and Malcata 1998).

Salinity is another crucial factor affecting the survival of bifidobacteria in traditional foods. Fortin et al. (2011) investigated the impact of salt addition on the survival of *Bifidobacterium longum* during cheddar cheese production and found that salting resulted in a 13% reduction in cell count in the whey during processing. Additionally, after three days of storage, a further 3 log cfu/mL loss in *B. longum* viability was observed.

Probiotic Preservation Strategies

Due to heterogeneity in the tolerance of bifidobacteria to stress factors, industrial production, and commercialization of many these bacteria is challenging. This has intensified the interest in understanding the stress physiology of these bacteria (Schöpping, Zeidan, and Franzén 2022). One strategy to keep the bacteria metabolically active during their passage through the gastrointestinal tract (GIT) is to include them in matrices that buffer the effects of acidic pH. Fermented products derived from milk are the main vehicles for *Lactobacillus* and *Bifidobacterium*, where milk proteins are used (Table 1). Currently, new food matrices are being implemented to increase tolerance to low pH conditions. These include products of plant origin such as fruits, vegetables, cereals, and beverages, among others (Castillo-Escandón et al. 2019).

In the case of drinks based on fruits and vegetables, whose acceptance in the market is widely known, probiotics can be added to the drink, without the need to ferment it, or they can be added to obtain fermented juices. In unfermented drinks, special care must be taken regarding the pH, since there are fruits such as kiwi and pineapple that have a degree of acidity that affects specific bacteria, while in fermented drinks temperature regulation (refrigeration) is a factor preponderant for its conservation (Ranadheera et al. 2017).

Edible films or coatings are an alternative to increase the shelf life of minimally processed foods, acting as a barrier that controls interaction with the environment, maintains humidity, and prevents lipid oxidation. These coatings are an excellent option for the immobilization and controlled release of probiotics while protecting them from environmental conditions. There are three types of coatings: hydrocolloids made up of proteins or carbohydrates, lipids composed of acylglycerols, fatty acids, or waxes, and combinations of the first two (Castillo-Escandón et al. 2019; Pavli et al. 2018).

Encapsulation is a way of coating that can improve the stability of probiotics, and it can be achieved through various techniques such as atomization, complex coacervation, interfacial polymerization, molecular inclusion, emulsification, lyophilization, liposomes, and ionic gelation. These techniques involve using different materials, such as lipids, proteins, dextrins, gums, alginates, and plant extracts, but the most common ones are polysaccharides that can form spherical macroparticles (Rodríguez, Rojas, and Rodríguez, 2016).

There is a wide range of options available to maintain the viability and stability of probiotic microorganisms in food and ensure that they reach their destination in sufficient numbers within the gastrointestinal tract. The choice of method depends on a thorough study of the species, as microorganisms within the same genus can exhibit highly variable behavior depending on the environmental conditions they are exposed to.

Production of Bioactive Compounds by Bifidobacteria

Traditional foods have benefits for gut health thanks to bioactive compounds produced by bifidobacteria, such as peptides, exopolysaccharides, conjugated linoleic acid, antioxidants, and short-chain fatty acids.

Bioactive Peptides

The *Bifidobacterium* genus is recognized to provide health benefits to the host (Chen, Chen, and Ho 2021), as numerous studies have shown that *Bifidobacterium* can release a wide range of bioactive compounds, such as short-chain fatty acids, bacteriocins, exopolysaccharides, vitamins, and bioactive peptides (Chugh and Kamal-Eldin 2020). Among biomolecules, bioactive peptides are noteworthy because they can meet basic nutritional requirements and provide beneficial effects for consumer health. Bioactive peptides are small fragments, typically comprising 2 to 20 amino acids, which are derived from proteins (Fan et al. 2022). They exhibit various bioactivities, including antihypertensive (Wang et al. 2019), immunomodulatory (Cai et al. 2022), antidiabetic (Wang et al. 2019), antimicrobial (Tkaczewska 2020), antioxidant (Fan et al. 2022), anti-inflammatory (Aursuwanna et al. 2022), hepatoprotective (Liu et al. 2018), cognitive (Katayama, Corpuz, and Nakamura 2021), and other activities. Regarding their impact on intestinal health, these peptides possess diverse properties, including anti-inflammatory, cytoimmunomodulatory, immunomodulatory, antimicrobial, anti-appetizing, and mineral-binding activities (Rafiq et al. 2021). Lactic acid bacteria, including *Bifidobacterium*, release bioactive peptides from parent proteins through a proteolytic system. This process involves three essential steps: (1) hydrolysis of the protein by proteases that are linked to the cell envelope of the microorganism, producing oligopeptides and some extracellular peptides; (2) transport of these nitrogenous compounds into the bacterium via various transport systems; and (3) intracellular hydrolysis of oligopeptides and peptides by peptidases, producing free amino acids. The first step of the process releases bioactive peptides (Juillard, Lopez-Kleine, and Monnet 2022). So far, the cell envelope proteolytic system (CEP) of the *Bifidobacterium* genus remains unknown. However, it is established that *Bifidobacterium* is auxotrophic and unable to synthesize some essential amino acids, making the use of proteolytic systems vital for survival (Chang et al. 2013). Additionally, *Bifidobacterium* releases bioactive peptides through the CEP. It is noteworthy that the bioactivity of these peptides is influenced by several factors, including the *Bifidobacterium* species, isolation source, and the protein source from which the peptides are released (Juillard, Lopez-Kleine, and Monnet 2022).

Several strains of *Bifidobacterium* have been reported to produce ACE-I inhibitory (Ha et al. 2015), antioxidant (Chang et al. 2013), antibacterial, antimutagenic (Heydari et al. 2023), immunomodulatory (Albenzio et al. 2017), and hypocholesterolemic (Ismail et al. 2019) peptides, as summarized in Table 2. However, reports of bioactive peptides released by *Bifidobacterium* strains remain scarce (Chen, Chen, and Ho 2021). Among lactic acid bacteria, *B. lactis* has been shown to have strong proteolytic activity, resulting in higher bioactivity compared to bacteria such as *Streptococcus thermophilus* and *Lactobacillus delbreuckii* ssp. *bulgaricus* (Heydari et al. 2023). Moreover, most *Bifidobacterium* strains are recognized as probiotics (Markowiak and Śliżewska 2017), which makes them an attractive source of bioactive peptides due to their GRAS status (Venegas-Ortega et al. 2019). Nonetheless, the bioactivity of peptides produced by *Bifidobacterium* strains can vary depending on factors such as the species, source of isolation, and the protein source from which the peptides are released.

The production of these peptides has been identified in traditional foods. For instance, in Scamorza cheese with probiotics, a mixture of

Bifidobacterium longum and *Bifidobacterium lactis* or *Lactobacillus acidophilus* were used as probiotic strains (Albenzio et al. 2015). Similarly, in ripened cheese, a combination of *Lactobacillus acidophilus* and bifidobacteria were used as starter cultures and bioactive peptides were obtained (Ryhänen, Pihlanto-Leppälä, and Pahkala 2001).

The use of *Bifidobacterium* strains to produce bioactive peptides is an area of opportunity to obtain new amino acid sequences with potential biological effects. Further research with this genus is needed. Since it is known that the proteolytic system of LAB is strain-dependent (Cruz-Casas et al. 2023).

Table 2. *Bifidobacterium* species producing peptides with different bioactivities

***Bifidobacterium* species**	**Peptide sequence**	**Bioactivity**	**Source**	**Reference**
B. longum KACC91563	VLSLSQSKVLPVPQK, VLSLSQSKVLPVPQKAVPYPQRDMPIQA	Antioxidant	Bovine casein	Chang et al. 2013
B. lactis	NI	Antioxidant Antimutagenic Antibacterial	Yoghurt	Heydari et al. 2023
B. bifidum	LVYPFP	ACE-I inhibitory	Fermented milk	Gonzalez-Gonzalez, Gibson, and Jauregi 2013
B. longum *B. lactis*	VLGPVRGPFPI, RPKHPIKHQGLPQEVLNENLLRF, KAGAESGGMEMS, SAEPTVHSTPTTE, RPKHPI, ETHLEAQPTVASAQ, LALLFSILVLFIMPM, RGGGAGEEE	ACE-I inhibitory Antimicrobial Immunomodulating	Pasta filata Scamorza ovine cheeses	Albenzio et al. 2015

NI: Not identified.

Exopolysaccharides

Exopolysaccharides (EPS) are secondary metabolites excreted into the growth medium by some gram-positive bacteria. EPS are natural polymers of varying composition and molecular weight, which impart unique physicochemical and biological properties. The design of EPS depends on the conformation of different types of monosaccharides and whether the molecules are linear or branched (Yang et al. 2023; Xu et al. 2019). EPS are classified into homopolysaccharides (hoPS) and heteropolysaccharides (hePS), based on their chemical composition and polysaccharide synthesis route. HoPS are characterized by the presence of a single type of monosaccharide in the structure, with an average molecular weight of 10^6 Da and α and β bonds. The prominent hoPS are glucans, fructans, and galactans (Zhou et al. 2019; Tiwari et al. 2021). Heteropolysaccharides (hePS), on the other hand, have the characteristic of presenting in their structure three or more types of monosaccharides that make up the polysaccharide with a molecular weight range of 10^4 to 10^6 Da. The hePS have α and β bonds, are mainly branched, and are made of glucose, galactose, and rhamnose. They also contain a smaller percentage of other monosaccharides such as fucose, arabinose, mannose, N-acetylglucosamine, N-acetylgalactosamine, and glucuronic acid, as well as non-carbohydrates such as pyruvate, acetate, succinate, and phosphate, which are intermediate products of carbohydrate metabolism (Yang et al. 2023; Zhou et al. 2019; Daba, Elnahas, and Elkhateeb 2021). Because they are safe, hePS can be used as natural food additives to improve texture, acting as thickeners, emulsifiers, and stabilizers of traditional foods (Xu et al. 2019).

EPS are not only known for their rheological properties but also for their beneficial biological activities, including antioxidant, immunomodulatory, anticancer, antibacterial effects, control of glycemic indexes, blood pressure, and cholesterol, as well as their ability to induce the colonization of probiotics in the host intestine (Tiwari et al. 2021; Schmid, Sieber, and Rehm 2015; Angelin and Kavitha 2020). Among the EPS properties, molecular weight (MW) plays a crucial role. High MW EPS generates high viscosity, making it an ideal thickener and possesses anti-inflammatory activity. In contrast, low MW EPS is better soluble, waterproof, and has anticancer effects (colon) (Schmid, Sieber, and Rehm 2015; Soumya and Nampoothiri 2021). Modifications such as phosphorylation, sulfation, acetylation, and depolymerization of EPS enhance their bioactivities, including anticancer, antioxidant, antibacterial, and toxin antagonistic effects. Moreover, EPS exhibits high digestion tolerance and can support the colonization of probiotics in the intestine, making it an excellent prebiotic agent (Schmid, Sieber, and Rehm 2015; Salazar et al. 2009; Xu et al. 2017).

Ten *Bifidobacterium* species have been reported to synthesize EPS, primarily HePS, with a molecular weight range lower than that of HoPS (Xu et al. 2019; Derrien et al. 2022). The synthesis pathway of HoPS involves enzymes for polymerizing glucose units, namely transglucosidases (dextransucrases, mutansucrases, and reuteransucrases), and for polymerizing fructose units using transfructosidases (levansucrases and inulosucrases). The genes encoding transglucosidases and transfructosidases are *gtf* and *ftf*, respectively (Xu et al. 2019; Schmid, Sieber, and Rehm 2015; Soumya and Nampoothiri 2021). The synthesis pathway of HePS is more complex, owing to the greater diversity of monosaccharides and organic molecules that can comprise the EPS structure. The biosynthesis of HePS is proposed to occur in four stages: (1) transport and phosphorylation of monosaccharides, (2) formation of sugar-nucleotides from glucose-1-phosphate (UDP-glucose, UDP-galactose, and dTDP-rhamnose) and the glycolysis intermediate fructose-6-phosphate (GDP-fucose, GDP-mannose, UDP-N-acetylglucosamine, and UDP-N-acetylgalactosamine), (3) formation of EPS repeat units, and (4) polymerization of the repeating units to form the EPS chain (Soumya and Nampoothiri 2021; Altmann et al. 2016). The correct formation of HePS genes involves those that participate in housekeeping genes and those that are specific for EPS (eps genetic cluster). These genes are related to the regulation, synthesis of the repetitive units, determination of the degree of polymerization, and the formation and export of the EPS. Approximately 24 enzymes participate in HePS biosynthesis (Xu et al. 2019; Soumya and Nampoothiri 2021; Castro-Bravo et al. 2018).

Production of Bifidobacterium EPS

Bifidobacterium animalis RH produces a HePS consisting of a linear region made up of glucose, galactose, and mannose, and a branched region consisting of glucose and arabinose. The monosaccharides are linked by α 1→3, 1→4, and 1→6 glycosidic bonds. The neutral HePS has a molecular weight of 2.31 x 10^4 Da. *B. animalis* was cultured in PTYG (Peptone-tryptone-yeast extract-glucose) medium for 48 h, and the HePS was precipitated with ethanol. The HePS was then purified using ion exchange chromatography (DEAE-Sepharose column) and gel filtration (Sepharose CL-6B column). Structural characterization was determined using gas chromatography-mass spectrometry (GC-MS), and the immunomodulatory activity was evaluated using specific pathogen-free Kunming murine models (Xu et al. 2017; Shang, Xu, and Li 2013). *Bifidobacterium longum* subsp. *longum* 35624 was cultured in MRS medium for 60 hours, followed by ethanol precipitation to recover HePS from the medium. The purification process involved size exclusion chromatography using a PL aquagel-OH MIXED-H 8 column and anion exchange using an EconoPac-Q cartridge column. The structure of the HePS synthesized by *B. longum* includes glucose, galactose, galacturonic acid, and 6-deoxy-talose in a ratio of approximately 2:2:1:1, respectively. The HePS has an approximate molecular weight of 1 x 10^4. It exhibits biological activities such as inhibition of osteoclast formation and dampening of host proinflammatory response. *B. longum* subsp. *infantis* CCUG 52486 and *B. infantis* NCIMB 702205 were cultured in milk for 24 hours, and the EPS was recovered using TCA and later ethanol precipitation.

The EPS was partially purified by gel filtration chromatography. The HePS of *B. longum* and *B. infantis* comprises glucose and galactose, giving a MW of 7.48 x 10^4 and 1.36 x 10^6, respectively. Due to their rheological properties, such as high solution viscosity and emulsifying activity, these EPS can be applied in the food industry (Prasanna et al. 2012). *B. animalis* subsp. *lactis* BB12 was cultured in milk permeate for 48 h, and the EPS was precipitated with ethanol. It was then purified by dialysis (MW cut-off of 14 kDa). The structural characterization was carried out by GC-MS, showing the presence of glucose, galactose, glucuronic acid, rhamnose, and xylose. This HePS exhibits antioxidant activity, which makes it suitable as a food additive (Amiri et al. 2019). *B. longum* subsp. *longum* IPLA E44 and *B. animalis* subsp. *lactis* IPLA R1 were cultured in MRSc medium for 24 h. After the incubation time, the EPS was precipitated with ethanol, and partially purified by dialysis (12-14 kDa MW cutoff) for three days (Salazar et al. 2009). The EPS of *B. longum* subsp. *longum* IPLA E44 is composed of glucose and galactose monosaccharides with a molecular weight of 11.1 x 10^6 Da. This EPS has been found to exhibit prebiotic activity (Salazar et al. 2009). In another study, *B. bifidum* WBBI01, WBIN03, *B. breve* WBBR04, *B. infantis* WBAN07, and *B. longum* WBLO01 were grown in MRS medium for 48 h. The resulting EPS was recovered by ethanol precipitation and purified by dialysis using a pore size of 3.5 kDa. The purified EPS showed regulatory activity in anaphylaxis in mice (Luo et al. 2020). Similarly, *B. bifidum* WBIN03 was grown in MRSc medium for 24 h, and the EPS was recovered by ethanol precipitation and purified by gel filtration chromatography using a Bio-Gel P-30 column. This EPS exhibits attractive antibacterial and antioxidant activity and has potential applications (Li et al. 2014). *B. animalis* subsp. *lactis* A1dOxR was cultured in MRSc medium for three days, and the EPS was recovered by ethanol precipitation and partially purified by dialysis. This EPS presents immunomodulatory activity in blood and gut-associated lymphoid tissue (Hidalgo-Cantabrana et al. 2014). *B. breve* strains also synthesize EPS in MRS medium, which can block dendritic cell maturation and activate CD4+ T cells

(Hickey et al. 2021). Furthermore, the EPS synthesized by *B. breve* UCC2003 exhibits immunomodulatory activity and offers protection against pathogens (Fanning et al. 2012).

B. animalis subsp. *lactis* DSM10140 and S89L can also synthesize EPS, which interacts with TLR4 in intestinal epithelial cells (Castro-Bravo et al. 2018). Finally, *B. longum* BCRC 14634 was cultured in MRS medium for 48 h, and the synthesized EPS was precipitated with ethanol. This EPS has been found to immunomodulate macrophages and can be used as an antimicrobial additive in food (Wu et al. 2010).

Optimizing the fermentation process is important for obtaining exopolysaccharides from probiotics. For example, Amiri et al. (2021) used the Box-Behnken design to optimize the fermentation process of whey supplemented with *Bifidobacterium lactis* BB12. This approach resulted in the production of conjugated linoleic acid (CLA), exopolysaccharides (EPSs), and bacteriocins (BACs).

Conjugated Linoleic Acid

Probiotic bacteria produce a wide range of bioactive molecules that offer health benefits, including bioactive lipids such as conjugated linoleic acid (CLA). Researchers have shown great interest in harnessing the potential of probiotic lactobacilli and bifidobacteria as CLA producers. *Bifidobacterium lactis* is a commonly used probiotic strain in the production of fermented milk products and has been extensively studied for its CLA biosynthetic capabilities. Given that most species within these genera can produce CLA and have been generally recognized as "safe" (GRAS), they present promising options for CLA production (Amiri et al. 2020).

Bifidobacteria are considered one of the most important probiotics due to their ability to promote health. By maintaining homeostasis between the microbiota in the human gut, stimulating intestinal immunity, activity against pathogens such as *Salmonella* spp., suppressing the expression of oncogenic genes, and preventing certain chronic diseases (Mei et al. 2022).

Conjugated linoleic acid (CLA) refers to the positional and geometric isomers of linoleic acid (LA; c9c12-C18:2) and alpha-linolenic acid (LNA; c9c12c15-C18:3) show in Figure 1. (Dahiya and Puniya 2017; Gorissen et al. 2015; B. Yang et al. 2014). Conjugated linoleic acid is a group of 18 conjugated carbons, where carbons in different positions form different geometric isomers. CLA has various activities within these anti-inflammatory, antihypertensive, anticancer, antioxidant, anti-atherosclerotic, and anti-obesity properties, among others (Mei et al. 2022).

The enzyme linoleate isomerase (LAI) is necessary to produce CLA and CLNA from linoleic acid and alpha-linolenic acid, respectively. This enzyme has been found in several types of bacteria, including bifidobacterial (Gorissen et al. 2012). *Bifidobacterium* has been reported to have a high bioconversion rate and higher CLA production. It is also recognized as one of the best producers of CLA among microorganisms (Mei et al. 2022). Several studies have investigated the potential of food-grade bacteria to produce CLA and CLNA isomers using milk-based media. Also *B. breve, B. dentium* and *Bifidobacterium lactis* have been reported to have good conversion of LA (0.55 mg/l) to CLA in MRS medium (Gorissen et al. 2012).

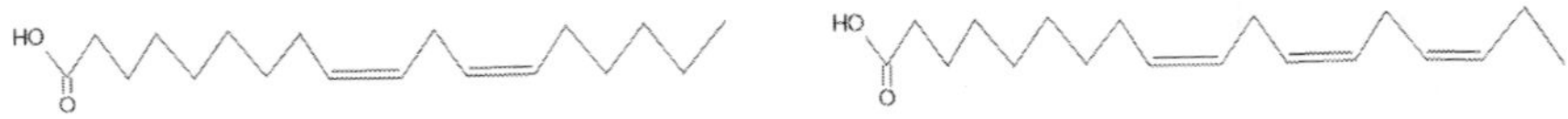

Figure 1. Structures of LA left (c9c12-C18:2) and LNA right (c9c12c15-C18:3).

Antioxidants

The presence of high concentrations of reactive oxygen species (ROS), such as superoxide anion, peroxide, hydrogen, and hydroxyl radicals, can cause damage to an organism through oxidative stress, leading to damage to proteins, DNA, and lipids, decreasing cell viability and resulting in cell death. Therefore, alternative methods are being sought to limit this type of effect through the consumption of antioxidants (AO) (Feng and Wang 2020). Various studies have proposed different ways of obtaining these AO compounds, and one current alternative is the use of microorganisms, which is increasing in both the food and pharmaceutical industries. This approach offers advantages such as rapid production, low toxicity, and biodegradability compared to synthetic antioxidants. Additionally, microorganisms present a therapeutic alternative due to their anti-inflammatory, anticancer, antidiabetic, and antineurodegenerative effects (Kim et al. 2020; Martorell et al. 2021; Rani et al. 2021; Yang Wang et al. 2017; Yao et al. 2021). Among the microorganisms proposed to produce antioxidants are bifidobacteria and various probiotics.

Table 3. Previous work on the production of antioxidants with multiple effects from bifidobacterial

Culture	Model	Effect	Reference
B. animalis 01	Cell culture supernatant // Aged mice	Free radical scavenging, increased antioxidant enzyme activity, MDA, lipofuscin, and MAO reduction	Shen, Shang, and Li 2011
B. animalis, B. breve y *B. longum*	Fermented lupine, quinoa, and wheat	Increased antioxidant capacity, polyphenolic content, inhibition of α-glucosidase, cytotoxicity of Caco-2 and MCF-7 cells.	Ayyash et al. 2018
B. longum CUETM 172	Fermented milk	High antioxidant capacity with high oxygen radical absorbance capacity (ORAC).	Gagnon, Savard, Rivière, LaPointe, et al. 2015
B. longum CCFM 752	Cell culture supernatant	Inhibition of NADPH oxidase, altered transcriptomic profile, increased CAT activity.	Yusheng Wang et al. 2021
B. longum KACC 91563	Bovine casein hydrolysate	Increased antioxidant activity due to the presence of bioactive peptides.	Chang et al. 2013
B. longum	Fermented goat's milk	High antioxidant potential by scavenging free radicals, regulating lactic acid bacteria numbers, and altered pH and lactic acid values.	Hanum, Yurliasni, and Seutia 2022
B. bifidum	Encapsulated supplement with probiotics	Increased plasma antioxidant capacity, reduction of C-reactive protein, plasma malondialdehyde and plasma glucose.	Soleimani et al. 2017
B. bifidum	Fermented blackberry juice	Promote changes in the phytochemical profile by increasing the antioxidant capacity after the fermentation process.	Wu et al. 2021
B. lactis	Fermented milk	High antioxidant capacity.	Gagnon et al. 2015
B. infantis	Cell-free culture supernatant // Topical use	DPPH, ABTS, -OH and O_2 radical scavenger, reduction of intracellular ROS, malondialdehyde and enhanced antioxidant enzyme activities (CAT, SOD and GSH-Px) in H_2O_2treated HaCaT cells.	Ma et al. 2022
B. lactis	Yoghurt	Improve antioxidant capacity and bioactive peptide content.	Heydari et al. 2023

These microorganisms possess different antioxidant processes and mechanisms that interact with the environment, as has been demonstrated in various reports (see Table 3). The application of these microorganisms in food fermentation processes has been shown to improve food production due to the benefits they provide (Feng and Wang 2020). These bacteria possess genetic characteristics that allow them to produce different metabolites with antioxidant activity (Oberg and Broadbent 2016), which enable the elimination of free radicals and limit oxidative stress in cells by increasing oxygen tolerance. Bifidobacteria employ various antioxidant mechanisms, including the production of enzymes with antioxidant properties (see Table 4), such as pseudocatalase (Mn-Kat) and heme-dependent catalase (Heme-Kat), which limit the toxicity of H_2O_2. Additionally, the production of ferredoxin enables the reduction of Fe^{2+} levels by iron chelation, and the activation of other antioxidant methods such as the reduction of O^{2-} by superoxide dismutases (SOD), which reduces the concentration of free metal cations and thus the damage caused by oxidation (Feng and Wang 2020; Oberg et al. 2015; Satoh et al. 2019).

In addition to the enzymes mentioned above, it has also been reported the presence of different bioactive peptides which may contribute to the reduction of oxidative stress by contributing to the antioxidant potential and presenting different biological properties from the reduction of free radicals to cytotoxic effects on cancer cells (Alwendawi 2019; Chang et al. 2013). On the other hand, previous reports have shown that fermentation with this type of bacteria allows the production of various organic acids which may have different antioxidant activities (Guo et al. 2022). For example, it has been reported that the fermentation of milk with *Bifidobacterium animalis* increases the content of conjugated linoleic acid, as well as other polyunsaturated fatty acids and various organ acids, which can contribute to the production of foods with bioactive properties that allow the treatment of different pathologies (Mei et al. 2022; Moghadam et al. 2022). In addition to the metabolites with antioxidant potential, bifidobacteria can produce exopolysaccharides which have several technological applications due to their potential on human health (Hidalgo-Cantabrana et al. 2012; Xu et al. 2019), an example is the production of these from dairy effluents by means of *B. lactis* (Amiri et al. 2021; Yuan et al. 2021), *B. animalis* and *B. longum* which have been shown to have high antioxidant potential as additives with bioactive activities that can promote protection against different pathogens as protectors, restore cell morphology of cells in the environment as well as the intestinal microbiota, which makes them attractive in the food and nutraceutical industry (Amiri et al. 2019;

Angelin and Kavitha 2020; Inturri et al. 2017; Kang et al. 2023; Liu et al. 2019; Yuan et al. 2021).

In general, bifidobacteria have several mechanisms to produce antioxidant agents which can be used to produce different food or pharmacological products which, when interacting with the host, could exert different beneficial effects on health.

Table 4. Antioxidant enzymes present in bifidobacteria and function

Strain	Enzyme	Function	Reference
B. bifidum	Ferredoxin ADP reductase	Iron chelating activity	Marcos-Fernández et al. 2023
B. bifidum	Alkyl hydroperoxide reductase (AhpCF)	Detoxification and degradation of organic peroxide	Marcos-Fernández et al. 2023; Satoh et al. 2019
B. dentium	γ-glutamylcysteine	Reduces ROS generated by stressors in the endoplasmic reticulum, increases glutathione levels and suppresses NF-κB activation and IL-8 secretion	Engevik et al. 2021
B. longum NCC2705	Ferredoxin ADP reductase	It has a high antioxidant capacity through the chelation of Fe^{2+} or Cu^{2+}	Feng and Wang 2020
B. longum y *B. lactis*	Peroxiredoxins and thioredoxin reductase	Protects against H_2O_2 induced stress.	Oberg and Broadbent 2016

Short-Chain Fatty Acids

Short-chain fatty acids (SCFAs) are carboxylic acids obtained from bacterial fermentation of non-digestible carbohydrates in the gut. The formation of SCFAs is determined by the intestinal microflora, which consists of 50 genera and more than 400 species of bacteria, among which we find bifidobacteria and lactobacilli. The principal SCFAs in the intestine are butyrate, acetate, and propionate; however, we can also find valproate, caproate, isocaproate, succinate, valerate, and iso-valerate in small amounts (O'Riordan et al. 2022; Wong et al. 2006). There are different enzymatic pathways to produce SCFAs depending on the species of bacteria involved in the process. The glycolic pathway is the most common; however, bifidobacteria use other pathways such as the pentose phosphate and fructose-6-phosphate phosphoketolase pathways (Macfarlane and Macfarlane 2003). SCFAs have various functions in the body, including acting as a fuel source for intestinal epithelial cells, absorbing water, and electrolytes, and playing a critical role in intestinal immune function. Furthermore, when present in optimal amounts, they can prevent pathologies such as colon cancer, inflammatory bowel disease, obesity, and diabetes (Vinolo et al. 2011).

The favorable impact of short-chain fatty acids (SCFAs) on gut health has been demonstrated in traditional food consumption. For example, a study administering Queso Blanco cheese containing *Bifidobacterium longum* KACC 91563 to companion dogs for 8 weeks showed beneficial effects on gut microbiota and metabolites. This intervention resulted in an increase in beneficial gut bacteria, such as *Bifidobacterium*, and a decrease in harmful bacteria, such as Enterobacteriaceae and *Clostridium*. Additionally, SCFAs, along with acetic and propionic acid, were significantly increased in these dogs (Park et al. 2018). Consuming traditional foods supplemented with bifidobacteria also leads to an improvement in the intestinal environment. In a study conducted on adults, yogurt containing *B. longum* BB53 was given for a duration of two weeks. The study found that the proportion of beneficial bacteria, including *Bifidobacterium* and *Lactobacillus*, increased in the fecal microbiota, while the levels of harmful bacteria such as *Clostridium* sp. and total aerobic bacteria decreased. Moreover, the consumption of this yogurt led to a significant increase in the levels of short-chain and volatile fatty acids, while reducing the levels of some putrefactive substances such as ammonia, indole, and p-cresol. Furthermore, the activity of urease, an enzyme responsible for ammonia production, decreased along with the decrease in ammonia levels (Ogata, Kingaku, and Yaeshima 1999).

Short Chain Fatty Acids in Gut Health

SCFAs have a positive impact on various aspects of gut health. They play a crucial role in maintaining the integrity of the gut and tight junction permeability, facilitate the proper digestion and absorption of food, aid in the production of gastrointestinal secretions, and help regulate motility and intestinal transit, which can affect stool pattern and consistency (Blaak et al. 2020).

Gut and Tight Junction's Permeability

The intestinal mucosal barrier is a protective layer consisting of the intestinal epithelium and mucous layer that shields the human body from the contents of the gut. The tight junction proteins, situated between the epithelial cells, are a vital component in maintaining the barrier's integrity by binding the cells together, and are responsible of controlling the size of macromolecules that can pass through the intestinal barrier. The barrier has two key functions: to selectively absorb nutrients from the diet and to prevent harmful microbes and toxins from entering the circulation. If the barrier is weakened or impaired, intestinal permeability increases, allowing certain molecules to bypass the protective regulations of the barrier, thereby exposing the circulation to harmful pathogens, inflammatory mediators, and uremic toxins (Snelson et al. 2021; Lee 2015).

Several factors, including tissue pH, insulin, insulin-like growth factors, protein kinase C activators, nitric oxide, and cytokines, have been shown to affect the permeability of the gastrointestinal epithelial layer, particularly the tight junctions. Ohata, Usami, and Miyoshi (2005) found that short-chain fatty acids (SCFAs), particularly butyrate and propionate, had a concentration-dependent effect on tight junction permeability. The study used different concentrations of butyrate (0.5 to 2 mM), propionate (8 to 16 mM), and acetate (8 to 32 mM) on an intestinal cell line and found a significant decrease in tight junction permeability after 48 hours. In addition, Huang et al. (2021) observed that butyrate can mitigate the negative effects of cytokines on intestinal barrier function by regulating levels of claudin-2 on Caco-2, a colonic epithelial cell line. Butyrate also helps maintain gut health by promoting the expression of colonic mucin, as demonstrated by Gaudier et al. (2004) using human polarized colonic goblet cell lines. Furthermore, animal research suggests that acetate can directly activate NLRP3 inflammasome in gut epithelial cells, leading to the release of IL-18, which can activate the IL-18 receptor on mice's epithelial cells and support intestinal barrier function (Macia et al. 2015). In addition, administering SCFAs orally or introducing probiotic bacteria that produce SCFAs through transplantation can reinforce the strength of the intercellular junctions between colon cells (Pohl, Moodley, and Dhanda 2022).

Mucus Production

The gut epithelium is protected by a layer of mucus, which serves to keep bacteria separated from the mucosa, thereby preventing infections. The gut microbiota and diet are two essential components for maintaining a normal structure and production of intestinal mucus. When the gut microbiota is altered due to a low-fiber diet, it can severely damage the mucus layer, increasing susceptibility to infections and the development of chronic inflammatory diseases. Dietary fibers and SCFAs, mostly acetate and butyrate, play a significant role in stimulating mucus production and secretion (Makki et al. 2018). A deficiency of dietary fibers can harm the mucus barrier and is linked to an increased presence of bacteria that degrade mucin, such as *Akkermansia muciniphila* (Desai et al. 2016). Animal studies have also shown that a low-fiber diet can lead to decreased growth rate and increased permeability of the inner mucus layer, making it more susceptible to infections. This increased permeability may result in a weakened mucus layer that is easily penetrated (Schroeder et al. 2018). Furthermore, in the absence of dietary fibers, certain gut bacteria adjust their metabolic processes to utilize mucin glycans by activating the expression of genes that encode mucin-degrading enzymes (Sonnenburg et al. 2005).

Motility and Transit

The microbiota utilizes SCFAs for both growth and maintaining proper host cell function. In the human colon, SCFAs are found in concentrations of up to 150 mmol/L, making them the primary organic anions. SCFAs have a significant role in regulating colon motility; however, the effects of SCFAs are dependent on various factors such as the specific type of SCFA, the segment of the colon, the animal species, and experimental models used (Shaidullov et al. 2021). Fukomoto et al. investigated the impact of SCFAs on colonic transit and intestinal motility in conscious rats. Their research revealed that the intraluminal application of SCFA at concentrations ranging from 100 to 200 mM in the proximal colon had a notable effect on the acceleration of colonic transit (Fukumoto et al. 2003). Similarly, Cherbut et al. (1998) found that SCFAs alter colonic motility patterns and increase transit rates in a murine model. They also observed that this effect was dependent on hormones, with PYY playing a crucial role.

Antimicrobial Effect of Bifidobacteria

The balance of intestinal microbiota includes the inhibition of pathogens. The antimicrobial activity of probiotics is achieved by the production of antimicrobial substances such as organic acids, bacteriocins, and antimicrobial peptides, as well as competitive exclusion and the modulation of the host immune system (Igbafe et al. 2020).

The antimicrobial substances produced by bifidobacteria generate pore formation and permeabilization, causing cell lysis and preventing cell wall biosynthesis. As these substances are of protein origin, they are susceptible to proteinases. It has been reported that the maximum inhibitory effect is shown in the late logarithmic phase of growth (Sarkar and Mandal 2016). Moreover, the mechanisms of competitive exclusion of pathogens by bifidobacteria are strain dependent; some strains present inhibitory activity on enterotoxigenic and enteropathogenic bacterial growth, while others inhibit the adhesion of pathogens in the intestinal tract (Uraipan and Hongpattarakere 2015). Probiotics exhibit molecular models that recognize transmembrane receptors as pathogens, blocking pathogen access sites through competitive exclusion, and occasionally moving already bound pathogens (Madsen 2012). Bifidobacteria are efficient ion sequesters in the gut, developing a mechanism of nutrient competition against enteropathogenic bacteria (Vazquez-Gutierrez et al. 2015).

Table 5. Inhibitory activity of Bifidobacteria strains against food borne pathogens

***Bifidobacterium* Strain**	**Study objective**	**Results**	**Reference**
Bifdobacterium spp	Evaluate antibacterial activity and probiotic features of *Bifdobacterium* spp. for its potential application in functional food/feed products.	Due to the inhibition test against *S. aureus* and *E. coli*, as well as probiotic characterization such as resistance to low pH, bile salts and sensitivity to antibiotics, *Bifdobacterium pseudolongum* DSM 20099, and *Bifdobacterium animalis* DSM 20105 appear as probiotic candidates for the development of functional food/feed.	Cizeikiene and Jagelaviciute 2021
Bifidobacterium longum	Prove probiotic potential and antimicrobial activity of *Bifidobacterium longum* against pathogens in poultry (*E. coli* O157:H7, *Salmonella Typhimurium* and *L. monocytogenes*)	*B. longum* presented probiotic potential for controlling *E. coli* O157:H7, *Salmonella* and *L. monocytogenes* in poultry.	Igbafe et al. 2020
Bifidubacterum lactis BB-12	Demonstrate that the culture of *B. lactis* BB-12 with *Lactobacillus acidophilus* LA-5 can lead to the production of a new fermentation product with antimicrobial properties.	The antimicrobial substances produced by LA-5, BB-12, and their mixture culture had inhibitory activity against both G+ and G− bacteria being higher the effect against *L. monocytogenes*	Amiri et al. 2022

Table 5. (Continued)

***Bifidobacterium* Strain**	**Study objective**	**Results**	**Reference**
Bifidobacteria isolated from monkey and chicken faeces	Characterization of bifidobacteria by evaluating technological and inhibition of gram-positive and -negative pathogens to be used as probiotics.	Bifidobacteria isolated from monkey presented higher inhibitory capacity than the reference strains, being Listeria monocytogenes ATCC 15313 the pathogen with a higher rate of inhibition.	Sarquis et al. 2019
Bifidobacterium spp.	Study the effect of silver nanoparticles (AgNPs) synthesized by probiotic bacteria (Bifidobacterium spp.) on pathogenic bacteria isolated from Ready-To-Eat (RTE) salads.	Antagonism effect of AgNPs was found on S. aureus, P. aeruginosa and E. coli.	Jafar et al. 2022
B. longum *B. pseudolongum* *B. bifidum* *B. thermophilum* *B. boum* *B. merycicum* *B. ruminantium*	Characterize the biological potencial of bacteriocins produced by *Bifidobacterium* spp. isolated from ruminants.	Minimum inhibitory concentration (MIC) values varied from 300 µl/ml to 500 µl/ml and minimum bactericidal concentration (MBC) values ranged from 500 µl/ml to >500 µl/ml for *E. coli* and *S. aureus* respectively. indicated that bifidobacterial bacteriocins have considerable potential to be used as biopreservative.	Zafar et al. 2022

Bifidobacterium species are commonly used as probiotics in traditional foods due to their ability to inhibit pathogenic microorganisms. Table 5 summarizes several studies where bifidobacteria have been demonstrated to be effective inhibitors of foodborne pathogens (Nguyen et al. 2019).

The studies presented in Table 5 indicate that bifidobacteria have the potential to act as inhibitory agents when added to food. However, further research is needed to fully understand the mechanisms underlying their inhibitory activity as well as their behavior in the food matrix.

Interrelation of Bifidobacteria in Tradition Food and Parasites and Their Impact on Gut Health

The consumption of traditional foods containing bifidobacteria has been suggested to improve parasitic diseases. In one study, administration of bifidobacteria in yogurt to mice infected with *C. parvum* led to cessation of oocyst shedding on the eighth day of treatment (Mohammed, Jabur, and Aja 2017). Although there are limited reports on the effect of traditional food consumption on parasitic diseases, this section provides an overview of studies investigating the interaction between bifidobacteria and pathogenic parasites, with particular emphasis on modulatory effects on the immune response, alterations in the microbiota, and antiparasitic effects of bifidobacteria.

Bifidobacterium Modulates the Immune Response in Parasitic Infections

The impact of ascariasis on human health is significant, making it a global disease of concern. The roundworms *Ascaris lumbricoides* and *Ascaris suum* are the etiological agents responsible for human and swine infections, respectively (Eamsobhana et al. 2022). The efficacy of probiotic intervention using *Bifidobacterium animalis* subspecies *lactis* (Bb12) was investigated against *A. suum*-infected pigs. The parasite was found to increase the mucosal response to histamine and 5-HT, which was attenuated in pigs fed with Bb12. Conversely, *Bifidobacterium* administration improved glucose absorption, which was adversely affected by the worm infection. In terms of immune responses, Bb12 treatment resulted in increased levels of anti-*Ascaris* antibodies IgG1 and IgG2 (ileum fluid) and IgA (serum). In addition, treatment with bifidobacteria has been shown to inhibit eosinophil levels and modulate the expression of genes related to Th1/Th2 cells, Treg cells, and mast cells, suggesting that bifidobacteria may be a promising agent for ameliorating responses caused by dysregulated type-2 diseases, such as allergies or chronic inflammation (Solano-Aguilar et al. 2018). *Bifidobacterium* has also been associated with the host's response to combat toxoplasmosis, a protozoan infection with a global impact on health that can cause massive ileum necrosis and death in mice. In a murine model of toxoplasmosis, the absence of bifidobacteria was observed in TLR-9-/- mice with acutely induced ileum inflammation (ileitis) but not in WT mice. Bifidobacteria have anti-inflammatory activity and the capacity to stimulate dendritic cells that enhance the population of CD25+ FOXP3+ Tregs, and the absence of bifidobacteria has been linked to a lack of increase in FOXP3+ Treg population. Similar observations were made in a study using a model of *T. gondii* ileitis in NOD2-/- mice, where the absence of bifidobacteria resulted in a diminished anti-inflammatory response and incapacity to combat the protozoa infection, possibly due to the role of nucleotide-binding oligomerization domain (NOD)-like receptors in microbial product recognition and host immune regulation (Bereswill et al. 2014; Heimesaat et al. 2014). Bifidobacteria have been proposed to regulate the abundance of parasites through competitive exclusion or immunomodulation. An experimental infection with *Leishmania infantum*, the causative agent of visceral leishmaniasis, was conducted in hamsters to assess the changes in bifidobacteria levels. During the eight-month monitoring period, a significant increase in bifidobacteria levels was observed during the infection. This increase was correlated with a lower number of parasites and histological alterations in the colon of the infected animals. These findings suggest that bifidobacteria may have a protective role in infected hosts, potentially preventing severe disease (Passos et al. 2020).

Parasitic Diseases Affect the Microbiota

A recent study demonstrated the modulatory effect of *A. suum* infection on pig's microbiota. The researchers analyzed fecal and ingesta samples to compare the impact of single or trickle-dose infection. The results showed that the trickle-infected group exhibited an increased abundance of taxonomic composition of microbiota in the early stage of infection, including *Bifidobacterium*, *Fibrobacter*, an unclassified *Clostridia* genus (day 3), and an unclassified *Prevotellaceae* genus (day 7). However, the abundance of bifidobacteria decreased during days 28 to 49 post-infection, particularly *B. boum* and *B. thermophilum* in fecal samples, and lower levels in ingesta samples from the ileum, caecum, and colon at day 49 were also observed. The results indicated that this parasitic disease prevents microbiota colonization, and the investigators concluded that the reduction in bifidobacteria might be considered a parasite survival strategy (Springer et al. 2022). Jensen and colleagues (2011) studied the impact of diet on both microbiota and intestinal helminths. Specifically, they investigated the effects of a fructan-rich diet of chicory as a probiotic on infections caused by *A. suum* and *Trichuris suis*, a swine whipworm that can cause intestinal disease. The researchers found that the percentage of *A. suum* worms in the small intestine decreased by 64%, while the number of *T. suis* helminths in the large intestine increased. Furthermore, the consumption of chicory led to an increase in bifidobacteria levels in the pigs' microbiota. These findings suggest that a chicory-fed diet can lead to complex changes in both the microbiota and parasite communities in the intestinal tract. Recently, the effects of *H. contortus* infection were investigated in goats, where microbiota alterations were found in the jejunum and ileum, affecting families such as Bifidobacteriaceae, Lachnospiraceae, Enterobacteriaceae, and Micrococcaceae, among others. The nematode infection also caused changes in amino acid metabolism and the expression of related transporters, potentially impacting the distribution and abundance of gut bacteria (Chen et al. 2023).

On the other hand, the intestinal microbiota composition was altered by using a mixture of probiotics in a model of helminthic infection. In pigs infected with the worm *Oesophagostomum dentatum*, the combined administration of *Lactobacillus rhamnosus* LGG and Bb12 caused an increase in the diversity of bacteria in fecal and large intestine samples over the course of infection. Moreover, it appears that these effects are also modulated by helminth infection. Additionally, the probiotic mixture caused changes in the levels of SCFA and lactic acid in the intestine. These are metabolites that can strongly influence the dynamics of infection and participate in the response against intestinal parasites (Myhill et al. 2022).

In human population studies, the interaction between parasites and the microbiota has also been reported. In a case-control study in Iran, the gut bacteria of asymptomatic individuals infected with *Blastocystis* sp., an intestinal protozoan, was analyzed. Results showed that the expression of *Bifidobacterium* was upregulated in comparison to the control group, suggesting that asymptomatic protozoa infection alters the gut bacteria composition (Behboud et al. 2022). Another investigation in Thailand tested the influence of *Strongyloides stercoralis* infection on gut microbiota. Subjects who were carriers of the nematode showed high quantities of *Escherichia-Shigella* and *Bacteroides* but low abundances of *Bifidobacterium*, *Lactobacillus*, and *Blautia* genera. This also had an impact on the level of bacterial metabolites such as SCFA and acetic acid, which were decreased in infected individuals. These events indicate that S. stercoralis could manipulate the gut microbiota structure and functionality (Nguyen et al. 2022).

Therapeutic or Preventive Effects of Bifidobacterium in Parasitic Diseases

Cryptosporidium spp. are important intestinal protozoa that infect humans and other animals worldwide, causing clinical manifestations such as diarrhea, growth retardation, weight loss, and, in some cases, death (Jang et al. 2023). The *in vitro* effects of bifidobacteria against the infective stage of *C. parvum* were reported by Foster et al. (2003). They used oocysts of the parasite from infected calves that were exposed to probiotic bacteria, including *B. breve* and *B. longum*. Only the treatment with *B. longum* slightly reduced the viability of the protozoa, probably because this bacterium produces little or no antimicrobial substances that are toxic to *C. parvum*. The need for *Bifidobacterium* to associate with other lactic acid bacteria may also be related to the substances produced and the observed effects (Foster et al. 2003).

The preventive effects of bifidobacteria against parasitic infections have been studied in various animal models. In a mouse model of giardiasis, a common gastrointestinal disease, *B. bifidum* has shown promising results as a potential control agent. Pre-administration of bifidobacteria reduced the protozoan infection and improved histological changes. Thus, probiotic bacteria can be a safe alternative to promote intestinal health and prevent or treat parasitic diseases (Al-Megrin et al. 2021).

Similarly, in a murine model of malaria, the administration of *B. longum* reduced parasitemia and modulated immunity. *Plasmodium* spp. infect erythrocytes, causing dysbiosis in various organs, including the gastrointestinal tract. The impact of bifidobacteria was analyzed in *P. berghei*-infected mice. The pre-administration of bacteria reduced the number of parasites and systemic levels of proinflammatory cytokines (TNFα and IFNγ) by increasing expression of CD103 and FOXP3. Moreover, the administration of bacteria also improved the colon damage observed in histopathological examination. These results indicate that *B. longum* exerts a protective effect against *Plasmodium* infection *in vivo* (Fitri et al. 2023).

Bifidobacteria Present in Traditional Food as Potential Therapeutic Agents in Gut Disorders

Abnormal changes in the composition of the gut microbiota, a phenomenon known as dysbiosis, are directly involved in the pathophysiology of several diseases, including inflammatory bowel disease, type 2 diabetes mellitus, neurodegenerative diseases, and depression (Álvarez et al. 2021; Kandpal et al. 2022). The consumption of traditional foods modifies the structure of this microbiota, stimulating the immune response, either by the presence of microbial cell wall components or by molecules released by these microorganisms during fermentation processes such as metabolites, peptides, and exopolysaccharides (He et al. 2002). Similarly, the consumption of fermented foods can prevent the presentation of intestinal diseases, e.g., Ishikawa et al. (2003) observed that *B. breve* and *B. bifidum* present in fermented cow's milk prevented ulcerative colitis.

Bifidobacteria Present in Traditional Foods Modulate the Immune Response

Bifidobacteria Stimulate Immune Effector Functions

Various species of *Bifidobacterium* present in traditional foods have shown the ability to activate the immune system and induce inflammation. This increase in the amount and activity of proinflammatory cytokines in the mucosa can lead to damage of intestinal tissues (Yao et al. 2021). In a study where healthy dogs were fed white cheese with *B. longum*, there was an increase in the concentration of proinflammatory serum cytokines (TNFα and IL-6), which induced peripheral blood mononuclear cell proliferation (Park et al. 2020). However, cytokine production can vary depending on the bacterium, the cytokine, and the cell type being evaluated. For example, *B. bifidum* induces greater production of IL-2 in PMA-stimulated ELAIL2 lymphoblasts than *Streptococcus* and *Lactobacillus*. However, *B. adolescentis* and *B. bifidum* induce less TNFα in activated RAW 264.7 cells than *Lactobacillus* and *Streptococcus* (Marin et al. 1998). Likewise, the consumption of fermented foods in adults increases the phagocytic activity of monocytes and granulocytes, the presence of T lymphocytes, the concentration of IgA in feces, and serum IL-12 (Olivares et al. 2006). In another study, but in BALB/c mice, a similar effect was observed; the administration of commercial fermented milk for 98 consecutive days increased the number of IgA-secreting cells, the number of CD4 and CD8 lymphocytes in the small and large intestine, and the production of IL-2, TNFα, and IFNγ, thus increasing phagocytic capacity (de Moreno de LeBlanc et al. 2008). In inflammatory bowel diseases, immune cells become activated after receiving a stimulating signal. This leads to the secretion of a large number of inflammatory cytokines, including TNFα, interleukin IL-1β, IL-6, and reactive oxygen species (ROS) (Yao et al. 2021). *B. breve* can exacerbate this situation, as observed in individuals with chronic inflammatory diseases infected with adherent-invasive *Escherichia coli* (AIEC). In people with ulcerative colitis and Crohn's disease, *B. breve* increases TNFα production in AIEC-infected macrophages and decreases IL-10 production in macrophages from Crohn's disease patients, thus aggravating the inflammatory effect (Leccese et al. 2020).

Bifidobacteria Induce Immune Regulation Functions

There is interest in the immunomodulatory properties of probiotic bacteria since the intestinal microbiota is essential for the development of the immune system (Mazmanian et al. 2005). It has been observed that consumption of fermented foods in adults increases the production of anti-inflammatory cytokines such as IL-10 and IL-4 (Olivares et al. 2006). For example, the consumption of functional kimchi for 12 weeks was found to decrease TNFα and IL-12 expression and increase *B. adolescentis* production in subjects with irritable bowel syndrome (Kim et al. 2022). Similarly, cheese consumption has been observed to decrease the prevalence of food allergies in 6-year-old children (Nicklaus et al. 2019).

Bifidobacterium longum can protect intestinal epithelial cells through various mechanisms. For example, it can decrease myeloperoxidase activity and production of ROS, obstruct the NF-κB pathway, which results in a decrease of inflammatory cytokines, and generate diverse metabolites that enhance the adherence to the intestinal tract and hinder harmful bacteria (Yao et al. 2021). In a study on ethanol-induced steatosis, oral administration of *B. longum* LC67 to mice reduced blood liver enzymes, inhibited NF-κB expression, increased intestinal tight junction protein expression, and restored the microbiota composition (Kim et al. 2018). Similarly, in mice with high-fat diet-induced obesity, *B. longum* alleviated colitis by inhibiting lipopolysaccharide production from the microbiota (In Kim et al. 2019).

Bifidobacterium longum subsp. *infantis* can produce indole-3-lactic acid (ILA), which reduces the IL-8 response upon IL-1β stimulation in immature enterocytes (Meng et al. 2020). In another study, it was observed that administration of this bacterium, together with the prebiotic "Synergy 1," reduced the production of defensins 2, 3, and 4, as well as TNFα and IL-1α in people with ulcerative colitis (Furrie et al. 2005). *B. infantis* has also been shown to decrease the expression of CRP, IL-6, and TNFα in ulcerative colitis (Groeger et al. 2013). Similarly, *B. longum* has been shown to reduce signs of inflammation in BALB/c mice with food allergy, resulting in a decrease in infiltration of inflammatory cells in intestinal tissues (Liu et al. 2017).

Bifidobacterial-induced reduction of proinflammatory cytokines has been observed during infections. For instance, *Bifidobacterium breve* has been shown to reduce secretion of IL-8 in HT29 cells (intestinal epithelial cells) infected with adherent-invasive *Escherichia coli* (Leccese et al. 2020). Consumption of yogurt can restore the microbiota by incorporating *Bifidobacterium lactis*, which increases IgA and reduces IL-6 in children infected with *Helicobacter pylori* (Yang and Sheu 2012).

Regarding food allergies, *Bifidobacterium longum* has been shown to induce apoptosis in mast cells, thereby relieving allergy symptoms in BALB/c mice (Kim et al. 2016). In C3H/H3J mice with food allergy, *Bifidobacterium lactis* decreased the production of IgG and IgE, as well as mast cells and intestinal eosinophils, while increasing IgA (Kim, Choi, and Ji 2008). Oral administration of Dahi, a food prepared from buffalo milk containing *Bifidobacterium bifidum*, reduces IgE and suppresses allergic response in mice immunized with pasteurized milk (Shandilya et al. 2016).

Fermented food brine drink shows site-specific restructuring of the gut microbiome and promotion of tolerogenic barrier immunity. Lactate produced by microbiota increases regulatory T-cells (Treg cells) in the small intestine (Spencer et al. 2022). Similarly, fermented milk containing probiotics has the potential to stimulate the mucosal response and regulate cytokine production, while promoting the growth of CD4+, CD8+, and IgA+ cells (Santiago-López et al. 2018). For example, bifidobacteria can control food allergy by inducing Treg cell growth (Zhang et al. 2010).

Short-chain fatty acids (SCFAs) secreted by bifidobacteria have been shown to regulate the immune system. The activation of free fatty acid receptor 2 (FFA2) and inhibition of histone deacetylase (HDAC) lead to the inhibition of the NF-κB signaling pathway and anti-inflammatory effects. HDACs are generally expressed on immune, endothelial, and vascular smooth muscle cells. When they are inhibited, an open DNA/chromatin structure is created, which facilitates the regulation of the expression of transcription factors such as NF-κB and FOXP3 (Yao et al. 2021).

Impact of Bifidobacterial Present in Traditional Foods on Gut Health: Evidence from Animal Studies

Several reports have used animal models to determine the benefits of *Bifidobacterium* genus bacteria on various diseases. The application of gnotobiotic animal models provides a valuable method for investigating the contributions of bacterial species or strains to the pathogenesis of intestinal inflammation (Onderdonk 2000).

Inflammatory bowel disease (IBD) is a chronic, recurrent, non-specific, and multifactorial disease. One of its possible causes is an alteration in the intestinal microbiome that triggers immune imbalance and intestinal inflammatory responses (Jakubczyk, Leszczyńska, and Górska 2020).

Animal models, such as those induced with dextran sodium sulfate (DSS) or 2,4,6-trinitrobenzene sulfonic acid (TNBS), have been employed to investigate intestinal diseases such as colitis. Studies utilizing these models have suggested that consumption of traditional foods may have the potential to improve symptoms and management of inflammatory bowel disease (IBD). Sprong, Schonewille, and van der Meer (2010) demonstrated that administering cheese whey protein to rats protects against mild colitis induced by dextran sulfate sodium. This protection was attributed to the threonine and cysteine content of the whey protein, which increased the counts of lactobacilli and bifidobacteria in the feces. The protective effect is likely due to both the stimulation of intestinal mucin synthesis and the alteration of the composition of the gut microbiota.

Employing the colitis model, it has been observed that administering probiotics through traditional foods may represent a potential therapeutic approach for managing IBD. Veiga et al. (2010) reported that ingestion of a fermented milk product containing *Bifidobacterium animalis* subsp. *lactis* strain DN-173010 resulted in a reduction in cecal pH and changes in short-chain fatty acid profiles. These changes were accompanied by an increase in the abundance of select bacteria that consume lactate and produce butyrate. The resulting metabolic environment was unfavorable for the emergence of colitogenic Enterobacteriaceae in a T-bet-/-Rag2-/- mouse model of ulcerative colitis. In a study by Satish Kumar et al. (2017), the therapeutic potential of oral administration of *Bifidobacterium bifidum* at a dose of 1.4×10^{11} CFU/day for 14 days was investigated in a TNBS colitis model in rats. The study revealed an anti-inflammatory effect, as indicated by a reduction in the presence of macroscopic lesions in the colon and less damage to the mucosa, reflected by less infiltration of macrophages and neutrophils at the probiotic adherence site. Additionally, the study found that *B. bifidum* reduced oxidative stress in the intestinal mucosa by in increasing the presence of reduced glutathione and decreasing the levels of peroxidized lipids and nitric oxide compared to the colitis control group. Furthermore, the administration of probiotics modulated cytokine levels, with reduced levels of the inflammatory cytokine IL-1β and increased levels of the anti-inflammatory cytokine IL-10. Several studies have reported the beneficial effects of *Bifidobacterium bifidum* on colitis (Satish Kumar et al. 2017; Din et al. 2020). In one study, mice were administered the probiotic at a dose of 2×10^8 CFU/day for 27 days, and colitis was induced with DSS from days 21-27. The study found that animals treated with bifidobacteria presented less cell infiltration and disruption of the epithelial structure, as well as lower activity of the myeloperoxidase enzyme, which is an indicator of neutrophil infiltration in tissues. Furthermore, the expression of scavenger genes for reactive oxygen species (SOD1, SOD2, CAT, and GPX2), anti-inflammatory cytokines (IL-10, PPARγ, IL-6), and cell adhesion molecules (ZO-1, MUC-2, Claudin-3, and E Cadherin-1) were upregulated in the Bifido group (Din et al. 2020). In another study, the therapeutic potential of *B. bifidum* was investigated in a TNBS colitis model in rats. The study revealed an anti-inflammatory effect, as indicated by a reduction in the presence of macroscopic lesions in the colon and less damage to the mucosa, reflected by less infiltration of macrophages and neutrophils at the probiotic adherence site. Additionally, the study found that *B. bifidum* reduced oxidative stress in the intestinal mucosa by increasing the presence of reduced glutathione and decreasing the levels of peroxidized lipids and nitric oxide compared to the colitis control group. Furthermore, the administration of probiotics modulated cytokine levels, with reduced levels of the inflammatory cytokine IL-1β and increased levels of the anti-inflammatory cytokine IL-10 (Satish Kumar et al. 2017).

Bifidobacterium infantis has also been found to be beneficial in the DSS model of colitis. Zhou et al. (2019) administered different doses of *B. infantis* ($1x10^7$, $1x10^8$, and $1x10^9$ CFU/day) to mice during the 7 days of colitis induction. They found that the groups treated with bifidobacteria had less damage to the intestinal mucosa and observed an increase in the expression of IL-10 and TGF-β1, as well as the FOXP3 transcription factor. The authors suggest that this increase is related to an increase in Treg cells and thus creates an anti-inflammatory microenvironment in the colon. Additionally, the use of products derived from bifidobacteria in colitis models has also been evaluated. The study conducted by Yan et al. (2020) showed that fermented milk containing *Bifidobacterium longum* had a positive impact on mice with DSS colitis by reducing inflammation and improving the mucosal barrier, ultimately leading to a decrease in pathogenic bacteria such as Enterobacteriaceae. This suggests that products derived from bifidobacteria may also have therapeutic potential in the treatment of colitis (Figure 2).

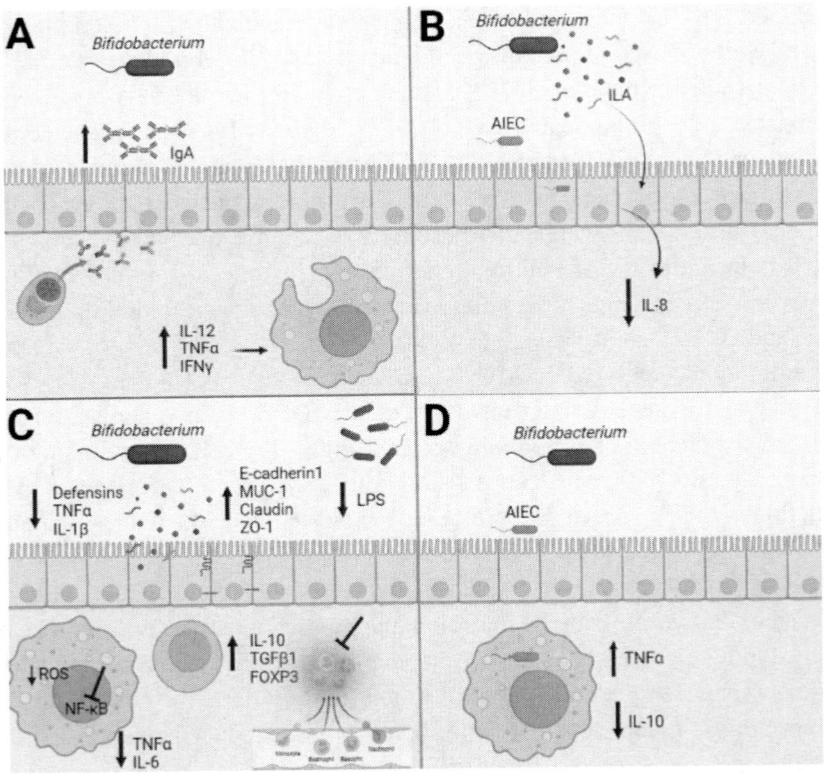

Figure 2. Effect of bifidobacteria present in traditional foods on intestinal health. A. Normal intestine: Bifidobacteria induce increased secretion of IgA, IL-12, TNFα, and IFNγ, thereby inducing macrophage activation. B. Intestine infected with AIEC: *Bifidobacterium* secretes ILA by reducing the expression of IL-8 by enterocytes. C. IBD gut: *Bifidobacterium* induces a decrease in defensins, TNFα, IL-1β, and an increase in tight junction proteins by enterocytes. It also results in a decreased production of LPS by the microbiota, an increase in IL-10, TGFβ1, and FOXP3 by lymphocytes, and a blockade of inflammatory cell infiltration. D. IBD intestine infected with AIEC: Bifidobacteria increase TNFα production and decrease IL-10 production by AIEC-infected macrophages, exacerbating the inflammatory effects.

The effects of the microbiota are not restricted to its beneficial effects on the gastrointestinal tract. Recently, there has been an emphasis on the influence of the intestinal microbiota on brain and behavioral functions, which has led to the establishment of the microbiota-gut-brain axis (Herselman, Bailey, and Bobrovskaya 2022). Depression, which is commonly comorbid with anxiety, is a heterogeneous neuropsychiatric disorder. The serotonin (5-HT) system in the brain is key for both the development of depression and its treatment. In recent years, data has revealed that the gut microbiota in patients with major depression disorders is altered (Hu et al. 2019). Studies have shown that the intestinal microbiota can influence depressive-type behaviors by regulating the metabolism of glycerophospholipids and tryptophan (a serotonin precursor), controlling the response to stress, and the synthesis of neurotrophic factors (Li et al. 2019). For example, in a mouse model of depression induced by unpredictable chronic mild stress (UCMS), Tian et al. (2020) found that the administration of *Bifidobacterium breve* at a dose of 1×10^9 CFU/mL/day for 5 weeks reduced anxiety and depressive behaviors. The potential mechanism of action might involve mitigating HPA-axis hyperactivity and inflammation by regulating the expression of glucocorticoid receptors, upregulating brain-derived neurotrophic factor (BDNF), downregulating c-Fos levels, and enhancing the serotonergic system in both the gut and brain. Fecal short chain fatty acid (SCFA) and *Bifidobacterium breve* levels were positively correlated with the beneficial effects (Tian et al. 2020). In a study by Huang et al. (2022), the administration of probiotics such as *Bifidobacterium animalis* subsp. *lactis* was found to alleviate anxiety and depression caused by a model of unpredictable chronic mild stress (UCMS) in rats. Rats were exposed to two different stressors daily for six weeks, followed by oral administration of bifidobacteria (10^9 CFU/day) for the next 6 weeks while continuing UCMS stimulation. Treatment with probiotics increased exploration and movement behaviors in tests such as the open field and elevated-plus maze, and normalized levels of various neurotransmitters, metabolites, and cytokines in UCMS rats, including 5-HT, dopamine, noradrenaline, homovanillic acid, 3,4-dihydroxyphenylacetic acid, 5-hydroxyindole acetic acid, TNF-α, IL-6, IL-18, and IL-1β.

In another study, Guo et al. (2019) investigated the effect of pretreatment with *Bifidobacterium adolescentis* on the behavioral performance of mice using a chronic restraint stress model. Mice were administered 0.25×10^9 CFU/kg *B. adolescentis* for 21 days, the same duration as the chronic restraint stress procedure. The administration of *Bifidobacteria* resulted in anxiolytic and antidepressant effects, as evidenced by an increase in the time spent in the center of the open field apparatus and a decrease in immobility time in the tail suspension and forced swim tests. Additionally, the study found an increase in

BDNF levels and a decrease in inflammatory cytokines TNF-α and IL-1β in the hippocampal region of the brain, as well as a decrease in the activation of NF-κB, responsible for the development of inflammatory processes, and a decrease in the microglia activation marker Iba-1.

These studies suggest that probiotics, particularly *Bifidobacterium* strains, may have a beneficial effect on anxiety and depression-like behaviors in animal models of stress. These effects may be mediated through the modulation of the gut-brain axis, regulation of the HPA-axis and inflammatory pathways, and changes in neurotransmitter and neurotrophic factor levels in key regions of the brain. While further research is needed to determine the specific mechanisms involved and the potential for translation to human populations, these findings offer promising insights into the potential use of probiotics as a complementary therapy for stress-related mental health disorders.

Future Trends

Isolation

There are currently various methods for isolating bifidobacteria from different sources, including breast milk, fruits, fermented foods, and cheeses. However, there is still a need for the isolation of bifidobacteria from sources that are rich in these microorganisms, such as the intestines of newborns and infants. Zhang et al. (2023) demonstrated that employing 20-fucosyllactose (20-FL) as the sole carbon source enabled them to isolate different *Bifidobacterium* strains with better probiotic capacities. This is because 20-fucosyllactose is a key compound that promotes the growth of bifidobacteria in the intestines of newborns.

Technological advancements are necessary for ensuring the viability of probiotic strains during processing and storage. To this end, researchers have investigated the use of various compounds such as lactulose, milk proteins, inulin, and plant phytochemicals, as well as different encapsulation methods to maintain a high viability rate of probiotic strains (Shori 2022). However, there is a paucity of information regarding the optimal physical properties and mechanical stability of the polymers utilized for encapsulation.

Relief of Disease Symptoms

Bifidobacteria are among the dominant microorganisms in the human intestine during infancy and play a critical role in newborns. Studies have shown that infants with lower levels of bifidobacteria are at a higher risk of various diseases, including neurodevelopmental disorders, inflammatory bowel disease, late-onset sepsis, necrotizing enterocolitis, and allergies that may persist into adulthood (Sadeghpour Heravi and Hu 2023; Saturio et al. 2021). These observations suggest the importance of identifying the role of specific bifidobacterial strains, profiles, and levels in the health of newborns and early childhood, as well as the potential impact of reduced bifidobacteria levels on the health of adults and the elderly.

During the COVID-19 epidemic, it was observed that hospitalized patients with moderate/severe SARS-CoV-2 who received an oral booster of a single strain probiotic bifidobacteria showed reduced levels of mortality and interleukin-6, and a shorter hospital stay (Bozkurt and Bilen 2021). Although these findings suggest a potential therapeutic use for bifidobacteria, the underlying mechanisms by which they reduce the symptoms of serious diseases still need to be investigated.

Understanding Metabolic Pathways

It has been suggested that different species of bifidobacteria can metabolize a variety of substrates. For example, in the absence of glucose, *B. dentium* can utilize different plant-based substrates by producing diverse proteins associated with various metabolic pathways (Engevik, Danhof, et al. 2021). However, not all species of bifidobacteria possess the same range of proteins, and there is still a lack of information about the key metabolic differences between different strains of bifidobacteria. For instance, (Devika and Raman 2019) indicated that acetate production is specific to the niche and strain. Therefore, further investigation is needed to gain a better understanding of the metabolic pathways of different *Bifidobacterium* strains.

The study of the role of bifidobacteria in regulating anti-inflammatory activity is of great interest. It has been reported that *Bifidobacterium* can mitigate intestinal immunopathology caused by the blockade of cytotoxic T lymphocyte antigen-4 (CTLA-4) by modifying the gut microbiota composition in a regulatory T cell (Treg)-dependent manner (Sun et al. 2020). The same authors indicated that the modified community increased mitochondrial fitness and IL-10-mediated suppressive functions of intestinal Tregs, which reflected in the amelioration of colitis during immune checkpoint blockade. In addition, probiotics (including *Bifidobacterium longum*) can alleviate Enterotoxigenic *Escherichia coli* (ETEC) K88-induced diarrhea by increasing the metabolism of starch, sucrose, galactose, fructose, and mannose, as well as ABC transporters. Furthermore, the expression of inflammatory cytokines, Toll-like receptor, and downstream genes (TLR4, MyD88, NF-κB) in the jejunum induced by ETEC was downregulated, restoring dysbiosis (Li et al. 2022). It is expected that soon, more mechanisms of action of bifidobacteria in processes such as inflammation and cancer will be identified and described.

Bifidobacteria and Psychological Conditions

Lactobacilli and bifidobacteria are referred to as "psychobiotics" because they have the potential to affect the host's mental health through endocrine, neural, and immune pathways. *Bifidobacterium* has been associated with the regulation of mood, anxiety, cognition, and pain. This microorganism can produce and deliver serotonin and GABA, which are neuroactive compounds that transfer signals between the gut and brain. Therefore, the consumption of psychobiotics to regulate mood disorders is an area of hopeful study (Altaib et al., 2021). However, further research is still needed to analyze different species and isolate bifidobacteria, as the effect is strain specific.

Genetic studies have revealed that the genetic diversity found in bifidobacteria seems to have evolved with their host. Strains isolated from different sources have shown differences in genome size and gene composition, especially in those related to amino acid production and the degradation of carbohydrates. Interestingly, bifidobacteria strains isolated from humans do not exhibit a phylogenetic signal or differences in amino acid biosynthesis genes and carbohydrate-active enzymes (CAZymes) (Rodriguez and Martiny 2020).

The genetic engineering of *Bifidobacterium* has the potential to improve the production of value-added compounds such as polyketides, fatty acids, and conjugated linoleic acids, thanks to its unique Bifid shunt pathway. Additionally, the use of bifidobacteria as an engineering chassis provides numerous advantages for metabolic engineers, synthetic biologists, and evolutionary biologists. However, not all *Bifidobacterium* species can be used as probiotics due to their lack of resistance to adverse conditions or potential to damage host mucin layers. These limitations can be addressed by supplementing, removing, or editing specific genes (Chen et al. 2021). However, most of the genetic engineering efforts to date have focused on *B. longum* and *B. breve*, highlighting the need to study and engineer other bifidobacterial genomes. The bifidobacteria genome also offers a potential source of constitutive and inducible promoters, as well as regulatory elements. Despite this, there is still a lack of research to determine the interactions between these genetic segments in other bifidobacteria genomes.

Conclusion

The presence of *Bifidobacterium* in traditional foods, such as milk, cheeses, meat, cocoa, and various plants, offers potential benefits due to the nutrients present in these foods, which support the growth of *Bifidobacterium*. Consequently, these foods are considered functional and prebiotic. Molecular techniques, including polymerase chain reaction (PCR) and next-generation sequencing (NGS) analysis, are commonly employed to identify *Bifidobacterium* strains. Among these techniques, 16S rRNA gene sequencing is most frequently used for this purpose. *Bifidobacterium* exhibits versatility and potential benefits in the production of traditional foods, particularly in the development of probiotic and functional food products. Its interaction with other ingredients can enhance bioavailability and nutritional properties. Nonetheless, to ensure the survival and viability of bifidobacteria in probiotic food products, it is crucial to consider environmental factors, such as temperature, pH, and oxygen levels, and implement appropriate conservation strategies. Research focusing on bioactive peptides and exopolysaccharides derived from *Bifidobacterium* and lactic acid bacteria has revealed promising biological effects. Further research is necessary to investigate strain-dependent proteolytic systems and modifications that enhance bioactivities, with potential applications in nutrition, health, and the development of feed additives.

Bifidobacterium species have the potential to produce conjugated linoleic acid (CLA), which finds various applications in the food industry, promotes intestinal health, and helps prevent diseases. The yield of CLA production can be increased by optimizing the fermentation processes employed. Furthermore, these bacteria present a promising opportunity to obtain antioxidants through diverse mechanisms, thereby promoting intestinal health and aiding in the prevention of certain diseases.

Short-chain fatty acids (SCFAs) produced by bifidobacteria contribute to intestinal health by preserving the integrity of tight junctions, promoting mucus production, and regulating motility and transit. A diet rich in dietary fiber or the introduction of SCFA-producing probiotics can enhance gut health and prevent gastrointestinal disorders. The antimicrobial properties exhibited by bifidobacteria make them potential probiotics for incorporation into traditional foods. Nevertheless, the interaction between bifidobacteria and parasites is complex, and further research is necessary to comprehensively understand these interactions and explore the potential of bifidobacteria in improving gut health within the context of parasitic diseases.

Bifidobacterium holds great promise as a therapeutic and preventive agent in parasitic diseases and intestinal disorders. Further research is necessary to elucidate the specific mechanisms involved and to evaluate the efficacy of *Bifidobacterium*-based interventions in clinical settings. Incorporating *Bifidobacterium*-containing foods or probiotic supplements into daily routines can foster gut health and contribute to the prevention and treatment of parasitic diseases and gut-related conditions. Animal studies provide valuable insights into the significant impact of *Bifidobacterium* on gut health and offer potential for its use as an adjunctive therapy for gut-related disorders, as well as stress-related mental health conditions.

The study of bifidobacteria spans various research areas, including isolation methods, technological advancements, disease relief, metabolic pathways, anti-inflammatory activity, psychological conditions, genetic diversity, and genetic engineering. Advancements in these areas will contribute to the understanding and utilization of bifidobacteria for various applications in the future.

References

Albenzio, M., A. Santillo, R. Marino, A. Della Malva, M. Caroprese, and A. Sevi. 2015. "Identification of Peptides in Functional Scamorza Ovine Milk Cheese." *Journal of Dairy Science* 98 (12): 8428–32. https://doi.org/10.3168/jds.2015-9844.

Albenzio, Marzia, Antonella Santillo, Mariangela Caroprese, Antonella della Malva, and Rosaria Marino. 2017. "Bioactive Peptides in Animal Food Products." *Foods* 6 (5): 1–14. https://doi.org/10.3390/foods6050035.

Allouche, Rania, Sébastien Dupont, Alexandre Charriau, Patrick Gervais, Laurent Beney, and Odile Chambin. 2018. "Optimized Tableting for Extremely Oxygen-Sensitive Probiotics Using Direct Compression." *International Journal of Pharmaceutics* 538 (1): 14–20. https://doi.org/10.1016/j.ijpharm.2018.01.010.

Al-Megrin, Wafa A., Shadia H. Mohamed, Moudy M. Saleh, and Hany M. Yehia. 2021. "Preventive Role of Probiotic Bacteria against Gastrointestinal Diseases in Mice Caused by *Giardia lamblia*." *Bioscience Reports* 41 (2): BSR20204114. https://doi.org/10.1042/BSR20204114.

Altmann, F., Kosma, P., O'Callaghan, A., Leahy, S., Bottacini, F., Molloy, E., Plattner, S., Schiavi, E., Gleinser, M., Groeger, D., Grant, R., Rodriguez Perez, N., Healy, S., Svehla, E., Windwarder, M., Hofinger, A., O'Connell Motherway, M., Akdis, C. A., Xu, J., … O'Mahony, L. 2016. "Genome Analysis and Characterisation of the Exopolysaccharide Produced by *Bifidobacterium longum* subsp. *longum* 35624™." *PLOS ONE* 11 (9): e0162983-. https://doi.org/10.1371/journal.pone.0162983.

Álvarez, Julia, José Manuel Fernández Real, Francisco Guarner, Miguel Gueimonde, Juan Miguel Rodríguez, Miguel Saenz de Pipaon, and Yolanda Sanz. 2021. "Gut Microbes and Health." *Gastroenterología y Hepatología (English Edition)* 44 (7): 519–35. https://doi.org/10.1016/j.gastre.2021.01.002.

Alwendawi, Shadan A. 2019. "*In Vitro* Assessment the Potential Antioxidant and Antitumor Activities of *Bifidobacterium* Derived Bacteriocins." *International Journal of Drug Delivery Technology* 9 (02). https://doi.org/10.25258/ijddt.9.2.15.

Amiri, Saber, Mahmoud Rezazadeh-Bari, Mohammad Alizadeh-Khaledabad, Reza Rezaei-Mokarram, and Mahmoud Sowti-Khiabani. 2021. "Fermentation Optimization for Co-Production of Postbiotics by *Bifidobacterium Lactis* BB12 in Cheese Whey." *Waste and Biomass Valorization* 12 (11): 5869–84. https://doi.org/10.1007/s12649-021-01429-7.

Amiri, Saber, Reza Rezaei Mokarram, Mahmoud Sowti Khiabani, Mahmoud Rezazadeh Bari, and Mohammad Alizadeh Khaledabad. 2019. "Exopolysaccharides Production by *Lactobacillus acidophilus* LA5 and *Bifidobacterium animalis* subsp. *lactis* BB12: Optimization of Fermentation Variables and Characterization of Structure and Bioactivities." *International Journal of Biological Macromolecules* 123: 752–65. https://doi.org/10.1016/j.ijbiomac.2018.11.084.

Amiri, Saber, Reza Rezaei Mokarram, Mahmoud Sowti Khiabani, Mahmoud Rezazadeh Bari, and Mohammad Alizadeh Khaledabad. 2020. "*In Situ* Production of Conjugated Linoleic Acid by *Bifidobacterium lactis* BB12 and *Lactobacillus acidophilus* LA5 in Milk Model Medium." *LWT* 132: 109933. https://doi.org/10.1016/j.lwt.2020.109933.

Amiri, Saber, Reza Rezaei Mokarram, Mahmoud Sowti Khiabani, Mahmoud Rezazadeh Bari, and Mohammad Alizadeh Khaledabad. 2022. "Characterization of Antimicrobial Peptides Produced by *Lactobacillus acidophilus* LA-5 and *Bifidobacterium lactis* BB-12 and Their Inhibitory Effect against Foodborne Pathogens." *LWT* 153: 112449. https://doi.org/10.1016/j.lwt.2021.112449.

An, S. B., Yang, B.-G., Jang, G., Kim, D.-Y., Kim, J., Oh, S.-M., Oh, N., Lee, S., Moon, J.-Y., Kim, J.-A., Kim, J.-H., Song, Y.-J., Hyun, H.-W., Kim, J., Lee, K., Lee, D., Kwak, M.-J., Kim, B. K., Park, Y.-K., … Jang, M. H. 2022. "Combined IgE Neutralization and *Bifidobacterium longum* Supplementation Reduces the Allergic Response in Models of Food Allergy." *Nature Communications* 13 (1): 5669. https://doi.org/10.1038/s41467-022-33176-1.

Angelin, J., and M. Kavitha. 2020. "Exopolysaccharides from Probiotic Bacteria and Their Health Potential." *International Journal of Biological Macromolecules* 162: 853–65. https://doi.org/10.1016/j.ijbiomac.2020.06.190.

Aursuwanna, Thanyaporn, Sajee Noitang, Papassara Sangtanoo, Piroonporn Srimongkol, Tanatorn Saisavoey, Songchan Puthong, Onrapak Reamtong, and Aphichart Karnchanatat. 2022. "Investigating the Cellular Antioxidant and Anti-Inflammatory Effects of the Novel Peptides in Lingzhi Mushrooms." *Heliyon* 8 (10): e11067. https://doi.org/10.1016/j.heliyon.2022.e11067.

Ayyash, Mutamed, Stuart K. Johnson, Shao-Quan Liu, Aysha Al-Mheiri, and Aisha Abushelaibi. 2018. "Cytotoxicity, Antihypertensive, Antidiabetic and Antioxidant Activities of Solid-State Fermented Lupin, Quinoa and Wheat by *Bifidobacterium* Species: *In Vitro* Investigations." *LWT* 95: 295–302. https://doi.org/10.1016/j.lwt.2018.04.099.

Behboud, Sahar, Kavous Solhjoo, Saiedeh Erfanian, Majid Pirestani, and Amir Abdoli. 2022. "Alteration of Gut Bacteria Composition among Individuals with Asymptomatic *Blastocystis* Infection: A Case-Control Study." *Microbial Pathogenesis* 169: 105639. https://doi.org/10.1016/j.micpath.2022.105639.

Bereswill, Stefan, Anja A. Kühl, Marie Alutis, André Fischer, Luisa Möhle, Daniela Struck, Oliver Liesenfeld, Ulf B. Göbel, Ildikò R. Dunay, and Markus M. Heimesaat. 2014. "The Impact of Toll-like-Receptor-9 on Intestinal Microbiota Composition and Extra-Intestinal Sequelae in Experimental *Toxoplasma gondii* Induced Ileitis." *Gut Pathogens* 6 (1): 19. https://doi.org/10.1186/1757-4749-6-19.

Bezkorovainy, Anatoly. 2001. "Probiotics: Determinants of Survival and Growth in the Gut1,2,3." *The American Journal of Clinical Nutrition* 73 (2): 399s–405s. https://doi.org/10.1093/ajcn/73.2.399s.

Blaak, E. E., Canfora, E. E., Theis, S., Frost, G., Groen, A. K., Mithieux, G., Nauta, A., Scott, K., Stahl, B., Van Harsselaar, J., Van Tol, R., Vaughan, E. E., & Verbeke, K. 2020. "Short Chain Fatty Acids in Human Gut and Metabolic Health." *Beneficial Microbes* 11 (5): 411–55. https://doi.org/10.3920/BM2020.0057.

Bocchi, Serena, Valeria Sagheddu, Marina Elli, Chong-Yoon Lim, and Lorenzo Morelli. 2020. "The Synergistic Interaction between Probiotics and Food Affects Their Beneficial Features." *Advances in Nutrition and Food Science* 2020 (02): 01–12. https://doi.org/10.37722/ANAFS.20202.

Bottacini, Francesca, Douwe van Sinderen, and Marco Ventura. 2017. "Omics of Bifidobacteria: Research and Insights into Their Health-Promoting Activities." *Biochemical Journal* 474 (24): 4137–52. https://doi.org/10.1042/BCJ20160756.

Bowey, E., H. Adlercreutz, and I. Rowland. 2003. "Metabolism of Isoflavones and Lignans by the Gut Microflora: A Study in Germ-Free and Human Flora Associated Rats." *Food and Chemical Toxicology* 41 (5): 631–36. https://doi.org/10.1016/S0278-6915(02)00324-1.

Boylston, Terri D., Celso G. Vinderola, Hamid B. Ghoddusi, and Jorge A. Reinheimer. 2004. "Incorporation of Bifidobacteria into Cheeses: Challenges and Rewards." *International Dairy Journal* 14 (5): 375–87. https://doi.org/10.1016/j.idairyj.2003.08.008.

Bozkurt, Hüseyin S., and Ömer Bilen. 2021. "Oral Booster Probiotic Bifidobacteria in SARS-COV-2 Patients." *International Journal of Immunopathology and Pharmacology* 35 (January): 205873842110596. https://doi.org/10.1177/20587384211059677.

Bunesova, Vera, Jiri Killer, Eva Vlkova, Sarka Musilova, Martin Tomaska, Vojtech Rada, and Vladimir Kmet. 2014. "Isolation and Characterization of Bifidobacteria from Ovine Cheese." *International Journal of Food Microbiology* 188: 26–30. https://doi.org/10.1016/j.ijfoodmicro.2014.07.001.

Cai, Bingna, Hua Chen, Peng Wan, Lianxiang Luo, Ziqing Ye, Jingtong Huang, Deke Chen, and Jianyu Pan. 2022. "Isolation and Identification of Immunomodulatory Peptides from the Protein Hydrolysate of Tuna Trimmings (*Thunnas albacares*)." *LWT* 164: 113614. https://doi.org/10.1016/j.lwt.2022.113614.

Castillo-Escandón, Valeria, Silvia Guadalupe Fernández-Michel, María Cristina Cueto-Wong, and Gabriela Ramos-Clamont Montfort. 2019. "Criterios y Estrategias Tecnológicas Para La Incorporación y Supervivencia de Probióticos En Frutas, Cereales y Sus Derivados." *TIP Revista Especializada En Ciencias Químico-Biológicas* 22 (May). https://doi.org/10.22201/fesz.23958723e.2019.0.173.

Castro-Bravo, Nuria, Jerry M. Wells, Abelardo Margolles, and Patricia Ruas-Madiedo. 2018. "Interactions of Surface Exopolysaccharides From *Bifidobacterium* and *Lactobacillus* Within the Intestinal Environment." *Frontiers in Microbiology* 9. https://doi.org/10.3389/fmicb.2018.02426

Chang, O. K., K.-H. Seol, S.-G. Jeong, M.-H. Oh, B.-Y. Park, C Perrin, and J.-S. Ham. 2013. "Casein Hydrolysis by *Bifidobacterium longum* KACC91563 and Antioxidant Activities of Peptides Derived Therefrom." *Journal of Dairy Science* 96 (9): 5544–55. https://doi.org/10.3168/jds.2013-6687.

Charteris, Kelly, Morelli, and Collins. 1998. "Development and Application of an in Vitro Methodology to Determine the Transit Tolerance of Potentially Probiotic *Lactobacillus* and *Bifidobacterium* Species in the Upper Human Gastrointestinal Tract." *Journal of Applied Microbiology* 84 (5): 759–68. https://doi.org/10.1046/j.1365-2672.1998.00407.x.

Chen, Jun, Xinyi Chen, and Chun Loong Ho. 2021. "Recent Development of Probiotic Bifidobacteria for Treating Human Diseases." *Frontiers in Bioengineering and Biotechnology* 9. https://doi.org/10.3389/fbioe.2021.770248

Chen, Shengshuang, Guoxin Huang, Weilin Liao, Shilin Gong, Jianbo Xiao, Jiao Bai, W. L. Wendy Hsiao, Na Li, and Jian-Lin Wu. 2021. "Discovery of the Bioactive Peptides Secreted by *Bifidobacterium* Using Integrated MCX Coupled with LC–MS and Feature-Based Molecular Networking." *Food Chemistry* 347: 129008. https://doi.org/10.1016/j.foodchem.2021.129008.

Chen, Wenxun, Qiongxian Yan, Rongzhen Zhong, and Zhiliang Tan. 2023. "Amino Acid Profiles, Amino Acid Sensors and Transporters Expression and Intestinal Microbiota Are Differentially Altered in Goats Infected with *Haemonchus contortus*." *Amino Acids* 55 (3): 371–84. https://doi.org/10.1007/s00726-023-03235-y.

Cherbut, Christine, Laurent Ferrier, Claude Rozé, Younès Anini, Hervé Blottière, Gérard Lecannu, and Jean-Paul Galmiche. 1998. "Short-Chain Fatty Acids Modify Colonic Motility through Nerves and Polypeptide YY Release in the Rat." *American Journal of Physiology-Gastrointestinal and Liver Physiology* 275 (6): G1415–22. https://doi.org/10.1152/ajpgi.1998.275.6.G1415.

Chugh, Bhawna, and Afaf Kamal-Eldin. 2020. "Bioactive Compounds Produced by Probiotics in Food Products." *Current Opinion in Food Science* 32: 76–82. https://doi.org/10.1016/j.cofs.2020.02.003.

Chung, Soo Hyun, In Hwan Kim, Hui Gyu Park, Hye Soon Kang, Chil Suk Yoon, Ha Yeon Jeong, Nag Jin Choi, Eung Gi Kwon, and Young Jun Kim. 2008. "Synthesis of Conjugated Linoleic Acid by Human-Derived *Bifidobacterium breve* LMC 017: Utilization as a Functional Starter Culture for Milk Fermentation." *Journal of Agricultural and Food Chemistry* 56 (9): 3311–16. https://doi.org/10.1021/jf0730789.

Cifuentes-Orjuela, Gloria. 2018. "Aislamiento, Identificación y Caracterización de Nuevos Probióticos Con Propiedades Funcionales Para Su Aplicación En Alimentación." Barcelona: Universitat Autonoma de Barcelona.

Cizeikiene, Dalia, and Jolita Jagelaviciute. 2021. "Investigation of Antibacterial Activity and Probiotic Properties of Strains Belonging to *Lactobacillus* and *Bifidobacterium* Genera for Their Potential Application in Functional Food and Feed Products." *Probiotics and Antimicrobial Proteins* 13 (5): 1387–1403. https://doi.org/10.1007/s12602-021-09777-5.

Cruz-Casas, Dora Elisa, Cristóbal N. Aguilar, Juan A. Ascacio-Valdés, Raúl Rodríguez-Herrera, Mónica L. Chávez-González, and Adriana C. Flores-Gallegos. 2023. "Bioactive Protein Hydrolysates Obtained from Amaranth by Fermentation with Lactic Acid Bacteria and *Bacillus* Species." *Heliyon* 9 (2): e13491. https://doi.org/10.1016/j.heliyon.2023.e13491.

Daba, Ghoson M., Marwa O. Elnahas, and Waill A. Elkhateeb. 2021. "Contributions of Exopolysaccharides from Lactic Acid Bacteria as Biotechnological Tools in Food, Pharmaceutical, and Medical Applications." *International Journal of Biological Macromolecules* 173 (March): 79–89. https://doi.org/10.1016/j.ijbiomac.2021.01.110.

Dahiya, Dinesh Kumar, and Anil Kumar Puniya. 2017. "Isolation, Molecular Characterization and Screening of Indigenous Lactobacilli for Their Abilities to Produce Bioactive Conjugated Linoleic Acid (CLA)." *Journal of Food Science and Technology* 54 (3): 792–801. https://doi.org/10.1007/s13197-017-2523-x.

Delgado, Susana, Lucía Guadamuro, Ana Belén Flórez, Lucía Vázquez, and Baltasar Mayo. 2019. "Fermentation of Commercial Soy Beverages with Lactobacilli and Bifidobacteria Strains Featuring High β-Glucosidase Activity." *Innovative Food Science & Emerging Technologies* 51 (January): 148–55. https://doi.org/10.1016/j.ifset.2018.03.018.

Derrien, Muriel, Francesca Turroni, Marco Ventura, and Douwe van Sinderen. 2022. "Insights into Endogenous *Bifidobacterium* Species in the Human Gut Microbiota during Adulthood." *Trends in Microbiology* 30 (10): 940–47. https://doi.org/10.1016/j.tim.2022.04.004.

Desai, M. S., Seekatz, A. M., Koropatkin, N. M., Kamada, N., Hickey, C. A., Wolter, M., Pudlo, N. A., Kitamoto, S., Terrapon, N., Muller, A., Young, V. B., Henrissat, B., Wilmes, P., Stappenbeck, T. S., Núñez, G., & Martens, E. C. 2016. "A Dietary Fiber-

Deprived Gut Microbiota Degrades the Colonic Mucus Barrier and Enhances Pathogen Susceptibility." *Cell* 167 (5): 1339-1353.e21. https://doi.org/10.1016/j.cell.2016.10.043.

Devika, N. T., and Karthik Raman. 2019. "Deciphering the Metabolic Capabilities of Bifidobacteria Using Genome-Scale Metabolic Models." *Scientific Reports* 9 (1): 18222. https://doi.org/10.1038/s41598-019-54696-9.

Dias, Desirrê Morais, Nikolai Kolba, Jon J. Hart, Michelle Ma, Sybil T. Sha, Naveena Lakshmanan, Marilia Regini Nutti, Hércia Stampini Duarte Martino, Raymond P. Glahn, and Elad Tako. 2019. "Soluble Extracts from Carioca Beans (*Phaseolus vulgaris* L.) Affect the Gut Microbiota and Iron Related Brush Border Membrane Protein Expression in Vivo (*Gallus gallus*)." *Food Research International* 123 (September): 172–80. https://doi.org/10.1016/j.foodres.2019.04.060.

Din, Ahmad Ud, Adil Hassan, Yuan Zhu, Kun Zhang, Yi Wang, Tianhan Li, Yang Wang, and Guixue Wang. 2020. "Inhibitory Effect of *Bifidobacterium bifidum* ATCC 29521 on Colitis and Its Mechanism." *The Journal of Nutritional Biochemistry* 79 (May): 108353. https://doi.org/10.1016/j.jnutbio.2020.108353.

Dyachkova, Marina S., Evgeny V. Chekalin, and Valery N. Danilenko. 2019. "Positive Selection in *Bifidobacterium* Genes Drives Species-Specific Host–Bacteria Communication." *Frontiers in Microbiology* 10 (October). https://doi.org/10.3389/fmicb.2019.02374.

Eamsobhana, Praphathip, Hoi-Sen Yong, Sudarat Boonyong, Darawan Wanachiwanawin, and Anchalee Tungtrongchitr. 2022. "Genetic Diversity and Identity of *Ascaris* Worms from Human and Pig Hosts in Thailand." *Veterinary Parasitology: Regional Studies and Reports* 33 (August): 100752. https://doi.org/10.1016/j.vprsr.2022.100752.

Engevik, M. A., Danhof, H. A., Hall, A., Engevik, K. A., Horvath, T. D., Haidacher, S. J., Hoch, K. M., Endres, B. T., Bajaj, M., Garey, K. W., Britton, R. A., Spinler, J. K., Haag, A. M., & Versalovic, J. 2021. "The Metabolic Profile of *Bifidobacterium dentium* Reflects Its Status as a Human Gut Commensal." *BMC Microbiology* 21 (1): 154. https://doi.org/10.1186/s12866-021-02166-6.

Engevik, M. A., Herrmann, B., Ruan, W., Engevik, A. C., Engevik, K. A., Ihekweazu, F., Shi, Z., Luck, B., Chang-Graham, A. L., Esparza, M., Venable, S., Horvath, T. D., Haidacher, S. J., Hoch, K. M., Haag, A. M., Schady, D. A., Hyser, J. M., Spinler, J. K., & Versalovic, J. 2021. "*Bifidobacterium dentium* -Derived y-Glutamylcysteine Suppresses ER-Mediated Goblet Cell Stress and Reduces TNBS-Driven Colonic Inflammation." *Gut Microbes* 13 (1). https://doi.org/10.1080/19490976.2021.1902717.

Escutia-Gutiérrez, Rebeca, Mónica Almeida-López, and Ana Sandoval-Rodríguez. 2023. "Alimentos Tradicionales de Origen Mexicano: ¿Cómo Contribuyen Para Combatir La Obesidad a Través de La Microbiota Intestinal?" *Revista de Divulgación Científica IBIO* 5 (1): CO119. http://revistaibio.com/ojs33/index.php/main/article/view/119.

Fan, Hongxiu, Hongcheng Liu, Yanrong Zhang, Shanshan Zhang, Tingting Liu, and Dawei Wang. 2022a. "Review on Plant-Derived Bioactive Peptides: Biological Activities, Mechanism of Action and Utilizations in Food Development." *Journal of Future Foods* 2 (2): 143–59. https://doi.org/10.1016/j.jfutfo.2022.03.003.

Fan, Hongxiu, Hongcheng Liu, Yanrong Zhang, Shanshan Zhang, Tingting Liu, and Dawei Wang. 2022b. "Review on Plant-Derived Bioactive Peptides: Biological Activities, Mechanism of Action and Utilizations in Food Development." *Journal of Future Foods* 2 (2): 143–59. https://doi.org/10.1016/j.jfutfo.2022.03.003.

Fanning, S., Hall, L. J., Cronin, M., Zomer, A., MacSharry, J., Goulding, D., O'Connell Motherway, M., Shanahan, F., Nally, K., Dougan, G., & Van Sinderen, D. 2012. "Bifidobacterial Surface-Exopolysaccharide Facilitates Commensal-Host Interaction through Immune Modulation and Pathogen Protection." *Proceedings of the National Academy of Sciences* 109 (6): 2108–13. https://doi.org/10.1073/pnas.1115621109.

FAO/WHO. 2006. "Probiotics in Food. Health and Nutritional Properties and Guidelines for Evaluation." In *Food and Nutrition Paper*, 85:4–5.

Feng, Tao, and Jing Wang. 2020. "Oxidative Stress Tolerance and Antioxidant Capacity of Lactic Acid Bacteria as Probiotic: A Systematic Review." *Gut Microbes* 12 (1): 1801944. https://doi.org/10.1080/19490976.2020.1801944.

Fitri, Loeki Enggar, Teguh Wahju Sardjono, Nuning Winaris, Aulia Rahmi Pawestri, Agustina Tri Endharti, Eviana Norahmawati, Dian Handayani, Shahdevi Nandar Kurniawan, Syafiatul Azizah, Lustyafa Inassani Alifia, Rokhmatul Asiyah, Tita Rachma Ayuningtyas. 2023. "*Bifidobacterium longum* Administration Diminishes Parasitemia and Inflammation During Plasmodium Berghei Infection in Mice." *Journal of Inflammation Research* Volume 16 (March): 1393–1404. https://doi.org/10.2147/JIR.S400782.

Fortin, Marie-Hélène, Claude P. Champagne, Daniel St-Gelais, Michel Britten, Patrick Fustier, and Monique Lacroix. 2011. "Effect of Time of Inoculation, Starter Addition, Oxygen Level and Salting on the Viability of Probiotic Cultures during Cheddar Cheese Production." *International Dairy Journal* 21 (2): 75–82. https://doi.org/10.1016/j.idairyj.2010.09.007.

Foster, James C., Matthew D. Glass, Polly D. Courtney, and Lucy A. Ward. 2003. "Effect of *Lactobacillus* and *Bifidobacterium* on *Cryptosporidium parvum* Oocyst Viability." *Food Microbiology* 20 (3): 351–57. https://doi.org/10.1016/S0740-0020(02)00120-X.

Fukumoto, Satoshi, Makoto Tatewaki, Tadanori Yamada, Mineko Fujimiya, Chris Mantyh, Miranda Voss, Steve Eubanks, Mary Harris, Theodore N. Pappas, and Toku Takahashi. 2003. "Short-Chain Fatty Acids Stimulate Colonic Transit via Intraluminal 5-HT Release in Rats." *American Journal of Physiology-Regulatory, Integrative and Comparative Physiology* 284 (5): R1269–76. https://doi.org/10.1152/ajpregu.00442.2002.

Furrie, E., S. Macfarlane, A. Kennedy, J. H. Cummings, S. V. Walsh, D. A. O´Neil, and G. T. Macfarlane. 2005. "Synbiotic Therapy (*Bifidobacterium longum*/Synergy 1) Initiates Resolution of Inflammation in Patients with Active Ulcerative Colitis: A Randomised Controlled Pilot Trial." *Gut* 54 (2): 242–49. https://doi.org/10.1136/gut.2004.044834.

Gagnon, Mérilie, Patricia Savard, Audrey Rivière, Gisèle LaPointe, and Denis Roy. 2015. "Bioaccessible Antioxidants in Milk Fermented by *Bifidobacterium Longum* Subsp. *Longum* Strains." *BioMed Research International* 2015: 1–12. https://doi.org/10.1155/2015/169381.

Gaudier, E., A. Jarry, H. M. Blottière, P. de Coppet, M. P. Buisine, J. P. Aubert, C. Laboisse, C. Cherbut, and C. Hoebler. 2004. "Butyrate Specifically Modulates *MUC* Gene Expression in Intestinal Epithelial Goblet Cells Deprived of Glucose." *American Journal of Physiology-Gastrointestinal and Liver Physiology* 287 (6): G1168–74. https://doi.org/10.1152/ajpgi.00219.2004.

Gavini, F., V. Delcenserie, K. Kopeinig, S. Pollinger, H. Beerens, C. Bonaparte, and M. Upmann. 2006. "*Bifidobacterium* Species Isolated from Animal Feces and from Beef and Pork Meat." *Journal of Food Protection* 69 (4): 871–77. https://doi.org/10.4315/0362-028X-69.4.871.

Gaya, Pilar, Ángela Peirotén, and José Mª Landete. 2017. "Transformation of Plant Isoflavones into Bioactive Isoflavones by Lactic Acid Bacteria and Bifidobacteria." *Journal of Functional Foods* 39 (December): 198–205. https://doi.org/10.1016/j.jff.2017.10.029.

Gaya, Pilar, Ángela Peirotén, Margarita Medina, and José Maria Landete. 2016. "Isoflavone Metabolism by a Collection of Lactic Acid Bacteria and Bifidobacteria with Biotechnological Interest." *International Journal of Food Sciences and Nutrition* 67 (2): 117–24. https://doi.org/10.3109/09637486.2016.1144724.

Ghedini, C. P., N. L. Whitehouse, D. C. Moura, A. S. Oliveira, and A. F. Brito. 2017. "Short Communication: The Mammalian Lignan Enterolactone Is Absorbed by Newborn Dairy Calves Fed Enterolactone-Enriched Milk." *Journal of Dairy Science* 100 (10): 8170–75. https://doi.org/10.3168/jds.2017-13093.

Gholami-Shabani, Mohammadhassan, Masoomeh Shams-Ghahfarokhi, and Mehdi Razzaghi-Abyaneh. 2023. "Food Microbiology: Application of Microorganisms in Food Industry." In *Health Risks of Food Additives - Recent Developments and Trends in Food Sector*, edited by Dr. Muhammad Sajid Arshad and Mr. Waseem Khalid, Ch. 2. Rijeka: IntechOpen. https://doi.org/10.5772/intechopen.109729.

Gomes, Ana M. P., and F. Xavier Malcata. 1998. "Development of Probiotic Cheese Manufactured from Goat Milk: Response Surface Analysis via Technological Manipulation." *Journal of Dairy Science* 81 (6): 1492–1507. https://doi.org/10.3168/jds.S0022-0302(98)75715-7.

Gonzalez-Gonzalez, Cid, Trevor Gibson, and Paula Jauregi. 2013. "Novel Probiotic-Fermented Milk with Angiotensin I-Converting Enzyme Inhibitory Peptides Produced by *Bifidobacterium bifidum* MF 20/5." *International Journal of Food Microbiology* 167 (2): 131–37. https://doi.org/10.1016/j.ijfoodmicro.2013.09.002.

Gorissen, Lara, Frédéric Leroy, Luc De Vuyst, Stefaan De Smet, and Katleen Raes. 2015. "Bacterial Production of Conjugated Linoleic and Linolenic Acid in Foods: A Technological Challenge." *Critical Reviews in Food Science and Nutrition* 55 (11): 1561–74. https://doi.org/10.1080/10408398.2012.706243.

Gorissen, Lara, Luc De Vuyst, Katleen Raes, Stefaan De Smet, and Frédéric Leroy. 2012. "Conjugated Linoleic and Linolenic Acid Production Kinetics by Bifidobacteria Differ among Strains." *International Journal of Food Microbiology* 155 (3): 234–40. https://doi.org/10.1016/j.ijfoodmicro.2012.02.012.

Groeger, David, Liam O'Mahony, Eileen F. Murphy, John F. Bourke, Timothy G. Dinan, Barry Kiely, Fergus Shanahan, and Eamonn M. M. Quigley. 2013. " *Bifidobacterium infantis* 35624 Modulates Host Inflammatory Processes beyond the Gut." *Gut Microbes* 4 (4): 325–39. https://doi.org/10.4161/gmic.25487.

Guo, Shuai, Meixuan Chen, Ting Wu, Kailong Liu, Heping Zhang, and Jicheng Wang. 2022. "Probiotic *Bifidobacterium animalis* sp. *lactis* Probio-M8 Improves the Properties and Organic Acid Metabolism of Fermented Goat Milk." *Journal of Dairy Science* 105 (12): 9426–38. https://doi.org/10.3168/jds.2022-22003.

Guo, Y., Xie, J.-P., Deng, K., Li, X., Yuan, Y., Xuan, Q., Xie, J., He, X.-M., Wang, Q., Li, J.-J., & Luo, H.-R. 2019. "Prophylactic Effects of *Bifidobacterium adolescentis* on Anxiety and Depression-Like Phenotypes After Chronic Stress: A Role of the Gut Microbiota-Inflammation Axis." *Frontiers in Behavioral Neuroscience* 13 (June). https://doi.org/10.3389/fnbeh.2019.00126.

Ha, Go Eun, Oun Ki Chang, Su-Mi Jo, Gi-Sung Han, Beom-Young Park, Jun-Sang Ham, and Seok-Geun Jeong. 2015. "Identification of Antihypertensive Peptides Derived from Low Molecular Weight Casein Hydrolysates Generated during Fermentation by *Bifidobacterium longum* KACC 91563." *Korean Journal for Food Science of Animal Resources* 35 (6): 738–47. https://doi.org/10.5851/kosfa.2015.35.6.738.

Hanum, Zuraida, Yurliasni Yurliasni, and Fadella Haqqi Seutia. 2022. "Antioxidant Activity of Fermented Goat's Milk with the Use of *Bifidobacterium Longum.*" In . https://doi.org/10.2991/absr.k.220309.073.

He, Fang, Hirotsugu Morita, Arthur C. Ouwehand, Masataka Hosoda, Masaru Hiramatsu, Jun-ichi Kurisaki, Erika Isolauri, Yoshimi Benno, and Seppo Salminen. 2002. "Stimulation of the Secretion of Pro-Inflammatory Cytokines by *Bifidobacterium* Strains." *Microbiology and Immunology* 46 (11): 781–85. https://doi.org/10.1111/j.1348-0421.2002.tb02765.x.

Heimesaat, Markus M., Ildiko R. Dunay, Marie Alutis, André Fischer, Luisa Möhle, Ulf B. Göbel, Anja A. Kühl, and Stefan Bereswill. 2014. "Nucleotide-Oligomerization-Domain-2 Affects Commensal Gut Microbiota Composition and Intracerebral Immunopathology in Acute *Toxoplasma gondii* Induced Murine Ileitis." *PLoS ONE* 9 (8): e105120. https://doi.org/10.1371/journal.pone.0105120.

Herselman, Mauritz F., Sheree Bailey, and Larisa Bobrovskaya. 2022. "The Effects of Stress and Diet on the 'Brain–Gut' and 'Gut–Brain' Pathways in Animal Models of Stress and Depression." *International Journal of Molecular Sciences* 23 (4): 2013. https://doi.org/10.3390/ijms23042013.

Heydari, Somayeh, Seyed Ebrahim Hosseini, Amir M. Mortazavian, and Salman Taheri. 2023. "Extraction of Bioactive Peptides Produced in Probiotic Yoghurt and Determination of Their Biological Activities." *International Dairy Journal* 139 (April): 105544. https://doi.org/10.1016/j.idairyj.2022.105544.

Hickey, A., Stamou, P., Udayan, S., Ramón-Vázquez, A., Esteban-Torres, M., Bottacini, F., Woznicki, J. A., Hughes, O., Melgar, S., Ventura, M., Van Sinderen, D., Rossini, V., & Nally, K.. 2021. "*Bifidobacterium breve* Exopolysaccharide Blocks Dendritic Cell Maturation and Activation of CD4+ T Cells." *Frontiers in Microbiology* 12 (June). https://doi.org/10.3389/fmicb.2021.653587.

Hidalgo-Cantabrana, Claudio, Milica Nikolic, Patricia López, Ana Suárez, Marija Miljkovic, Milan Kojic, Abelardo Margolles, Natasa Golic, and Patricia Ruas-Madiedo. 2014. "Exopolysaccharide-Producing *Bifidobacterium animalis* subsp.

lactis Strains and Their Polymers Elicit Different Responses on Immune Cells from Blood and Gut Associated Lymphoid Tissue." *Anaerobe* 26 (April): 24–30. https://doi.org/10.1016/j.anaerobe.2014.01.003.

Hidalgo-Cantabrana, Claudio, Patricia López, Miguel Gueimonde, Clara G. de los Reyes-Gavilán, Ana Suárez, Abelardo Margolles, and Patricia Ruas-Madiedo. 2012. "Immune Modulation Capability of Exopolysaccharides Synthesised by Lactic Acid Bacteria and Bifidobacteria." *Probiotics and Antimicrobial Proteins* 4 (4): 227–37. https://doi.org/10.1007/s12602-012-9110-2.

Hu, S., Li, A., Huang, T., Lai, J., Li, J., Sublette, M. E., Lu, H., Lu, Q., Du, Y., Hu, Z., Ng, C. H., Zhang, H., Lu, J., Mou, T., Lu, S., Wang, D., Duan, J., Hu, J., Huang, M., … Xu, Y. 2019. "Gut Microbiota Changes in Patients with Bipolar Depression." *Advanced Science* 6 (14): 1900752. https://doi.org/10.1002/advs.201900752.

Huang, L., Lv, X., Ze, X., Ma, Z., Zhang, X., He, R., Fan, J., Zhang, M., Sun, B., Wang, F., & Liu, H. 2022. "Combined Probiotics Attenuate Chronic Unpredictable Mild Stress-Induced Depressive-like and Anxiety-like Behaviors in Rats." *Frontiers in Psychiatry* 13 (September). https://doi.org/10.3389/fpsyt.2022.990465.

Huang, Xinyi, Tadayuki Oshima, Toshihiko Tomita, Hirokazu Fukui, and Hiroto Miwa. 2021. "Butyrate Alleviates Cytokine-Induced Barrier Dysfunction by Modifying Claudin-2 Levels." *Biology* 10 (3): 205. https://doi.org/10.3390/biology10030205.

Huang, Xiya, Weixi Cai, and Baojun Xu. 2014. "Kinetic Changes of Nutrients and Antioxidant Capacities of Germinated Soybean (*Glycine max* L.) and Mung Bean (*Vigna radiata* L.) with Germination Time." *Food Chemistry* 143 (January): 268–76. https://doi.org/10.1016/j.foodchem.2013.07.080.

Igbafe, Joy, Agnes Kilonzo-Nthenge, Samuel N. Nahashon, Abdullah Ibn Mafiz, and Maureen Nzomo. 2020. "Probiotics and Antimicrobial Effect of *Lactiplantibacillus plantarum*, *Saccharomyces cerevisiae*, and *Bifidobacterium longum* against Common Foodborne Pathogens in Poultry." *Agriculture* 10 (9): 368. https://doi.org/10.3390/agriculture10090368.

In Kim, Hye, Jeon-Kyung Kim, Jae-Young Kim, Se-Eun Jang, Myung Joo Han, and Dong-Hyun Kim. 2019. "*Lactobacillus plantarum* LC27 and *Bifidobacterium longum* LC67 Simultaneously Alleviate High-Fat Diet-Induced Colitis, Endotoxemia, Liver Steatosis, and Obesity in Mice." *Nutrition Research* 67 (July): 78–89. https://doi.org/10.1016/j.nutres.2019.03.008.

Inturri, Rosanna, Antonio Molinaro, Flaviana Di Lorenzo, Giovanna Blandino, Barbara Tomasello, Claudio Hidalgo-Cantabrana, Cristina De Castro, and Patricia Ruas-Madiedo. 2017. "Chemical and Biological Properties of the Novel Exopolysaccharide Produced by a Probiotic Strain of *Bifidobacterium longum*." *Carbohydrate Polymers* 174 (October): 1172–80. https://doi.org/10.1016/j.carbpol.2017.07.039.

Ishikawa, Hideki, Ikuko Akedo, Yoshinori Umesaki, Ryuichiro Tanaka, Akemi Imaoka, and Toru Otani. 2003. "Randomized Controlled Trial of the Effect of Bifidobacteria-Fermented Milk on Ulcerative Colitis." *Journal of the American College of Nutrition* 22 (1): 56–63. https://doi.org/10.1080/07315724.2003.10719276.

Ismail, Amin, Azrina Azlan, Mohd Manap, and Sadeq Hasan Al-Sheraji. 2019. "Nutrigenomic Effects of Fermented Milk Containing *Bifidobacterium longum* Bb536 on Hepatic Cholesterologenic Genes in Hypercholesterolemic Rats." *Advances in Dairy Research* 7 (220).

Jafar, Nehan Bahaaldden, Zainab Hussein Fadhil, Evan Mohammed Mustafa, and Ali Mohammed Saadi. 2022. "Investigation the Inhibitory Effects of AgNPs Generated by *Bifidobacterium* spp. on Bacteria Isolated from Ready-to-Eat Foods." *Food Science and Technology* 42. https://doi.org/10.1590/fst.88721.

Jakubczyk, Dominika, Katarzyna Leszczyńska, and Sabina Górska. 2020. "The Effectiveness of Probiotics in the Treatment of Inflammatory Bowel Disease (IBD)—A Critical Review." *Nutrients* 12 (7): 1973. https://doi.org/10.3390/nu12071973.

Jang, Dong-Hun, Hyung-Chul Cho, Yu-Jin Park, Jinho Park, and Kyoung-Seong Choi. 2023. "First Report of *Cryptosporidium andersoni* and Risk Factors Associated with the Occurrence of *Cryptosporidium* spp. in Pre-Weaned Native Korean Calves with Diarrhea." *Frontiers in Veterinary Science* 10 (March). https://doi.org/10.3389/fvets.2023.1145096.

Jensen, A. N., Mejer, H., Mølbak, L., Langkjær, M., Jensen, T. K., Angen, Ø., Martinussen, T., Klitgaard, K., Baggesen, D. L., Thamsborg, S. M., & Roepstorff, A. 2011. "The Effect of a Diet with Fructan-Rich Chicory Roots on Intestinal Helminths and Microbiota with Special Focus on Bifidobacteria and *Campylobacter* in Piglets around Weaning." *Animal* 5 (6): 851–60. https://doi.org/10.1017/S175173111000251X.

Juillard, Vincent, Liliana Lopez-Kleine, and Véronique Monnet. 2022. "Lactic Acid Bacteria: Proteolytic Systems." In *Encyclopedia of Dairy Sciences*, 249–55. Elsevier. https://doi.org/10.1016/B978-0-08-100596-5.00862-3.

Kandpal, Meenakshi, Omkar Indari, Budhadev Baral, Shweta Jakhmola, Deeksha Tiwari, Vasundhra Bhandari, Rajan Kumar Pandey, Kiran Bala, Avinash Sonawane, and Hem Chandra Jha. 2022. "Dysbiosis of Gut Microbiota from the Perspective of the Gut–Brain Axis: Role in the Provocation of Neurological Disorders." *Metabolites* 12 (11): 1064. https://doi.org/10.3390/metabo12111064.

Kang, M. J., Jeong, H., Kim, S., Shin, J., Song, Y., Lee, B.-H., Park, H.-G., Lee, T.-H., Jiang, H.-H., Han, Y.-S., Lee, B.-G., Lee, H.-J., Park, M.-J., & Park, Y.-S. 2023. "Structural Analysis and Prebiotic Activity of Exopolysaccharide Produced by Probiotic Strain *Bifidobacterium bifidum* EPS DA-LAIM." *Food Science and Biotechnology* 32 (4): 517–29. https://doi.org/10.1007/s10068-022-01213-w.

Katayama, Shigeru, Henry M. Corpuz, and Soichiro Nakamura. 2021. "Potential of Plant-Derived Peptides for the Improvement of Memory and Cognitive Function." *Peptides* 142 (August): 170571. https://doi.org/10.1016/j.peptides.2021.170571.

Kim, Hee-Young, Eui-Seong Park, Young Sik Choi, Seun Ja Park, Jae Hyun Kim, Hee Kyung Chang, and Kun-Young Park. 2022. "Kimchi Improves Irritable Bowel Syndrome: Results of a Randomized, Double-Blind Placebo-Controlled Study." *Food & Nutrition Research* 66 (May). https://doi.org/10.29219/fnr.v66.8268.

Kim, Hyemin, Jin-Seong Kim, YongGyeong Kim, Yulah Jeong, Ji-Eun Kim, Nam-Soo Paek, and Chang-Ho Kang. 2020. "Antioxidant and Probiotic Properties of Lactobacilli and Bifidobacteria of Human Origins." *Biotechnology and Bioprocess Engineering* 25 (3): 421–30. https://doi.org/10.1007/s12257-020-0147-x.

Kim, J.-H., Jeun, E.-J., Hong, C.-P., Kim, S.-H., Jang, M. S., Lee, E.-J., Moon, S. J., Yun, C. H., Im, S.-H., Jeong, S.-G., Park, B.-Y., Kim, K.-T., Seoh, J.-Y., Kim, Y.-K., Oh,

S.-J., Ham, J.-S., Yang, B.-G., & Jang, M. H. 2016. "Extracellular Vesicle–Derived Protein from *Bifidobacterium longum* Alleviates Food Allergy through Mast Cell Suppression." *Journal of Allergy and Clinical Immunology* 137 (2): 507-516.e8. https://doi.org/10.1016/j.jaci.2015.08.016.

Kim, Ji Yeun, Young Ok Choi, and Geun Eog Ji. 2008. "Effect of Oral Probiotics (*Bifidobacterium lactis* AD011 and *Lactobacillus acidophilus* AD031) Administration on Ovalbumin-Induced Food Allergy Mouse Model." *Journal of Microbiology and Biotechnology* 18 (8): 1393–1400.

Kim, Won-Gyeong, Hye In Kim, Eun Kyung Kwon, Myung Joo Han, and Dong-Hyun Kim. 2018. "*Lactobacillus Plantarum* LC27 and *Bifidobacterium Longum* LC67 Mitigate Alcoholic Steatosis in Mice by Inhibiting LPS-Mediated NF-κB Activation through Restoration of the Disturbed Gut Microbiota." *Food & Function* 9 (8): 4255–65. https://doi.org/10.1039/C8FO00252E.

Kowalczyk, Magdalena, Agata Znamirowska-Piotrowska, Magdalena Buniowska-Olejnik, and Małgorzata Pawlos. 2022. "Sheep Milk Symbiotic Ice Cream: Effect of Inulin and Apple Fiber on the Survival of Five Probiotic Bacterial Strains during Simulated *In Vitro* Digestion Conditions." *Nutrients* 14 (21): 4454. https://doi.org/10.3390/nu14214454.

Landete, J. M., J. Arqués, M. Medina, P. Gaya, B. de Las Rivas, and R. Muñoz. 2016. "Bioactivation of Phytoestrogens: Intestinal Bacteria and Health." *Critical Reviews in Food Science and Nutrition* 56 (11): 1826–43. https://doi.org/10.1080/10408398.2013.789823.

Leccese, Gabriella, Alessia Bibi, Stefano Mazza, Federica Facciotti, Flavio Caprioli, Paolo Landini, and Moira Paroni. 2020. "Probiotic *Lactobacillus* and *Bifidobacterium* Strains Counteract Adherent-Invasive Escherichia coli (AIEC) Virulence and Hamper IL-23/Th17 Axis in Ulcerative Colitis, but Not in Crohn's Disease." *Cells* 9 (8): 1824. https://doi.org/10.3390/cells9081824.

Lee, Sung Hee. 2015. "Intestinal Permeability Regulation by Tight Junction: Implication on Inflammatory Bowel Diseases." *Intestinal Research* 13 (1): 11. https://doi.org/10.5217/ir.2015.13.1.11.

Li, Huawei, Peng Wang, Luqiao Huang, Ping Li, and Dianliang Zhang. 2019. "Effects of Regulating Gut Microbiota on the Serotonin Metabolism in the Chronic Unpredictable Mild Stress Rat Model." *Neurogastroenterology & Motility* 31 (10). https://doi.org/10.1111/nmo.13677.

Li, Long-Qing, Xu Chen, Jie Zhu, Shuyan Zhang, Si-Qian Chen, Xiaozhen Liu, Lin Li, and Jing-Kun Yan. 2023. "Advances and Challenges in Interaction between Heteroglycans and *Bifidobacterium*: Utilization Strategies, Intestinal Health and Future Perspectives." *Trends in Food Science & Technology* 134 (April): 112–22. https://doi.org/10.1016/j.tifs.2023.02.018.

Li, Shengjie, Renhui Huang, Nagendra P. Shah, Xueying Tao, Yonghua Xiong, and Hua Wei. 2014. "Antioxidant and Antibacterial Activities of Exopolysaccharides from *Bifidobacterium bifidum* WBIN03 and *Lactobacillus plantarum* R315." *Journal of Dairy Science* 97 (12): 7334–43. https://doi.org/10.3168/jds.2014-7912.

Li, Wentao, Lixia Kai, Zipeng Jiang, Huan He, Mingzhi Yang, Weifa Su, Yizhen Wang, Mingliang Jin, and Zeqing Lu. 2022. "*Bifidobacterium longum, Lactobacillus plantarum* and *Pediococcus acidilactici* Reversed ETEC-Inducing Intestinal Inflammation in Mice." *Microorganisms* 10 (12): 2350. https://doi.org/10.3390/microorganisms10122350.

Liu, Guiyang, Huahai Chen, Junkui Chen, Xin Wang, Qing Gu, and Yeshi Yin. 2019. "Effects of Bifidobacteria-Produced Exopolysaccharides on Human Gut Microbiota *in Vitro*." *Applied Microbiology and Biotechnology* 103 (4): 1693–1702. https://doi.org/10.1007/s00253-018-9572-6.

Liu, M.-Y., Yang, Z.-Y., Dai, W.-K., Huang, J.-Q., Li, Y.-H., Zhang, J., Qiu, C.-Z., Wei, C., Zhou, Q., Sun, X., Feng, X., Li, D.-F., Wang, H.-P., & Zheng, Y.-J. 2017. "Protective Effect of *Bifidobacterium infantis* CGMCC313-2 on Ovalbumin-Induced Airway Asthma and β-Lactoglobulin-Induced Intestinal Food Allergy Mouse Models." *World Journal of Gastroenterology* 23 (12): 2149. https://doi.org/10.3748/wjg.v23.i12.2149.

Liu, Weiwei, Tao Hou, Wen Shi, Danjun Guo, and Hui He. 2018. "Hepatoprotective Effects of Selenium-Biofortified Soybean Peptides on Liver Fibrosis Induced by Tetrachloromethane." *Journal of Functional Foods* 50 (November): 183–91. https://doi.org/10.1016/j.jff.2018.09.034.

Llamas-Arriba, María Goretti, Ángela Peirotén, Ana Isabel Puertas, Alicia Prieto, Paloma López, Miguel Á. Pardo, Eva Rodríguez, and María Teresa Dueñas. 2019. "Heteropolysaccharide-Producing Bifidobacteria for the Development of Functional Dairy Products." *LWT* 102 (March): 295–303. https://doi.org/10.1016/j.lwt.2018.12.044.

Luo, Meng, Min Gan, XiaoMin Yu, XiaoLi Wu, and Feng Xu. 2020. "Study on the Regulatory Effects and Mechanisms of Action of Bifidobacterial Exopolysaccharides on Anaphylaxes in Mice." *International Journal of Biological Macromolecules* 165 (December): 1447–54. https://doi.org/10.1016/j.ijbiomac.2020.09.224.

Luo, Wei, Zhangmin Zhao, Hepeng Pan, Lankun Zhao, Chuangao Xu, and Xiaobin Yu. 2018. "Feasibility of Butanol Production from Wheat Starch Wastewater by *Clostridium acetobutylicum*." *Energy* 154 (July): 240–48. https://doi.org/10.1016/j.energy.2018.04.125.

Ma, X., Pan, Y., Zhao, W., Sun, P., Zhao, J., Yan, S., Wang, R., Han, Y., Liu, W., Tan, S., & Hung, W. 2022. "*Bifidobacterium Infantis* Strain YLGB -1496 Possesses Excellent Antioxidant and Skin Barrier-enhancing Efficacy in Vitro." *Experimental Dermatology* 31 (7): 1089–94. https://doi.org/10.1111/exd.14583.

Macfarlane, Sandra, and George T. Macfarlane. 2003. "Regulation of Short-Chain Fatty Acid Production." *Proceedings of the Nutrition Society* 62 (1): 67–72. https://doi.org/10.1079/PNS2002207.

Macia, L., Tan, J., Vieira, A. T., Leach, K., Stanley, D., Luong, S., Maruya, M., Ian McKenzie, C., Hijikata, A., Wong, C., Binge, L., Thorburn, A. N., Chevalier, N., Ang, C., Marino, E., Robert, R., Offermanns, S., Teixeira, M. M., Moore, R. J., … Mackay, C. R. 2015. "Metabolite-Sensing Receptors GPR43 and GPR109A Facilitate Dietary Fibre-Induced Gut Homeostasis through Regulation of the Inflammasome." *Nature Communications* 6 (1): 6734. https://doi.org/10.1038/ncomms7734.

Madsen, Karen L. 2012. "Enhancement of Epithelial Barrier Function by Probiotics." *Journal of Epithelial Biology and Pharmacology* 5 (1): 55–59. https://doi.org/10.2174/1875044301205010055.

Makki, Kassem, Edward C. Deehan, Jens Walter, and Fredrik Bäckhed. 2018. "The Impact of Dietary Fiber on Gut Microbiota in Host Health and Disease." *Cell Host & Microbe.* 23 (6): 705–15. https://doi.org/10.1016/j.chom.2018.05.012.

Marcos-Fernández, Raquel, Aitor Blanco-Míguez, Lorena Ruiz, Abelardo Margolles, Patricia Ruas-Madiedo, and Borja Sánchez. 2023. "Towards the Isolation of More Robust next Generation Probiotics: The First Aerotolerant *Bifidobacterium bifidum* Strain." *Food Research International* 165 (March): 112481. https://doi.org/10.1016/j.foodres.2023.112481.

Marin, Maria L., Maria V. Tejada-Simon, Jong H. Lee, Jill Murtha, Zeynep Ustunol, and James J. Pestka. 1998. "Stimulation of Cytokine Production in Clonal Macrophage and T-Cell Models by *Streptococcus thermophilus*: Comparison with *Bifidobacterium* sp. and *Lactobacillus bulgaricus*." *Journal of Food Protection* 61 (7): 859–64. https://doi.org/10.4315/0362-028X-61.7.859.

Markowiak, Paulina, and Katarzyna Śliżewska. 2017. "Effects of Probiotics, Prebiotics, and Synbiotics on Human Health." *Nutrients* 9 (9): 1021. https://doi.org/10.3390/nu9091021.

Marteau, P., M. Minekus, R. Havenaar, and J. H. J. Huis In't Veld. 1997. "Survival of Lactic Acid Bacteria in a Dynamic Model of the Stomach and Small Intestine: Validation and the Effects of Bile." *Journal of Dairy Science* 80 (6): 1031–37. https://doi.org/10.3168/jds.S0022-0302(97)76027-2.

Martín, Rocío, Esther Jiménez, Hans Heilig, Leonides Fernández, María L. Marín, Erwin G. Zoetendal, and Juan M. Rodríguez. 2009. "Isolation of Bifidobacteria from Breast Milk and Assessment of the Bifidobacterial Population by PCR-Denaturing Gradient Gel Electrophoresis and Quantitative Real-Time PCR." *Applied and Environmental Microbiology* 75 (4): 965–69. https://doi.org/10.1128/AEM.02063-08.

Martínez-López, Ana L., Elizabeth Carvajal-Millan, Valérie Micard, Agustín Rascón-Chu, Francisco Brown-Bojorquez, Norberto Sotelo-Cruz, Yolanda L. López-Franco, and Jaime Lizardi-Mendoza. 2016. "*In Vitro* Degradation of Covalently Cross-Linked Arabinoxylan Hydrogels by Bifidobacteria." *Carbohydrate Polymers* 144 (June): 76–82. https://doi.org/10.1016/j.carbpol.2016.02.031.

Martorell, P., Alvarez, B., Llopis, S., Navarro, V., Ortiz, P., Gonzalez, N., Balaguer, F., Rojas, A., Chenoll, E., Ramón, D., & Tortajada, M. 2021. "Heat-Treated *Bifidobacterium longum* CECT-7347: A Whole-Cell Postbiotic with Antioxidant, Anti-Inflammatory, and Gut-Barrier Protection Properties." *Antioxidants* 10 (4): 536. https://doi.org/10.3390/antiox10040536.

Mayorga-Reyes, L., P. Bustamante-Camilo, A. Gutiérrez-Nava, E. Barranco-Florido, and A. Azaola-Espinosa. 2009. "Crecimiento, sobrevivencia y adaptación de *Bifidobacterium infantis* a condiciones ácidas." *Revista Mexicana de Ingeniería Química* 8 (3): 259–64. https://www.redalyc.org/articulo.oa?id=62016349003.

Mazmanian, Sarkis K., Cui Hua Liu, Arthur O. Tzianabos, and Dennis L. Kasper. 2005. "An Immunomodulatory Molecule of Symbiotic Bacteria Directs Maturation of the

Host Immune System." *Cell* 122 (1): 107–18. https://doi.org/10.1016/j.cell.2005.05.007.

Mei, Yongchao, Haiqin Chen, Bo Yang, Jianxin Zhao, Hao Zhang, and Wei Chen. 2022. "Research Progress on Conjugated Linoleic Acid Bio-Conversion in *Bifidobacterium*." *International Journal of Food Microbiology* 369 (May): 109593. https://doi.org/10.1016/j.ijfoodmicro.2022.109593.

Meng, Di, Eduardo Sommella, Emanuela Salviati, Pietro Campiglia, Kriston Ganguli, Karim Djebali, Weishu Zhu, and W. Allan Walker. 2020. "Indole-3-Lactic Acid, a Metabolite of Tryptophan, Secreted by *Bifidobacterium longum* Subspecies *infantis* Is Anti-Inflammatory in the Immature Intestine." *Pediatric Research* 88 (2): 209–17. https://doi.org/10.1038/s41390-019-0740-x.

Modrackova, Nikol, Marie Makovska, Chahrazed Mekadim, Eva Vlkova, Vaclav Tejnecky, Petra Bolechova, and Vera Bunesova. 2019. "Prebiotic Potential of Natural Gums and Starch for Bifidobacteria of Variable Origins." *Bioactive Carbohydrates and Dietary Fibre* 20 (October): 100199. https://doi.org/10.1016/j.bcdf.2019.100199.

Moghadam, Behnam Esmaeilnejad, Zohreh Hasebi, Somayyeh Seyfzadeh, Vahideh Talebi, Fatemeh Keivaninahr, Masoumeh Fouladi, and Reza Rezaei Mokarram. 2022. "Barley β-Glucan for Conjugated Linoleic Acid (CLA) Production by *Bifidobacterium animalis* subsp. *lactis*: Fatty Acid Variation and Bacterial Viability Study." *Bioactive Carbohydrates and Dietary Fibre* 28 (November): 100321. https://doi.org/10.1016/j.bcdf.2022.100321.

Mohammed, S. T., K. Jabur, and Ha Aja. 2017. "Effect of Yogurt and *Bifidobacterium* on *Cryptosporidium parvum* Infection In Experiential Infected Mice." *Ibn AL-Haitham Journal For Pure and Applied Science* 24 (3).

Moreno de LeBlanc, A. de, S. Chaves, E. Carmuega, R. Weill, J. Antóine, and Gabriela Perdigón. 2008. "Effect of Long-Term Continuous Consumption of Fermented Milk Containing Probiotic Bacteria on Mucosal Immunity and the Activity of Peritoneal Macrophages." *Immunobiology* 213 (2): 97–108. https://doi.org/10.1016/j.imbio.2007.07.002.

Moreno, Izildinha, Elza Teresinha Grael Marasca, Patrícia Blumer Zacarchenco Rodrigu de Sá, Josiane de Souza Moitinho, Miriam Gonçalves Marquezini, Márcia Regina Cucatti Alves, and Renata Bromberg. 2018. "Evaluation of Probiotic Potential of Bacteriocinogenic Lactic Acid Bacteria Strains Isolated from Meat Products." *Probiotics and Antimicrobial Proteins* 10 (4): 762–74. https://doi.org/10.1007/s12602-018-9388-9.

Mutai, Masahiko, Higashi Yamato, Mitsuo Mada, Kodaira Kiyohiro Shimada, and all of Japan Kabushiki Kaisha Yakult Honsha. 1980. Method for producing foods and drinks containing bifidobacteria. 4187321, issued 1980.

Myhill, L. J., Stolzenbach, S., Mejer, H., Krych, L., Jakobsen, S. R., Kot, W., Skovgaard, K., Canibe, N., Nejsum, P., Nielsen, D. S., Thamsborg, S. M., & Williams, A. R. 2022. "Parasite-Probiotic Interactions in the Gut: *Bacillus* sp. and *Enterococcus faecium* Regulate Type-2 Inflammatory Responses and Modify the Gut Microbiota of Pigs During Helminth Infection." *Frontiers in Immunology* 12 (January). https://doi.org/10.3389/fimmu.2021.793260.

Nguyen, Bao Toan, Erika Bujna, Noemi Fekete, Anh T. M. Tran, Judit M. Rezessy-Szabo, Ram Prasad, and Quang D. Nguyen. 2019. "Probiotic Beverage From Pineapple Juice Fermented With *Lactobacillus* and *Bifidobacterium* Strains." *Frontiers in Nutrition* 6 (May). https://doi.org/10.3389/fnut.2019.00054.

Nguyen, H. T., Hongsrichan, N., Intuyod, K., Pinlaor, P., Yingklang, M., Chaidee, A., Sengthong, C., Pongking, T., Dangtakot, R., Banjong, D., Anutrakulchai, S., Cha'On, U., & Pinlaor, S. 2022. "Investigation of Gut Microbiota and Short-Chain Fatty Acids in *Strongyloides stercoralis*-Infected Patients in a Rural Community." *Bioscience of Microbiota, Food and Health* 41 (3): 2021–54. https://doi.org/10.12938/bmfh.2021-054.

Nicklaus, S., Divaret-Chauveau, A., Chardon, M., Roduit, C., Kaulek, V., Ksiazek, E., Dalphin, M., Karvonen, A. M., Kirjavainen, P., Pekkanen, J., Lauener, R., Schmausser-Hechfellner, E., Renz, H., Braun-Fahrländer, C., Riedler, J., Vuitton, D. A., Mutius, E. V., Dalphin, J., & Pasture Study Group. 2019. "The Protective Effect of Cheese Consumption at 18 Months on Allergic Diseases in the First 6 Years." *Allergy* 74 (4): 788–98. https://doi.org/10.1111/all.13650.

Nzingula, Olivier, Junior Disashi, José Mulwahali, Pius Kabututu, Paola Biakas, and Justin Masumu. 2023. "Identification of *Lactobacillus* and *Bifidobacterium* 16S RRNA Gene in Breast Milk of Some Healthy Women in Kinshasa (DR Congo)." *Journal of Biosciences and Medicines* 11 (02): 275–86. https://doi.org/10.4236/jbm.2023.112022.

O'Riordan, Kenneth J., Michael K. Collins, Gerard M. Moloney, Emily G. Knox, María R. Aburto, Christine Fülling, Shane J. Morley, Gerard Clarke, Harriët Schellekens, and John F. Cryan. 2022. "Short Chain Fatty Acids: Microbial Metabolites for Gut-Brain Axis Signalling." *Molecular and Cellular Endocrinology* 546 (April): 111572. https://doi.org/10.1016/j.mce.2022.111572.

Oberg, Taylor S., and Jeff R. Broadbent. 2016. "Hydrogen Peroxide Resistance in *Bifidobacterium animalis* subsp. *lactis* and *Bifidobacterium longum*." In *Stress and Environmental Regulation of Gene Expression and Adaptation in Bacteria*, 638–46. Hoboken, NJ, USA: John Wiley & Sons, Inc. https://doi.org/10.1002/9781119004813.ch61.

Oberg, Taylor S., Robert E. Ward, James L. Steele, and Jeff R. Broadbent. 2015. "Transcriptome Analysis of *Bifidobacterium longum* Strains That Show a Differential Response to Hydrogen Peroxide Stress." *Journal of Biotechnology* 212 (October): 58–64. https://doi.org/10.1016/j.jbiotec.2015.06.405.

Ogata, T., M. Kingaku, and T. Yaeshima. 1999. "Effect of *Bifidobacterium longum* BB536 Yogurt Administration on the Intestinal Environment of Healthy Adults." *Microbial Ecology in Health and Disease* 11 (1): 41–46. https://doi.org/10.1080/089106099435916.

Ohata, Atsushi, Makoto Usami, and Makoto Miyoshi. 2005. "Short-Chain Fatty Acids Alter Tight Junction Permeability in Intestinal Monolayer Cells via Lipoxygenase Activation." *Nutrition* 21 (7–8): 838–47. https://doi.org/10.1016/j.nut.2004.12.004.

Olivares, Mónica, Ma Paz Díaz-Ropero, Nuria Gómez, Saleta Sierra, Federico Lara-Villoslada, Rocío Martín, Juan Miguel Rodríguez, and Jordi Xaus. 2006. "Dietary Deprivation of Fermented Foods Causes a Fall in Innate Immune Response. Lactic

Acid Bacteria Can Counteract the Immunological Effect of This Deprivation." *Journal of Dairy Research* 73 (4): 492–98. https://doi.org/10.1017/S0022029906002068.

Onderdonk, B. W. 2000. "Intestinal Microflora and Inflammatory Bowel Disease." In *Inflammatory Bowel Disease*, edited by JB Krisner, 5th ed., 144–52. Philadelphia: Saunders.

Park, Ho-Eun, Ye Jin Kim, Kyung-Hyo Do, Jae Kwang Kim, Jun-Sang Ham, and Wan-Kyu Lee. 2018. "Effects of Queso Blanco Cheese Containing *Bifidobacterium longum* KACC 91563 on the Intestinal Microbiota and Short Chain Fatty Acid in Healthy Companion Dogs." *Korean Journal for Food Science of Animal Resources* 38 (6): 1261–72. https://doi.org/10.5851/kosfa.2018.e62.

Park, Ho-Eun, Ye Jin Kim, Minseok Kim, HyeRan Kim, Kyung-Hyo Do, Jae Kwang Kim, Jun-Sang Ham, and Wan-Kyu Lee. 2020. "Effects of Queso Blanco Cheese Containing *Bifidobacterium longum* KACC 91563 on Fecal Microbiota, Metabolite and Serum Cytokine in Healthy Beagle Dogs." *Anaerobe* 64 (August): 102234. https://doi.org/10.1016/j.anaerobe.2020.102234.

Passos, Fabine Correia, Marcelo Biondaro Gois, Adenilma Duranes Sousa, Ananda Isis Lima de Marinho, Laura Corvo, Manoel Soto, Manoel Barral-Netto, Aldina Barral, and Gyselle Chrystina Baccan. 2020. "Investigating Associations between Intestinal Alterations and Parasite Load According to *Bifidobacterium* spp. and *Lactobacillus* spp. Abundance in the Gut Microbiota of Hamsters Infected by *Leishmania infantum.*" *Memórias Do Instituto Oswaldo Cruz* 115. https://doi.org/10.1590/0074-02760200377.

Patel, Priya, Krishna Butani, Akash Kumar, Sudarshan Singh, and Bhupendra G. Prajapati. 2023. "Effects of Fermented Food Consumption on Non-Communicable Diseases." *Foods* 12 (4): 687. https://doi.org/10.3390/foods12040687.

Pavli, F., A. A. Argyri, G.-J. E. Nychas, C. Tassou, and N. Chorianopoulos. 2018. "Use of Fourier Transform Infrared Spectroscopy for Monitoring the Shelf Life of Ham Slices Packed with Probiotic Supplemented Edible Films after Treatment with High Pressure Processing." *Food Research International* 106 (April): 1061–68. https://doi.org/10.1016/j.foodres.2017.12.064.

Paz-Samaniego, Rita, Norberto Sotelo-Cruz, Jorge Marquez-Escalante, Agustín Rascon-Chu, Alma C. Campa-Mada, and Elizabeth Carvajal-Millan. 2019. "Nixtamalized Maize Flour By-Product as a Source of Health-Promoting Ferulated Arabinoxylans (AX)." In *Flour and Breads and Their Fortification in Health and Disease Prevention*, 225–35. Elsevier. https://doi.org/10.1016/B978-0-12-814639-2.00018-6.

Peirotén, Ángela, Daniel Bravo, and José M. Landete. 2020. "Bacterial Metabolism as Responsible of Beneficial Effects of Phytoestrogens on Human Health." *Critical Reviews in Food Science and Nutrition* 60 (11): 1922–37. https://doi.org/10.1080/10408398.2019.1622505.

Pérez, Indira, Aura Falco, María Soledad Tapia, and Guillermina Alonso. 2012. "Aislamiento e Identificación de Cepas Del Género *Bifidobacterium* Presentes En Productos Lácteos Fermentados Tipo Yogur." *Revista de La Sociedad Venezolana de Microbiología* 32: 29–36.

Perez-Chabela, M. Lourdes, Angelica Cerda-Tapia, Juan Diaz-Vela, P. Claudia Delgadillo, M. Margarita Diaz, and Gabriela Aleman. 2015. "Physiological Effects of

Agroindustrial Co-Products: Cactus (*Opuntia ficus*) Pear Peel Flour and Stripe Apple (*Malus domestica*) Marc Flour on Wistar Rats (*Rattus norvegicus*)." *Pakistan Journal of Nutrition* 14 (6): 346–52. https://doi.org/10.3923/pjn.2015.346.352.

Pochart, P., P. Marteau, Y. Bouhnik, I. Goderel, P. Bourlioux, and J. C. Rambaud. 1992. "Survival of Bifidobacteria Ingested via Fermented Milk during Their Passage through the Human Small Intestine: An *in Vivo* Study Using Intestinal Perfusion." *The American Journal of Clinical Nutrition* 55 (1): 78–80. https://doi.org/10.1093/ajcn/55.1.78.

Pohl, Keith, Prebashan Moodley, and Ashwin Dhanda. 2022. "The Effect of Increasing Intestinal Short-chain Fatty Acid Concentration on Gut Permeability and Liver Injury in the Context of Liver Disease: A Systematic Review." *Journal of Gastroenterology and Hepatology* 37 (8): 1498–1506. https://doi.org/10.1111/jgh.15899.

Prasanna, P. H. P., A. Bell, A. S. Grandison, and D. Charalampopoulos. 2012. "Emulsifying, Rheological and Physicochemical Properties of Exopolysaccharide Produced by *Bifidobacterium longum* subsp. *infantis* CCUG 52486 and *Bifidobacterium infantis* NCIMB 702205." *Carbohydrate Polymers* 90 (1): 533–40. https://doi.org/10.1016/j.carbpol.2012.05.075.

Rafiq, Saima, Nabila Gulzar, Aysha Sameen, Nuzhat Huma, Imran Hayat, and Raina Ijaz. 2021. "Functional Role of Bioactive Peptides with Special Reference to Cheeses." *International Journal of Dairy Technology* 74 (1): 1–16. https://doi.org/10.1111/1471-0307.12732.

Ranadheera, Chaminda, Janak Vidanarachchi, Ramon Rocha, Adriano Cruz, and Said Ajlouni. 2017. "Probiotic Delivery through Fermentation: Dairy vs. Non-Dairy Beverages." *Fermentation* 3 (4): 67. https://doi.org/10.3390/fermentation3040067.

Rani, Alka, Khem Saini, Felix Bast, Sanjeet Mehariya, Shashi Bhatia, Roberto Lavecchia, and Antonio Zuorro. 2021. "Microorganisms: A Potential Source of Bioactive Molecules for Antioxidant Applications." *Molecules* 26 (4): 1142. https://doi.org/10.3390/molecules26041142.

Rodríguez R., Yeimy Alejandra, Andrés Felipe Rojas G., and Sneyder Rodríguez B. 2016. "Encapsulación de Probióticos Para Aplicaciones Alimenticias." *Biosalud* 15 (2): 106–15. https://doi.org/10.17151/biosa.2016.15.2.10.

Rodriguez, Cynthia I., and Jennifer B. H. Martiny. 2020. "Evolutionary Relationships among Bifidobacteria and Their Hosts and Environments." *BMC Genomics* 21 (1): 26. https://doi.org/10.1186/s12864-019-6435-1.

Roselli, M., Natella, F., Zinno, P., Guantario, B., Canali, R., Schifano, E., De Angelis, M., Nikoloudaki, O., Gobbetti, M., Perozzi, G., & Devirgiliis, C. 2021. "Colonization Ability and Impact on Human Gut Microbiota of Foodborne Microbes From Traditional or Probiotic-Added Fermented Foods: A Systematic Review." *Frontiers in Nutrition* 8 (July). https://doi.org/10.3389/fnut.2021.689084.

Ruiz de la Bastida, Ana, Ángela Peirotén, Susana Langa, Inmaculada Álvarez, Juan Luis Arqués, and José Mª Landete. 2021. "Metabolism of Flavonoids and Lignans by Lactobacilli and Bifidobacteria Strains Improves the Nutritional Properties of Flaxseed-Enriched Beverages." *Food Research International* 147 (September): 110488. https://doi.org/10.1016/j.foodres.2021.110488.

Ryhänen, Eeva-Liisa, Anne Pihlanto-Leppälä, and Eero Pahkala. 2001. "A New Type of Ripened, Low-Fat Cheese with Bioactive Properties." *International Dairy Journal* 11 (4–7): 441–47. https://doi.org/10.1016/S0958-6946(01)00079-6.

Sadeghpour Heravi, Fatemah, and Honghua Hu. 2023. "*Bifidobacterium*: Host–Microbiome Interaction and Mechanism of Action in Preventing Common Gut-Microbiota-Associated Complications in Preterm Infants: A Narrative Review." *Nutrients* 15 (3): 709. https://doi.org/10.3390/nu15030709.

Salazar, N., A. Prieto, J. A. Leal, B. Mayo, J. C. Bada-Gancedo, C. G. de los Reyes-Gavilán, and P. Ruas-Madiedo. 2009. "Production of Exopolysaccharides by *Lactobacillus* and *Bifidobacterium* Strains of Human Origin, and Metabolic Activity of the Producing Bacteria in Milk." *Journal of Dairy Science* 92 (9): 4158–68. https://doi.org/10.3168/jds.2009-2126.

Santiago-López, Lourdes, Adrián Hernández-Mendoza, Verónica Mata-Haro, Belinda Vallejo-Cordoba, and Aarón F. González-Córdova. 2018. "Immune Response Induced by Fermented Milk with Potential Probiotic Strains Isolated from Artisanal Cocido Cheese." *Food and Agricultural Immunology* 29 (1): 911–29. https://doi.org/10.1080/09540105.2018.1485632.

Sarkar, Amrita, and Santanu Mandal. 2016. "Bifidobacteria—Insight into Clinical Outcomes and Mechanisms of Its Probiotic Action." *Microbiological Research* 192 (November): 159–71. https://doi.org/10.1016/j.micres.2016.07.001.

Sarquis, M. A., L. Siroli, M. Modesto, F. Patrignani, R. Lanciotti, P. Mattarelli, J. Reinheimer, and P. Burns. 2019. "Novel Bifidobacteria Strains Isolated from Nonconventional Sources. Technological, Antimicrobial and Biological Characterization for Their Use as Probiotics." *Journal of Applied Microbiology* 127 (4): 1207–18. https://doi.org/10.1111/jam.14367.

Satish Kumar, C. S. V., K. Kondal Reddy, G. Boobalan, A. Gopala Reddy, C. H. Sudha Rani Chowdhary, A. Vinoth, K. Jayakanth, and G. Srinivasa Rao. 2017. "Immunomodulatory Effects of *Bifidobacterium bifidum* 231 on Trinitrobenzenesulfonic Acid-Induced Ulcerative Colitis in Rats." *Research in Veterinary Science* 110 (February): 40–46. https://doi.org/10.1016/j.rvsc.2016.10.010.

Satoh, Takumi, Mitsunori Todoroki, Kazuya Kobayashi, Youichi Niimura, and Shinji Kawasaki. 2019. "Purified Thioredoxin Reductase from O2-Sensitive *Bifidobacterium bifidum* Degrades H2O2 by Interacting with Alkyl Hydroperoxide Reductase." *Anaerobe* 57 (June): 45–54. https://doi.org/10.1016/j.anaerobe.2019.03.012.

Saturio, Silvia, Alicja M. Nogacka, Guadalupe M. Alvarado-Jasso, Nuria Salazar, Clara G. de los Reyes-Gavilán, Miguel Gueimonde, and Silvia Arboleya. 2021. "Role of Bifidobacteria on Infant Health." *Microorganisms* 9 (12): 2415. https://doi.org/10.3390/microorganisms9122415.

Schmid, Jochen, Volker Sieber, and Bernd Rehm. 2015. "Bacterial Exopolysaccharides: Biosynthesis Pathways and Engineering Strategies." *Frontiers in Microbiology* 6 (May). https://doi.org/10.3389/fmicb.2015.00496.

Schöpping, Marie, Ahmad A. Zeidan, and Carl Johan Franzén. 2022. "Stress Response in Bifidobacteria." *Microbiology and Molecular Biology Reviews* 86 (4). https://doi.org/10.1128/mmbr.00170-21.

Schroeder, Bjoern O., George M. H. Birchenough, Marcus Ståhlman, Liisa Arike, Malin E. V. Johansson, Gunnar C. Hansson, and Fredrik Bäckhed. 2018. "Bifidobacteria or Fiber Protects against Diet-Induced Microbiota-Mediated Colonic Mucus Deterioration." *Cell Host & Microbe* 23 (1): 27-40.e7. https://doi.org/10.1016/j.chom.2017.11.004.

Shaidullov, Ilnar F., Dina M. Sorokina, Farit G. Sitdikov, Anton Hermann, Sayar R. Abdulkhakov, and Guzel F. Sitdikova. 2021. "Short Chain Fatty Acids and Colon Motility in a Mouse Model of Irritable Bowel Syndrome." *BMC Gastroenterology* 21 (1): 37. https://doi.org/10.1186/s12876-021-01613-y.

Shandilya, Umesh Kumar, Ankita Sharma, Rajeev Kapila, and Vinod Kumar Kansal. 2016. "Probiotic Dahi Containing *Lactobacillus Acidophilus* and *Bifidobacterium Bifidum* Modulates Immunoglobulin Levels and Cytokines Expression in Whey Proteins Sensitised Mice." *Journal of the Science of Food and Agriculture* 96 (9): 3180–87. https://doi.org/10.1002/jsfa.7497.

Shang, Nan, Rihua Xu, and Pinglan Li. 2013. "Structure Characterization of an Exopolysaccharide Produced by *Bifidobacterium animalis* RH." *Carbohydrate Polymers* 91 (1): 128–34. https://doi.org/10.1016/j.carbpol.2012.08.012.

Sharma, Muskan, Arunima Wasan, and Rakesh Kumar Sharma. 2021. "Recent Developments in Probiotics: An Emphasis on *Bifidobacterium*." *Food Bioscience* 41 (June): 100993. https://doi.org/10.1016/j.fbio.2021.100993.

Shen, Qian, Nan Shang, and Pinglan Li. 2011. "*In Vitro* and *In Vivo* Antioxidant Activity of *Bifidobacterium animalis* 01 Isolated from Centenarians." *Current Microbiology* 62 (4): 1097–1103. https://doi.org/10.1007/s00284-010-9827-7.

Shori, Amal Bakr. 2022. "Application of *Bifidobacterium* spp in Beverages and Dairy Food Products: An Overview of Survival during Refrigerated Storage." *Food Science and Technology* 42. https://doi.org/10.1590/fst.41520.

Snelson, Matthew, Cassandra de Pasquale, Elif I. Ekinci, and Melinda T. Coughlan. 2021. "Gut Microbiome, Prebiotics, Intestinal Permeability and Diabetes Complications." *Best Practice & Research Clinical Endocrinology & Metabolism* 35 (3): 101507. https://doi.org/10.1016/j.beem.2021.101507.

Solano-Aguilar, Gloria, Terez Shea-Donohue, Kathleen B. Madden, Alejandro Quinoñes, Ethiopia Beshah, Sukla Lakshman, Yue Xie, Harry Dawson, and Joseph F. Urban. 2018. "*Bifidobacterium animalis* subspecies *lactis* Modulates the Local Immune Response and Glucose Uptake in the Small Intestine of Juvenile Pigs Infected with the Parasitic Nematode Ascaris Suum." *Gut Microbes*, July, 1–15. https://doi.org/10.1080/19490976.2018.1460014.

Soleimani, Alireza, Malihe Zarrati Mojarrad, Fereshteh Bahmani, Mohsen Taghizadeh, Mohammad Ramezani, Maryam Tajabadi-Ebrahimi, Parvaneh Jafari, Ahmad Esmaillzadeh, and Zatollah Asemi. 2017. "Probiotic Supplementation in Diabetic Hemodialysis Patients Has Beneficial Metabolic Effects." *Kidney International* 91 (2): 435–42. https://doi.org/10.1016/j.kint.2016.09.040.

Sonnenburg, Justin L., Jian Xu, Douglas D. Leip, Chien-Huan Chen, Benjamin P. Westover, Jeremy Weatherford, Jeremy D. Buhler, and Jeffrey I. Gordon. 2005. "Glycan Foraging *in Vivo* by an Intestine-Adapted Bacterial Symbiont." *Science* 307 (5717): 1955–59. https://doi.org/10.1126/science.1109051.

Soumya, M. P., and K. Madhavan Nampoothiri. 2021. "An Overview of Functional Genomics and Relevance of Glycosyltransferases in Exopolysaccharide Production by Lactic Acid Bacteria." *International Journal of Biological Macromolecules* 184 (August): 1014–25. https://doi.org/10.1016/j.ijbiomac.2021.06.131.

Spencer, Sean Paul, Evelyn Giselle Lemus Silva, Elisa Benedetti Caffery, Matthew Merrill Carter, Rebecca Neal Culver, Min Wang, Rebecca Hope Gellman, Hannah Constance Wastyk, Steven Kyle Higginbottom, and Justin Laine Sonnenburg. 2022. "Fermented Foods Restructure Gut Microbiota and Promote Immune Regulation via Microbial Metabolites." *BioRxiv*, 2022–25.

Springer, Andrea, Liane Wagner, Sarina Koehler, Stefanie Klinger, Gerhard Breves, Dagmar A. Brüggemann, and Christina Strube. 2022. "Modulation of the Porcine Intestinal Microbiota in the Course of *Ascaris suum* Infection." *Parasites & Vectors* 15 (1): 433. https://doi.org/10.1186/s13071-022-05535-w.

Sprong, R. C., A. J. Schonewille, and R. van der Meer. 2010. "Dietary Cheese Whey Protein Protects Rats against Mild Dextran Sulfate Sodium–Induced Colitis: Role of Mucin and Microbiota." *Journal of Dairy Science* 93 (4): 1364–71. https://doi.org/10.3168/jds.2009-2397.

Sun, S., Luo, L., Liang, W., Yin, Q., Guo, J., Rush, A. M., Lv, Z., Liang, Q., Fischbach, M. A., Sonnenburg, J. L., Dodd, D., Davis, M. M., & Wang, F. 2020. "Bifidobacterium Alters the Gut Microbiota and Modulates the Functional Metabolism of T Regulatory Cells in the Context of Immune Checkpoint Blockade." *Proceedings of the National Academy of Sciences* 117 (44): 27509–15. https://doi.org/10.1073/pnas.1921223117.

Takahashi, Noritoshi, Jin-Zhong Xiao, Kazuhiro Miyaji, Tomoko Yaeshiima, Akinori Hiramatsu, Keiji Iwatsuki, Sadayuki Kokubo, and Akiyoshi Hosono. 2004. "Selection of Acid Tolerant Bifidobacteria and Evidence for a Low-PH-Inducible Acid Tolerance Response in *Bifidobacterium Longum*." *Journal of Dairy Research* 71 (3): 340–45. https://doi.org/10.1017/S0022029904000251.

Tian, Peijun, Kenneth J. O'Riordan, Yuan-kun Lee, Gang Wang, Jianxin Zhao, Hao Zhang, John F. Cryan, and Wei Chen. 2020. "Towards a Psychobiotic Therapy for Depression: *Bifidobacterium breve* CCFM1025 Reverses Chronic Stress-Induced Depressive Symptoms and Gut Microbial Abnormalities in Mice." *Neurobiology of Stress* 12 (May): 100216. https://doi.org/10.1016/j.ynstr.2020.100216.

Tiwari, Swati, Digambar Kavitake, Palanisamy Bruntha Devi, and Prathapkumar Halady Shetty. 2021. "Bacterial Exopolysaccharides for Improvement of Technological, Functional and Rheological Properties of Yoghurt." *International Journal of Biological Macromolecules* 183 (July): 1585–95. https://doi.org/10.1016/j.ijbiomac.2021.05.140.

Tkaczewska, Joanna. 2020. "Peptides and Protein Hydrolysates as Food Preservatives and Bioactive Components of Edible Films and Coatings - A Review." *Trends in Food Science & Technology* 106 (December): 298–311. https://doi.org/10.1016/j.tifs.2020.10.022.

Torres-Maravilla, Edgar, Vianey Méndez-Trujillo, Natalia C. Hernández-Delgado, Luis G. Bermúdez-Humarán, and Diana Reyes-Pavón. 2022. "Looking inside Mexican Traditional Food as Sources of Synbiotics for Developing Novel Functional Products." *Fermentation* 8 (3): 123. https://doi.org/10.3390/fermentation8030123.

Uraipan, Supansa, and Tipparat Hongpattarakere. 2015. "Antagonistic Characteristics Against Food-Borne Pathogenic Bacteria of Lactic Acid Bacteria and Bifidobacteria Isolated from Feces of Healthy Thai Infants." *Jundishapur Journal of Microbiology* 8 (5). https://doi.org/10.5812/jjm.8(5)2015.18264.

Valerino-Perea, Lara-Castor, Armstrong, and Papadaki. 2019. "Definition of the Traditional Mexican Diet and Its Role in Health: A Systematic Review." *Nutrients* 11 (11): 2803. https://doi.org/10.3390/nu11112803.

Vazquez-Gutierrez, Pamela, Christophe Lacroix, Tanja Jaeggi, Christophe Zeder, Michael Bruce Zimmerman, and Christophe Chassard. 2015. "Bifidobacteria Strains Isolated from Stools of Iron Deficient Infants Can Efficiently Sequester Iron." *BMC Microbiology* 15 (1): 3. https://doi.org/10.1186/s12866-014-0334-z.

Veiga, P., Gallini, C. A., Beal, C., Michaud, M., Delaney, M. L., DuBois, A., Khlebnikov, A., Van Hylckama Vlieg, J. E. T., Punit, S., Glickman, J. N., Onderdonk, A., Glimcher, L. H., & Garrett, W. S. 2010. "*Bifidobacterium animalis* Subsp. *lactis* Fermented Milk Product Reduces Inflammation by Altering a Niche for Colitogenic Microbes." *Proceedings of the National Academy of Sciences* 107 (42): 18132–37. https://doi.org/10.1073/pnas.1011737107.

Vélez, M. Perea, K. Hermans, T. L. A. Verhoeven, S. E. Lebeer, J. Vanderleyden, and S. C. J. De Keersmaecker. 2007. "Identification and Characterization of Starter Lactic Acid Bacteria and Probiotics from Columbian Dairy Products." *Journal of Applied Microbiology* 103 (3): 666–74. https://doi.org/10.1111/j.1365-2672.2007.03294.x.

Venegas-Ortega, María G., Adriana C. Flores-Gallegos, José L. Martínez-Hernández, Cristóbal N. Aguilar, and Guadalupe V. Nevárez-Moorillón. 2019. "Production of Bioactive Peptides from Lactic Acid Bacteria: A Sustainable Approach for Healthier Foods." *Comprehensive Reviews in Food Science and Food Safety* 18 (4): 1039–51. https://doi.org/10.1111/1541-4337.12455.

Ventura, Marco, Carlos Canchaya, Ziding Zhang, Valentina Bernini, Gerald F. Fitzgerald, and Douwe van Sinderen. 2006. "How High G+C Gram-Positive Bacteria and in Particular Bifidobacteria Cope with Heat Stress: Protein Players and Regulators." *FEMS Microbiology Reviews* 30 (5): 734–59. https://doi.org/10.1111/j.1574-6976.2006.00031.x.

Verruck, Silvani, Mariana Wolf de Carvalho, Gabriela Rodrigues de Liz, Edna Regina Amante, Cleide Rosana Werneck Vieira, Renata Dias de Mello Castanho Amboni, and Elane Schwinden Prudencio. 2017. "Survival of *Bifidobacterium* BB-12 Microencapsulated with Full-Fat Goat's Milk and Prebiotics When Exposed to Simulated Gastrointestinal Conditions and Thermal Treatments." *Small Ruminant Research* 153 (August): 48–56. https://doi.org/10.1016/j.smallrumres.2017.05.008.

Vinderola, C. G., W. Prosello, D. Ghiberto, and J. A. Reinheimer. 2000. "Viability of Probiotic (*Bifidobacterium*, *Lactobacillus acidophilus* and *Lactobacillus casei*) and Nonprobiotic Microflora in Argentinian Fresco Cheese." *Journal of Dairy Science* 83 (9): 1905–11. https://doi.org/10.3168/jds.S0022-0302(00)75065-X.

Vinolo, Marco A. R., Hosana G. Rodrigues, Renato T. Nachbar, and Rui Curi. 2011. "Regulation of Inflammation by Short Chain Fatty Acids." *Nutrients* 3 (10): 858–76. https://doi.org/10.3390/nu3100858.

Wang, Rongchun, Hongxing Zhao, Xiaoxi Pan, Caroline Orfila, Weihong Lu, and Ying Ma. 2019. "Preparation of Bioactive Peptides with Antidiabetic, Antihypertensive, and Antioxidant Activities and Identification of A-glucosidase Inhibitory Peptides from Soy Protein." *Food Science & Nutrition* 7 (5): 1848–56. https://doi.org/10.1002/fsn3.1038.

Wang, Yang, Yanping Wu, Yuanyuan Wang, Han Xu, Xiaoqiang Mei, Dongyou Yu, Yibing Wang, and Weifen Li. 2017. "Antioxidant Properties of Probiotic Bacteria." *Nutrients* 9 (5): 521. https://doi.org/10.3390/nu9050521.

Wang, Yusheng, Zhifeng Fang, Qixiao Zhai, Shumao Cui, Jianxin Zhao, Hao Zhang, Wei Chen, and Wenwei Lu. 2021. "Supernatants of *Bifidobacterium longum* and *Lactobacillus plantarum* Strains Exhibited Antioxidative Effects on A7R5 Cells." *Microorganisms* 9 (2): 452. https://doi.org/10.3390/microorganisms9020452.

Wong, Julia M. W., Russell de Souza, Cyril W. C. Kendall, Azadeh Emam, and David J. A. Jenkins. 2006. "Colonic Health: Fermentation and Short Chain Fatty Acids." *Journal of Clinical Gastroenterology* 40 (3): 235–43. https://doi.org/10.1097/00004836-200603000-00015.

Wu, Ming-Hsiu, Tzu-Ming Pan, Yu-Jen Wu, Sue-Joan Chang, Ming-Song Chang, and Chun-Yi Hu. 2010. "Exopolysaccharide Activities from Probiotic *Bifidobacterium*: Immunomodulatory Effects (on J774A.1 Macrophages) and Antimicrobial Properties." *International Journal of Food Microbiology* 144 (1): 104–10. https://doi.org/10.1016/j.ijfoodmicro.2010.09.003.

Wu, Yue, Sujin Li, Yang Tao, Dandan Li, Yongbin Han, Pau Loke Show, Guangzhong Wen, and Jianzhong Zhou. 2021. "Fermentation of Blueberry and Blackberry Juices Using Lactobacillus Plantarum, Streptococcus Thermophilus and *Bifidobacterium bifidum*: Growth of Probiotics, Metabolism of Phenolics, Antioxidant Capacity in Vitro and Sensory Evaluation." *Food Chemistry* 348 (June): 129083. https://doi.org/10.1016/j.foodchem.2021.129083.

Xu, Rihua, Qian Shen, Ruiyun Wu, and Pinglan Li. 2017. "Structural Analysis and Mucosal Immune Regulation of Exopolysaccharide Fraction from *Bifidobacterium Animalis* RH." *Food and Agricultural Immunology* 28 (6): 1226–41. https://doi.org/10.1080/09540105.2017.1333578.

Xu, Yuanmei, Yanlong Cui, Fangfang Yue, Lihua Liu, Yuanyuan Shan, Bianfang Liu, Yuan Zhou, and Xin Lü. 2019. "Exopolysaccharides Produced by Lactic Acid Bacteria and Bifidobacteria: Structures, Physiochemical Functions and Applications in the Food Industry." *Food Hydrocolloids* 94 (September): 475–99. https://doi.org/10.1016/j.foodhyd.2019.03.032.

Yan, Shuang, Bo Yang, R. Paul Ross, Catherine Stanton, Hao Zhang, Jianxin Zhao, and Wei Chen. 2020. "*Bifidobacterium longum* Subsp. *longum* YS108R Fermented Milk Alleviates DSS Induced Colitis via Anti-Inflammation, Mucosal Barrier Maintenance and Gut Microbiota Modulation." *Journal of Functional Foods* 73 (October): 104153. https://doi.org/10.1016/j.jff.2020.104153.

Yang, B., H. Chen, Z. Gu, F. Tian, R. P. Ross, C. Stanton, Y. Q. Chen, W. Chen, and H. Zhang. 2014. "Synthesis of Conjugated Linoleic Acid by the Linoleate Isomerase Complex in Food-Derived Lactobacilli." *Journal of Applied Microbiology* 117 (2): 430–39. https://doi.org/10.1111/jam.12524.

Yang, Shuo, Xiaoqing Xu, Qing Peng, Lan Ma, Yu Qiao, and Bo Shi. 2023. "Exopolysaccharides from Lactic Acid Bacteria, as an Alternative to Antibiotics, on Regulation of Intestinal Health and the Immune System." *Animal Nutrition* 13 (June): 78–89. https://doi.org/10.1016/j.aninu.2023.02.004.

Yang, Yao-Jong, and Bor-Shyang Sheu. 2012. "Probiotics-Containing Yogurts Suppress *Helicobacter pylori* Load and Modify Immune Response and Intestinal Microbiota in the *Helicobacter pylori*-Infected Children." *Helicobacter* 17 (4): 297–304. https://doi.org/10.1111/j.1523-5378.2012.00941.x.

Yao, Shunyu, Zixi Zhao, Weijun Wang, and Xiaolu Liu. 2021. "*Bifidobacterium longum*: Protection against Inflammatory Bowel Disease." *Journal of Immunology Research* 2021 (July): 1–11. https://doi.org/10.1155/2021/8030297.

Yasmin, I., Saeed, M., Khan, W. A., Khaliq, A., Chughtai, M. F. J., Iqbal, R., Tehseen, S., Naz, S., Liaqat, A., Mehmood, T., Ahsan, S., & Tanweer, S. 2020. "*In Vitro* Probiotic Potential and Safety Evaluation (Hemolytic, Cytotoxic Activity) of *Bifidobacterium* Strains Isolated from Raw Camel Milk." *Microorganisms* 8 (3): 354. https://doi.org/10.3390/microorganisms8030354.

Yuan, Lanxin, Bingxin Chu, Shiyan Chen, Yanan Li, Ning Liu, Yaohong Zhu, and Dong Zhou. 2021. "Exopolysaccharides from *Bifidobacterium animalis* Ameliorate *Escherichia coli*-Induced IPEC-J2 Cell Damage via Inhibiting Apoptosis and Restoring Autophagy." *Microorganisms* 9 (11): 2363. https://doi.org/10.3390/microorganisms9112363.

Zafar, Mahpara, Sadia Alam, Maimoona Sabir, Nusrat Saba, Ahmad Ud Din, Rafiq Ahmad, Muhammad Rafiullah Khan, Ali Muhammad, and Kenan Sinan Dayisoylu. 2022. "Isolation, Characterization, Bacteriocin Production and Biological Potential of Bifidobacteria of Ruminants." *Analytical Biochemistry* 658 (December): 114926. https://doi.org/10.1016/j.ab.2022.114926.

Zhang, Gongsheng, Hui Sun, Zihe Xu, Ze Tan, Lihong Xiao, Mingxue He, Jiaqi Shang, Anna N. Tsapieva, and Lili Zhang. 2023. "Screening of Bifidobacteria with Probiotic Potential from Healthy Infant Feces by Using 2′-Fucosyllactose." *Foods* 12 (4): 858. https://doi.org/10.3390/foods12040858.

Zhang, Li-Li, Xiao Chen, Peng-Yuan Zheng, Yu Luo, Gao-Feng Lu, Zhi-Qiang Liu, Huang Huang, and Ping-Chang Yang. 2010. "Oral Bifidobacterium Modulates Intestinal Immune Inflammation in Mice with Food Allergy." *Journal of Gastroenterology and Hepatology* 25 (5): 928–34. https://doi.org/10.1111/j.1440-1746.2009.06193.x.

Zhou, Linyan, Dongyan Liu, Ying Xie, Xinjie Yao, and Yan Li. 2019. "*Bifidobacterium Infantis* Induces Protective Colonic PD-L1 and Foxp3 Regulatory T Cells in an Acute Murine Experimental Model of Inflammatory Bowel Disease." *Gut and Liver* 13 (4): 430–39. https://doi.org/10.5009/gnl18316.

Zuo, Fanglei, Shangwu Chen, and Harold Marcotte. 2020. "Engineer Probiotic Bifidobacteria for Food and Biomedical Applications - Current Status and Future Prospective." *Biotechnology Advances* 45 (December): 107654. https://doi.org/10.1016/j.biotechadv.2020.107654.

Chapter 2

The Utilization of Postbiotics as Innovative Biological Compounds to Enhance Oral Health

Kimia Dehghan Sanej, MSc
Amin Abbasi, PhD
Samaneh Moradi, MSc
Saeedeh Shojaee-Aliabadi[*], PhD
and Hedayat Hosseini[†], PhD

Department of Food Science and Technology, National Nutrition and Food Technology Research Institute, Faculty of Nutrition Science and Food Technology, Shahid Beheshti University of Medical Sciences, Tehran, Iran

Abstract

Oral disorders are among the most frequent ailments that individuals throughout the globe experience during their lives. Tooth decay is a complex illness, and the makeup of the oral microbiota plays an important role in its progression. *Streptococcus mutans* is also regarded as the most major caries-causing species. Probiotics are predicted to exercise their health-giving benefits, particularly the anti-pathogenic impact, in the oral cavity, which is part of the human gastrointestinal system, since they alter the intestinal microbiota and lower the number of harmful bacteria in the human intestine. As a result, various *in vitro* and *in vivo* research on the effect of probiotics in tooth decay prevention have been done. While researching the effects of different strains of probiotic *Lactobacillus* and *Bifidobacteria* on oral diseases such as dental caries, *candida* yeast infections, periodontal diseases, and halitosis, we

* Corresponding Author's Email: hedayat@sbmu.ac.ir.
† Corresponding Author's Email: saeedeh.shojaee@gmail.com.

In: Exploring Microbiotics in Health and Disease
Editor: Edward L. Stillman
ISBN: 978-8-89113-410-2

also discussed the biological role of postbiotic compounds as a promising tool for improving oral health.

Keywords: biological activities, cell-free supernatant, gastrointestinal disorders, postbiotics

Introduction

The World Health Organization's estimation indicates that approximately 50% of the global population suffers from oral diseases. Permanent tooth decay affects about 2.4 billion people, and primary tooth decay affects 532 million children [1]. The expense of oral healthcare accounts for around 5% of the total cost of healthcare in high-income countries. In contrast, many other nations find it challenging to meet the financial demands associated with oral health [1].

There are a number of factors that can affect tooth decay. Environmental risk factors for tooth decay include things like a cariogenic diet, poor oral hygiene, high levels of cariogenic bacteria, dental plaque, insufficient fluoride exposure, and insufficient saliva flow [2]. Numerous studies have generally shown that the composition of the oral microbiota is directly related to oral health, and its disruption is a critical step in oral disease [3]. One of the oral microflora's bacteria, *S. mutans*, is known as the primary contributor to dental caries and one of the biofilm-forming bacteria [4, 5]. Numerous clinical research carried out on various community members have revealed a link between *S. mutans* levels and dental caries [6]. It should be mentioned that the relationship between *S. mutans* levels and caries in humans varies for a variety of reasons, including genetic variables in the etiopathogenesis of tooth decay [7]. Even though a number of factors can affect tooth decay, microbiological causes are the primary cause. Consequently, it is thought that bacteriotherapy may be a useful strategy for preventing oral illness [8]. It makes sense that probiotics would have an impact on the oral cavity and its microbiota as the oral cavity is the first section of the gastrointestinal system [9]. Probiotics are live microorganisms that, when taken in sufficient quantities, are beneficial to the health of the host [10]. The beneficial effects of many probiotic strains against oral infections have been demonstrated in in vitro investigations [11, 12]. The effects of probiotics in the prevention or treatment of tooth decay and periodontal diseases have also been addressed in in vivo investigations. Contradictory findings have been reported from several trials, though [8, 13].

The same processes highlighted in gastrointestinal research may also be responsible for probiotics' beneficial effects on dental health [14].

According to evidence, probiotics create chemicals such as bacteriocins, fatty acids, organic acids, and hydrogen peroxide, which may contribute to their antimicrobial activities [15, 16]. The use of their non-living components or metabolites (postbiotics) can be a novel and appropriate approach, taking into account some of the difficulties and restrictions associated with using probiotics in food products [17]. The challenges associated with the use of probiotics that can be solved by postbiotics include the emergence of clinical problems, especially in people with a weakened immune system [18], the emergence of antibiotic resistance and the likelihood of transmission of resistance genes to pathogenic microorganisms [19] and the need for high costs to provide a continuous cold chain from production to consumption [20]. Accordingly, in this chapter, we will examine the impact of postbiotics on oral and dental health.

Oral Microbiome

Numerous different bacteria live in the human mouth, where they depend on one another to keep the environment constant. Most of the time, these bacteria coexist peacefully with the host. This symbiosis is partly attributed to the local commensal flora, which includes planktonic bacteria, and inhabits the hard and mucous surfaces, and inhibits the growth of external microbes. The human aerodigestive tract is home to a total of 772 microbial species as of its most recent update, according to the enlarged Human Oral Microbiome Database (eHOMD; www.homd.org; accessed on December 9, 2022) [21]. The genome browser program allows users to see a total of 1570 genomes from 475 species. The oral microbiome is made up of bacteria, fungi, viruses, and archaea. As previously mentioned [22], 16S rRNA amplicon sequencing by targeted gene approach is the most used method for defining the oral microbiome. However, because there is no set method for gathering samples of the oral microbiome, sample collection can be challenging. The schedule of the day, whether it is before or after meals, the tools used to take the samples, and the storage conditions for the samples are some of the factors that can affect the collection. The sequencing analysis lacks standardization, much like the sample collection procedure did. These factors make it challenging to draw valid conclusions from the data. The mouth cavity is home to a large number of viruses, the majority of which are pathogens. All other living organisms on

Earth are outnumbered by viruses and phages, but the virome, or viral component of the microbiome, has not been well examined to determine its overall diversity in the mouth [23]. The impact of viruses on the oral microbiome has received very little attention in recent years due to the focus on bacteria and their function in the oral microbiome [24]. As new technical developments are made, old theories that were once considered to be common knowledge are refuted by fresh facts. Although it was originally believed that human blood was sterile, it now appears to contain both viruses and phages [23].

Bacteriophages, sometimes known as phages, are viruses that attack and replicate inside bacteria. Either the lytic cycle, in which the phage replicates using bacterial mechanisms before lysing the bacterial cells, or the lysogenic cycle, in which the phage inserts its DNA into the bacterial chromosome to be duplicated, can be used to do this. It has been demonstrated that phages make up a significant portion of the oral virome. Since lysogeny is one of the two ways previously described that phages can infect bacteria, it has been demonstrated that the majority of virus sequences discovered in the mouth cavity share similarities with phages [25]. Examples of viruses that enter the oral cavity through the oral mucosa and go into the upper respiratory tract to weaken the immune system include hepatitis viruses and HIV [26]. It has been demonstrated that the human papilloma virus (HPV) not only causes oral disease but also contributes significantly to HNSCC [27]. Gingival lesions have also been linked to the herpes simplex virus [28]. It is not surprising that the virome has a significant role in oral disease given the prevalence of viruses in the oral cavity. Archaea have been discovered to have a small role in the oral microbiome; however, given the variety of the community that constitutes the oral microbiome and the lack of knowledge about the interactions between bacteria at this time, Archaea should not be regarded as nonessential. The archaeal community discovered in the oral cavity is made almost entirely of methanogens, which means that the majority of their metabolic energy comes from the production of methane [29]. Methanosarcina mazeii, Methanobacterium curvum/congolense, and Methanobrevibacter oralis are the archaea with the highest incidence in periodontitis patients [30]. By encouraging the growth of bacteria that ferment food, Archea may be contributing to this sick state through interspecies hydrogen transfer. Recently, a link between colorectal cancer and methanogens was discovered [31]. Methanogens are capable of converting heavy metals into extremely poisonous methylated compounds. In order to pinpoint the precise role that these microorganisms play in oral disease, further research must be done to better understand the interactions between Archaea and other microorganisms. The mycobiome, which is a newly discussed concept, is the collective name for the fungi that live in the microbiome. It was discovered that the "basal" oral mycobiome had 85 genera—74 culturable and 11 non-culturable—during an analysis of the oral cavity of 20 healthy people [32]. More recent research indicates that the mouth cavity alone contains over 100 culturable types of fungi [33]. The fungus *Candida albicans* (*C. albicans*), which is frequently prevalent in the oral mucosa but can quickly acquire pathogenic characteristics, has been the subject of recent research [34]. Inducing alternate metabolic pathways such as fatty acid oxidation, gluconeogenesis, and the glyoxylate cycle, as well as promoting invasive filamentous development in a hypoxic environment, are some of these features [35, 36]. *Streptococci* and other members of the oral microbiome have been shown to provide *C. albicans* with useful things, like a place to stick to and a source of carbon [34]. However, studies in a rat model have shown that *C. albicans* and *S. mutans*, a recognized carcinogen, together increase the development of dental caries [37]. As a result, this may not be as beneficial to the host. Through these interactions, it has been demonstrated that *C. albicans* may serve as a conduit for bacteria, enabling them to cling to mucosal surfaces [38, 39]. Contrarily, *Streptococcus salivarius* has been demonstrated to inhibit *C. albicans'* adhesion to mucosal surfaces, raising the possibility of its use as a probiotic [40]. When *C. albicans* exists at pathogenic levels, both a late and an early host immune response take place. Macrophages, neutrophils, and dendritic cells are capable of early detection, but there is also an adaptive antifungal response [41]. The sum of these elements illustrates the significance of the mycobiome and its place in the oral microbiome. Bacteria are the most important component to the oral microbiome and are also the subject of the most research. Sex, race, age, and geography are only a few of the variables affecting this bacteria's composition. There was no discernible geographic variation among individuals' salivary microbiotas, according to a study of 120 people from 12 different places [29, 42]. The oral microbiome is made up of six primary phyla, which together make up 96% of the taxa: *Bacteroidetes*, *Firmicutes*, *Proteobacteria*, *Actinobacteria*, *Fusobacteria*, and *Spirochaetes*. *Chlamydia*, *phyla Euryarchaeota*, *Chloroflexi*, *SR1*, *Saccharibacteria*, *Tenericutes*, and *Synergistetes* make up the remaining 4% of the taxa [43, 44]. Even though they are all inherently commensal, some of the bacteria in these groups have also been thought of as pathogens. The amount of this bacteria present in the oral cavity's biofilms determines how frequently the switch from commensal to pathogenic occurs. *Porphyromonas gingivalis* (*P. gingivalis*) and *F. nucleatum* are two of the most important bacteria to possess pathogenic characteristics [45].

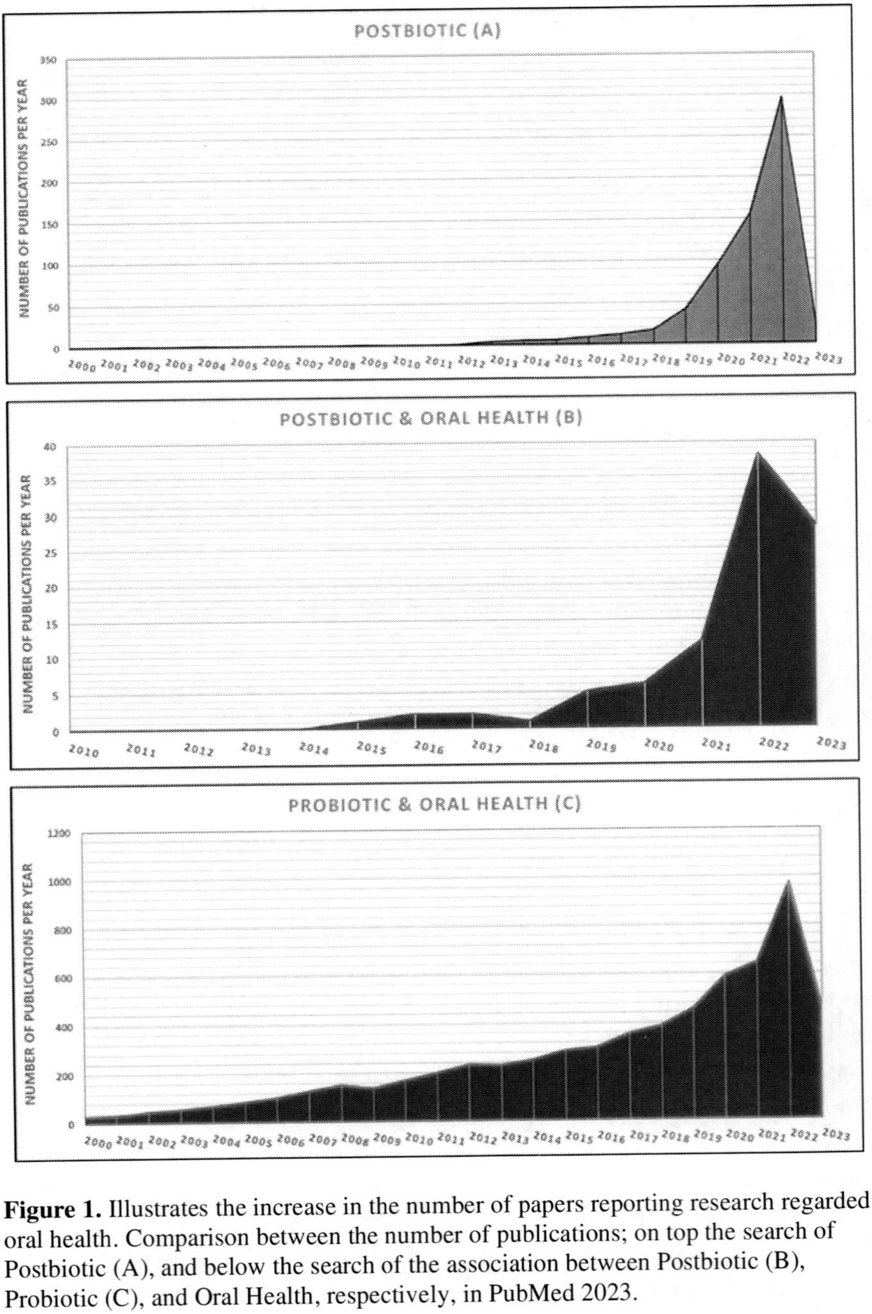

Figure 1. Illustrates the increase in the number of papers reporting research regarded oral health. Comparison between the number of publications; on top the search of Postbiotic (A), and below the search of the association between Postbiotic (B), Probiotic (C), and Oral Health, respectively, in PubMed 2023.

Compared to tobacco cigarette smokers or never smokers, e-cigarette users have been reported to have dysbiosis. Vapers had greater levels of *Veillonella* and *Porphyromonas* [46]. As was already indicated, the bacterium *S. mutans*, which is known to cause cancer, is found during the development of dental caries [37]. *Prevotella enoeca, Prevotella dentalis, Prevotella melaninogenica, Prevotella fusca, Prevotella denticola, Prevotella intermedia 17*, and *Prevotella intermedia 17-2* have all been linked to periodontitis [47]. Patients with various degrees of gingivitis have allowed for the isolation and recovery of *Leptotrichia buccalis* (*L. buccalis*) [48]. Since most of the bacteria in the oral microbiome are stringent anaerobes, which are more challenging to culture, samples must be handled and processed with the utmost care [34]. The following section will go through these bacteria in more detail. The thorough characterization of the bacterial taxa in the oral microbiome makes it clear that they play a key role in maintaining both oral and general health. To find new ways to combat the harmful impacts of these microorganisms, further research must be performed (Figure 1).

Lactobacillus Bacteria and Oral Health

Dental plaque, a bacterial build-up that is attached to the tooth surfaces and is comprised of a gelatinous material, is what causes tooth decay, which is a local demineralization of the hard tissues on the crown and root surfaces of the tooth [46]. Due to its strong acid production and excellent endurance in acidic environments, *S. mutans* has been designated as the primary species of caries-causing bacteria [49]. According to studies, people without caries often have between 10^4 and 10^5 CFU/mL of *S. mutans* in their saliva [50]. However, with 10^6 CFU/mL, the risk of developing caries dramatically rises [51]. Clinical research has established 10^5 CFU/mL as the threshold for caries in this regard [52, 53].

The microbial flora of people's mouth cavities may change chemically and physically as a result of probiotic microorganisms [54]. Probiotics can compete with infections for sticky surfaces and have potentially stronger adherence to oral tissues. This causes bacterial aggregation and co-aggregation, which then results in the development of a fresh biofilm [55]. Probiotics defend oral health by competing with pathogens and the oral microbial flora for adhesion sites, nutrition, and growth factors. By producing antimicrobial substances, including acids, peroxides, and bacteriocins, these bacteria agglomerate after adhering to the mouth cavity and stop pathogenic bacteria from adhering. Hence, probiotic bacteria may inhibit the development of periodontal and caries-causing bacteria, elicit an immune response towards pathogens, stop the deterioration of oral tissue, and reduce inflammation in the oral cavity [8, 55]. Many investigations have looked into how probiotic ingestion affects tooth decay. For instance, Wattanarat et al. (2015) [56] and Jindal et al. (2011) [57] came to the conclusion that using probiotics could reduce the amount of *S. mutans* and, thus, have a preventative effect on tooth decay. Probiotics, such as *Bifidobacterium*, *Lactobacillus*, and *Streptococcus*, could dramatically lower the count of *S. mutans* compared to control groups and prevent tooth decay, according to Nadelman et al.'s (2018) meta-analysis [58]. The findings of this meta-analysis are in line with systematic reviews that found that consuming probiotics significantly reduced the number of *S. mutans* in the body [8, 59].

It has been demonstrated that *L. rhamnosus*, *L. reuteri*, *L. casei* and some strains of *Bifidobacterium* spp. can alter the colonization of carious bacteria, thereby preventing tooth decay [60]. In their study on *Lactobacillus* strains, Kõll-Klais et al. (2005b) [61] found that 82% of the strains could suppress the growth of *Porphyromonas gingivalis* and 69% of the strains could inhibit the growth of *S. mutans*. According to Strahinic et al. (2007) [62], *L. fermentum* and *L. salivarius* both have antagonistic effects against the growth of *S. mutans*. Additionally, after co-cultivation, *L. salivarius* TI 2711, a human isolate from a healthy individual, inhibited the growth of *P. gingivalis*, *P. nigrescens*, and *P. intermedia* [63]. The potential of 3790 lactic acid bacteria (LAB) to prevent the growth of different oral infections was examined in a study by Sookkhee et al. (2001) [64], and it was found that *L. paracasei* and *L. rhamnosus* have a potent antibacterial impact on a number of oral pathogens. Meurman et al. (1995) [65] became the first researchers to demonstrate the inhibiting effect of this bacterium on a cariogenic pathogen, taking into account the digestive advantages of *Lactobacilli* as well as the fact that the *L. rhamnosus* GG strain is not cariogenic owing to being unable to consume lactose or sucrose (Homofermentative Lactobacilli). It follows that this bacterium should have benefited dental health [66]. According to this information, *L. rhamnosus* GG ATCC 53103 is said to create a substance that prevents *Streptococcus sobrinus* from growing, which may reduce the risk of tooth decay [67]. Another strain of *Lactobacilli* that is effective at preventing the colonization of harmful oral bacteria and regulating the oral microbiota is *Lactococcus lactis*. According to Comelli et al. (2002) [68], this bacterium has demonstrated the capacity to eradicate the colonization of bacteria like *V. dispar*, *Actinomyces*, *S. oralis*, and cariogenic *S. sobrinus*.

On the other hand *Lactobacillus* is linked to the beginning and progression of caries [69]. According to Huang et al. (2015) [70], *Lactobacilli* create acids throughout their metabolism that may raise the risk of caries. Shimada et al. (2015) [71] discovered that children with dental decay had considerably more *Lactobacilli* than those without disease. They came to the conclusion that the development of caries and the quantity of *Lactobacilli* in the oral cavity are related. Other studies have found evidence that *Lactobacilli* play a significant role in the progression of tooth decay and are more strongly connected with caries development than caries start [72, 73]. Additionally, it has been noted that there was no discernible difference in the number of Lactobacilli between the experimental and control groups after consuming probiotics [74]. According to a study, after taking oral probiotics, the count of *Lactobacilli* fell into one of the two probiotic groups [75]. Contrarily, it was found in two investigations [76, 77] that the number of *Lactobacilli* dramatically increased. Therefore, based on the findings of the majority of studies, it can be concluded that consuming probiotics does not cause tooth decay. According to an intervention study, children who consume *Lactobacilli* have a lower risk of developing dental decay and primary caries [78]. Several investigations have looked into the impact of consuming various probiotic strains on tooth decay to date. According to a review of the literature, the majority of research found that consuming probiotics effectively delays the onset of tooth decay and recommends doing so in moderation for the best results.

Bifidobacteria and Oral Health

The use of probiotic *Bifidobacteria* for the prevention and treatment of oral microbial illnesses is becoming more popular. However, the findings from clinical trials looking into the impact of bifidobacteria on the oral microbiome are contradictory and debatable. *Bifidobacteria* have been shown in certain research to have anti-cary properties, whereas other investigations have shown the opposite. There haven't been many studies looking at the impact of *bifidobacteria* on *S. mutans*, and some of these investigations have also looked at the combined impact of *bifidobacteria* and *lactobacilli*. It was demonstrated in a meta-analysis that *Bifidobacterium* does not significantly lower the number of *Lactobacilli* in saliva [8]. However, it significantly lowers the number of *S. mutans*. Furthermore, research using supplements of *Lactobacillus* and *Bifidobacterium* spp. found a decrease in the number of *S. mutans* in the oral cavity [52]. People who did not utilize fluoride also saw similar outcomes [52]. However, the utilization of *Bifidobacterium animalis* BB-12 and other species of the *Bifidobacterium* genus in individuals who did not take fluoride failed to demonstrate its therapeutic effects on decay of the teeth [79]. The difference between the number of *S. mutans* in saliva before and after ingesting *Bifidobacterium* was examined using a meta-analysis. The combined findings of four studies [80-83] did not reveal any appreciable changes. According to a study, *bifidobacteria* dramatically decreased the amount of *P. gingivalis* in the biofilm while having no discernible influence on the number of *S. mutans* [84]. However, Valdez et al. (2016) [85] demonstrated that *Bifidobacterium* can create an acidic environment and promote the creation of biofilm, which may cause caries in teeth. According to Haukioja et al. (2008) [86], *Bifidobacterium*'s synthesis of organic acids may contribute to tooth demineralization. Additionally, larger pH reductions will occur in dual-species biofilms made up of *Bifidobacteria* and *S. mutans* than in *S. mutans* biofilm alone [87]. The abundance of *Bifidobacterium* in the oral cavity and its link to childhood tooth decay were studied by Zhai et al. in 2009 [88]. According to the findings of this clinical trial, *Bifidobacterium* was present at a rate of 47.5% in patients with severe ECC and 0% in healthy individuals without caries. There isn't much research that has used *Bifidobacteria* by themselves or apart from *Lactobacilli*. This has made it difficult to determine how *Bifidobacteria* affect *S. mutans* count and tooth decay. Therefore, more research should be done in the future using dietary products that only contain *Bifidobacteria*.

Key Bacteria Involved in Oral Disease

L. buccalis is a common member of the oral flora and is a rod-shaped, facultatively anaerobic, gram-negative bacterium. It belongs to the family *Leptotrichiaceae* and the phylum *Fusobacteria*. By streaking bacteria onto a blood agar plate under anaerobic conditions, growth can be seen. Due to the similarity in shape and size across members of the *Leptotrichia* genus, identification is frequently accomplished using 16S rRNA gene sequencing [48].

Lactic acid is the by-product of the fermentation of carbohydrates, which *Leptotrichia* uses to survive [89]. By controlling the expression of pro-inflammatory interleukin (IL)-1, IL-6, IL-8, and the anti-inflammatory IL-10 [90], studies have demonstrated that *L. buccalis*, retrieved from gingivitis patients, may contribute to the inflammatory process [48]. *Leptotrichia* may be directly involved in the inflammatory process, although many oral bacteria have been linked to inflammatory response pathways; hence, it is more likely that a variety of microorganisms are at play. Ultimately, more research will be required to ascertain the precise function that each of the important bacteria performs.

Prevotella is a genus of bacteria, and several of its species have been linked to oral illness. *P. enoeca*, *P. dentalis*, *P. melaninogenica*, *P. fusca*, *P. denticola*, *P. intermedia 17*, and *P. intermedia 17-2* are a few of the species implicated [89]. anaerobic, Gram-negative *Prevotella* are typical oral microbiome constituents. They belong to the *Prevotellaceae* family and the phylum *Bacteroidetes*. Additionally, *Prevotella* has been found to be a commensal in the gut and vaginal microbiota [91]. *Prevotella* causes Toll-like receptor (TLR) 2 to begin to produce, which then causes the polarization of Th17, whereas the generation of inflammatory cytokines can result in a rise in the prevalence of periodontal disease [47]. *Prevotella* has been proven in studies on mice to encourage the clinical manifestations of human disease. *Lactobacillus* downregulation and *Prevotella* overexpression, two important lactic acid bacteria, have been linked to osteomyelitis in mice. Osteomyelitis protection has been demonstrated when *Prevotella* is decreased and *Lactobacillus* is elevated [92]. The clinical significance of *Prevotella*'s involvement in oral disease may be demonstrated by further research into this organism.

A microaerophilic, Gram-negative, helical bacteria called *Helicobacter pylori* (*H. pylori*) is frequently discovered in the stomach. Numerous illnesses, including gastric atrophy, duodenal ulcers, gastric ulcers, gastric cancer, and gastritis, have been linked to *H. pylori* [93]. There has recently been a lot of debate on whether *H. pylori* frequently co-habits in the oral cavity or only when it is sick [94, 95]. *H. pylori* is assumed to have evolved into its helical shape to assist it more easily enter the mucosal membrane of the stomach [96]. It shares characteristics with *Campylobacter*, including their corkscrew forms, and was formerly thought to be one of those species. Once infected, *H. pylori* is far more challenging to get rid of from the oral cavity than it is from the stomach. Antibacterial therapy is typically utilized to get rid of the bacteria. However, *H. pylori* will re-infect the stomach in a few weeks if therapy is insufficient [97]. Additionally, research has shown that better oral cleanliness and health won't likely increase the effectiveness of *H. pylori* removal from the stomach [98]. There is a need for more investigation into the connection between oral health and *H. pylori*, as long-term dental plaque control has been linked to preventing *H. pylori*-induced stomach illness or re-infection [115].

A facultatively anaerobic, gram-positive bacterium called *S. mutans* is present in the oral microbiome. The round bacteria can be found throughout the oral cavity; however, it is more frequently seen in the fissures and pits. This well-known carcinogen is now viewed as an opportunistic commensal of the oral cavity as a result of its interactions with specific fungi. *S. mutans* and certain fungi can communicate with one another to exchange chemical signals known as quorum sensing, which aids in the development of oral biofilms [99]. Early childhood caries (ECC) and dental caries in general have both been linked to the combination of *C. albicans* and *S. mutans* [100]. Due to bacterial colonization occurring as the teeth are developing and being vulnerable to demineralization, the bacterial etiology of ECC is complex [101]. Cospecies biofilms produce more biomass accumulation and raise the risk of periodontal disease [100]. There are now relatively few approved precision antibiotic treatments for avoiding dental caries, which is nevertheless regarded as the most prevalent chronic disease in the entire world. Recent research, however, suggests that synthetic compounds may be used in combination with antibiotics to target particular dental caries domains [102]. Although subsequent investigations will try to look at the method's long-term impacts, other studies have shown encouraging results employing *Lactobacillus salivarius* probiotics to reduce biofilm mass and pathogenic species [103]. Future research will continue to push the boundaries of how dental caries are managed globally.

P. gingivalis is one of the major microorganisms that cause periodontal disease [104]. This bacterium is a gram-negative, rod-shaped anaerobe that is a member of the *Porphyromonadaceae* family and the phylum *Bacteroidetes*. On blood agar, *P. gingivalis*, a pathogen that lives in the mouth cavity, may be seen developing black colonies. This bacterium benefits from a dysbiotic oral microbiome environment. *P. gingivalis* manipulates complement-TLR crosstalk, which triggers an inflammatory response, to create this dysbiosis. Periodontal disease develops as a result of the interaction of dysbiosis and inflammation [105]. According to research, *P. gingivalis* can infiltrate human fibroblasts in vitro and develop an antibiotic resistance level [106]. Fimbriae, or thin, long proteinaceous surface appendages, are present in the majority of *P. gingivalis* strains and serve crucial roles in the attachment and invasion of host cells [107]. According to one study, fimbriae type II have the capacity to bind to 51-integrin, which enhances the uptake of bacteria by dendritic and phagocyte cells while also allowing the actin cytoskeleton to be rearranged [108]. *P. gingivalis* infection has also been linked to an increased risk of developing gastric and oral malignancies, and oral squamous cell carcinoma frequently contains this bacterium [109]. This bacterium encourages PI3K/Akt signaling, which lowers apoptosis and increases host cell growth. Due to downregulation of GSK3-beta, decreased E-cadherin, and elevated pro-MMP9, tumorigenesis is further aided by *P. gingivalis*-facilitated EMT. Additionally, by blocking p53, this bacteria promotes tumor growth and metastasis [110]. *P. gingivalis* is a lethal infection that, due to a combination of these variables, increases the risk of oral cancer and causes extensive periodontal disease.

F. nucleatum may be the bacterium with the most impact on periodontal disease [111]. Originally thought of as an oral commensal, this anaerobic, Gram-negative bacterium is now more generally referred to as a pathogen. On a blood agar plate, *F. nucleatum* can grow anaerobically for observation. *F. nucleatum* is a member of the family *Fusobacteriaceae* and the phylum *Fusobacteria*. One of the most prevalent types of bacteria can be found in both healthy and sick people's oral cavities [112]. When disease conditions exist, *F. nucleatum* can be found in extra-oral sites and has been linked to illnesses like inflammatory bowel disease, Crohn's disease, colorectal cancer, appendicitis, rheumatoid arthritis, meningitis, and unfavorable pregnancy outcomes [113, 114]. Previously, it was believed that *F. nucleatum* existed almost exclusively in the oral cavity [115]. It has been documented that this species exhibits pathogenic characteristics when it is prevalent in the oral cavity or in extra-oral areas [116]. According to studies, *Fusobacterium* Adhesin A (FadA) signals to the IL-6-STAT3 axis, which in turn activates tumor growth [117]. The process in which FadA is engaged to emphasize the value of further research and additional bacteria with established pathogenic roles in periodontal disease, including the genera *Prevotella*, *Leptotrichia*, *Porphyromonas*, and *Streptococcus*, will also be discussed.

F. nucelatum is crucial to the structural connections of the polymicrobial biofilm in co-culture and is regarded as a secondary colonizer after initial colonizers like *Streptococcus* [118]. A potential pathway for the invasion of the anti-tumor immune response is suggested by the *fadA* gene, which is encoded by the fungus *F. nucleatum* [116]. This adhesin binds to host cells and is necessary for the binding of both normal and malignant cells. A galactose-sensitive adhesin called Fap2 is implicated in both the inflammatory process and cell adhesion [119]. Numerous host reactions are triggered by *F. nucleatum*, including the activation of IL-6, IL-8, and TNF [120]. The attachment of *F. nucleatum* to natural killer cells triggers the inflammatory responses related to periodontal disease [121]. The disorders associated with *F. nucleatum* range greatly in severity from mild types of gingivitis that are reversible to generalized aggressive forms of periodontitis [122]. Numerous extraoral locations have reported the presence of *F. nucleatum* [115], and it has been hypothesized that FadA's affinity for cadherins on endothelial and epithelial cells is probably the cause of this colonization [116].

Recent data indicate that the interaction between *Pseudomonas aeruginosa* and *F. nucleatum* via FadA may lead to antibiotic resistance [123]. Another recent study found that targeting TLR4 and certain microRNAs changed the chemotherapeutic response and promoted chemoresistance by activating the autophagy system [124]. Additional research has examined the function of *P. gingivalis* and *F. nucleatum* in the initiation and progression of oral cancer in mouse models. Together, these bacteria are frequently identified in oral cancer cells, where they cause the release of IL-6 and activate the STAT3 pathway. Additionally, mice infected with *P. gingivalis* and *F. nucleatum* had higher levels of pSTAT3 and IL-6 than mice that were not infected [125]. *F. nucleatum* will undoubtedly be discussed in the future due to all of its potential consequences in terms of disease, both serious and minor.

Evolving Research from Probiotics to Postbiotics

A "preparation of inanimate microorganisms and/or their components that confers a health benefit on the host" is referred to as a postbiotic [126, 127]. The International Scientific Association of Probiotics and Prebiotics (ISAPP) put forth this consensus definition in 2021 to take the place of various other earlier but conflicting definitions. The 2021 ISAPP consensus statement lists a number of examples, including (i) "soluble factors (products or metabolic byproducts), secreted by live bacteria, or released after bacterial lysis, such as peptides, enzymes, teichoic acids, polysaccharides, peptidoglycan-derived muropeptides, organic acids, and cell-surface proteins"; (ii) "non-viable metabolites produced by microorganisms In addition to the metabolites and/or secreted products of living bacteria, these definitions varied about the inclusion or exclusion of nonviable cells or cell components [128].

The ISAPP determined that postbiotics must contain inactivated cellular biomass, which consists of the parts of an inanimate microbe that are left over after a live microbe has been exposed to an inactivation process, in order to resolve this discrepancy [128]. Additionally, the ISAPP consensus statement makes it clear that postbiotic preparations must come from described microorganisms, excluding preparations from undefined bacteria [128, 129]. Along with these additional components, postbiotic formulations can also include metabolic and secretory metabolites made by bacteria during growth and fermentation in a medium before inactivation. These products include bacteriocins, teichoic acids, vitamins, short-chain fatty acids (SCFAs), exopolysaccharides (EPS), enzymes, and peptides [130]. Although live microorganisms produce these extracellular metabolites and secretions during fermentation in a medium or host environment, they aren't specifically mentioned in the definition of probiotics. The products left in a fermentation medium after cells have been removed using filtration or centrifugation, respectively, are referred to as "cell-free filtrate" or "cell-free supernatant" in the inaugural use of the term "postbiotics" [128, 131]. A cell-free medium-containing isolated product has also been referred to as a "postbiotic component" in this way. Prior to 2021, it's vital to keep this lexical sprawl caused by the absence of a widely accepted definition of postbiotics in mind when searching the literature on the subject. To date, the emphasis has been on food-safe microbes, particularly lactic acid bacteria, as the majority of postbiotic research has been a continuation of past probiotic research efforts. Postbiotics, which don't pose a risk of infection, are exempt from the rigorous laws limiting probiotic therapies for human application to food-safe GRAS or QPS since inactivation prevents the proliferation of administered postbiotics inside the body [132]. This postbiotic feature may make it possible to produce postbiotic preparations from a far wider variety of bacteria, including microbial taxa that haven't been used safely in the past and are thus disqualified from consideration for probiotic treatments.

For instance, *Faecalibacterium prausnitzii*, which is widely acknowledged to be a helpful endogenous gut microbe, cannot be supplied as a live microbe in probiotic therapy since it is not yet deemed safe to eat [133]. Although studies suggest that the production of butyrate by *Faecalibacterium prausnitzii* provides a health-promoting function within the gut, it may still be possible to achieve the same beneficial effects with postbiotic therapy based on an inactivated *Faecalibacterium prausnitzii* preparation including butyrate [133]. A microbial anti-inflammatory molecule (MAM), a protein that has been shown to have anti-inflammatory effects on mouse models with induced colitis, is another product that *Faecalibacterium prausnitzii* generates in addition to butyrate [134, 135].

Postbiotic research has gained more traction as a result of the discovery that endogenous microorganisms primarily interact with a host indirectly through the creation of different chemicals. Some of these substances work to reinforce the epithelial barrier that separates the internal host environment from the microbiome, while others can either pass through the epithelium (as in the case of metabolites) or cross it (as in the case of bigger molecules) to enter the body, where they have an impact on the internal host environment [136]. Since numerous species share the same metabolic pathways, neither metabolites nor secretory products are specialized to a single species. It is challenging to define a "normal healthy gut microbiome" due to the high level of functional redundancy seen within the gut microbiome and the significant heterogeneity in the makeup of gut microbiomes in "healthy individuals" [137, 138]. This emphasizes the need to change the emphasis from trying to identify particular microorganisms as biomarkers for a health or illness state to the preservation of health-associated functions [138]. As a result, in addition to focusing on the identification and existence of the endogenous microbial species themselves, microbiome research is increasingly giving more emphasis to the metabolic and secretory products created by the endogenous microorganisms.

According to the ISAPP consensus statement, it is crucial to establish that postbiotic products are safe for their intended application; hence, the microbial species from which postbiotics originate must be characterized [128]. Safety analyses are nevertheless necessary to make sure that postbiotic components themselves are not harmful, despite the fact that there is currently no regulatory framework specifically for postbiotic preparations for human application. The inactivation method must be taken into account in order to establish the safety profile of postbiotics because it is not restricted by the ISAPP postbiotics definition but may affect the kind and activity of postbiotic elements in a preparation [139]. The resulting inanimate postbiotic preparation might then be further processed to separate and analyze specific health-promoting components in order to facilitate the characterization of postbiotic products. Postbiotic research efforts that, to date, have been largely restricted to food-safe microbes targeting the gut microbiome could be expanded and broadened with the help of the characterization of the components within postbiotic preparations. This would allow postbiotic therapies to be developed using standardized concentrations.

Postbiotics as Novel Biological Compounds to Improve Oral Health

Organic acids are well recognized as a fundamental and noteworthy constituent of postbiotic metabolites. The production of lactic acid during bacterial fermentation may be a useful way to control the pathogenicity of microorganisms [140]. Bacteriocins are a class of peptides that have antibacterial properties. These chemicals exhibit resistance to high temperatures and varying pH levels, hence exerting inhibitory effects on the growth and proliferation of gastrointestinal infections. Bacteriocins exert their functional mechanism inside the cytoplasmic membrane, or cell wall, of bacteria [141]. Moreover, fatty acids, which constitute a vital component of postbiotic metabolites, have shown notable antibacterial properties. Eicosapentaenoic acid is one of the long-chain fatty acids that effectively combats gram-positive bacteria. Fatty acids demonstrate diverse antimicrobial functions toward bacteria, encompassing the augmentation of membrane permeability, interference with the electron transport chain, disruption of enzyme structure and activity, lysis of bacterial cells, and induction of morphological and functional alterations in susceptible protein elements [142, 143]. Hydrogen peroxide (H_2O_2) is an additional antimicrobial substance that is said to have antimicrobial properties as a result of its strong oxidizing activity on bacterial cells and its capacity to disrupt protein structures inside the cytoplasm [144] (Figure 2). Previously, the beneficial impacts of some probiotics on enhancing oral health and mitigating oral illnesses were discussed. The antimicrobial activities of probiotics are believed to be attributed to the synthesis of antibacterial chemicals, including organic acids and hydrogen peroxide, as well as antifungal components, such as fatty acids and bacteriocins [145, 146]. Furthermore, previous studies have shown that *L. reuteri* is capable of synthesizing water-soluble antimicrobial compounds such as reuterin [147] and reutericyclin [148], which exhibit antagonistic properties. According to El-Ziney and Debevere (1998) [149], these compounds exhibit resistance to lipolytic and proteolytic enzymes, and they retain their functionality throughout a broad pH spectrum [149]. According to the study conducted by López-López et al. (2017) [150], it was shown that the strain of *S. dentisani* obtained from individuals without dental caries has the ability to create bacteriocin. This finding suggests that this particular strain might potentially be regarded as a valuable probiotic species. Additionally, the findings from a clinical trial spanning a duration of three months indicated that the probiotic strain *S. salivarius* M18, known for its bacteriocin production, had the potential to mitigate the progression of dental caries in children [151, 152].

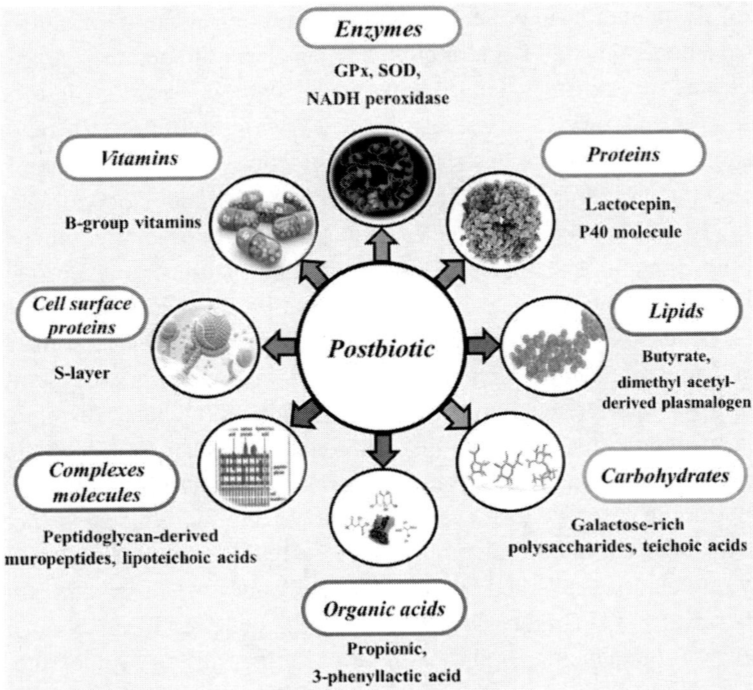

Figure 2. Main postbiotics with health-promoting effects. Postbiotics can be distinguished either by their fundamental components, such as enzymes, proteins, lipids, carbohydrates, organic acids, vitamins, cell surface proteins and complex molecules that indicate an extensive range of health-promoting effects through direct or indirect metabolic pathways.

Previous studies have shown the absence of certain bacterial species, including *S. sanguinis* [153] and *S. uberis*, in subgingival plaque samples collected from individuals diagnosed with refractory periodontitis and localized juvenile periodontitis. Simultaneously, they are detected inside the subgingival plaque specimens obtained from people exhibiting oral health. Previous studies have shown that these strains have inhibitory effects on the development of *A. actinomycetemcomitans* [154] as well as other pathogens associated with periodontal diseases [155] by means of hydrogen peroxide generation [156]. According to Kidd and Fejerskov (2004) [157], the reduction in pH levels and the process of tooth demineralization caused by bacteria such as *S. sobrinus*, *S. mutans*, and *Lactobacillus* spp. may be attributed to the organic acids generated inside the biofilm as metabolic byproducts during the fermentation process [158]. However, as previously stated, the creation of organic acids is one of the processes used by probiotics to inhibit the proliferation of harmful bacteria. Hence, one can inquire as to whether the existence of these acids leads to a subsequent decline in pH levels and an escalation in dental caries. Various investigations have shown that the salivary pH levels exhibited a statistically significant increase in the group receiving probiotic medication as compared to the control group. The findings of this investigation align with other research that has shown a rise in pH levels subsequent to the consumption of yogurt [159] and probiotics comprising curd [81]. The observed elevation in pH levels subsequent to probiotic ingestion may be attributed to their competitive interactions with pathogenic bacteria, resulting in a reduction in the abundance of the latter [160]. The decrease in the population of acid-producing bacteria leads to a reduction in acid production, thereby resulting in a rise in the pH level of saliva. Given the impact of pH imbalance on tooth decay, these results have significant importance. The issue of safeguarding and ensuring safety has garnered attention in recent years, mostly attributed to the widespread availability of probiotic food items. In order to effectively address a bacterial condition, a probiotic strain must possess certain discernible traits [161]. For instance, it is essential that probiotic bacteria do not induce pathogenicity or render the person more vulnerable to other illness conditions by disrupting of their residing habitat [162]. Furthermore, it is important to subject them to thorough examination and screening to ensure general safety, including the assessment of genes linked to antibiotic resistance and those associated with possible invasion [60].

Given the aforementioned difficulties surrounding the ingestion of live bacteria, it is imperative to explore a viable and secure substitute that offers equivalent physiological advantages akin to those provided by probiotics [163]. The findings obtained from pre-clinical and clinical investigations suggest that postbiotics possess a safety profile and exhibit advantageous and therapeutic effects when administered in suitable quantities and durations [164, 165]. Postbiotics provide many advantageous characteristics that make them viable alternatives to probiotics in the food and pharmaceutical sectors [166]. These include the presence of a secure profile, an extended shelf life of up to five years, the absence of harmful effects, standardization, and enhanced ease of transportation. Consequently, postbiotics offer a safe and cost-effective option for utilization in these industries. In this regard, *L. salivarius* subsp. *salicinius* AP-32, *L. plantarum* LPL28, and *L. paracasei* ET-66 postbiotic lozenges and heat-inactivated probiotic lozenges of *L. paracasei* ET-66, and *L. salivarius* subsp. *salicinius* AP-32 were examined by Chiao-Wen Lin et al. for their effects on oral health. A total of 75 persons who were in good health were randomly and blindly assigned to three groups: placebo, heat-inactivated probiotic lozenge, and postbiotic lozenge. Each group received the corresponding kind of lozenge for a duration of 4 weeks. The groups who received postbiotic and heat-inactivated probiotic lozenges exhibited antibacterial effects, leading to a significant rise in the population of *L. salivarius* in their oral cavity. In addition, there was an observed rise in salivary immunoglobulin A, as well as in the levels of *Bifidobacterium* spp. and *Lactobacillus* spp. The subjective questionnaires, which were completed by the participants, revealed that individuals in both experimental groups exhibited improved dental health and intestinal characteristics compared to those in the placebo group. In summary, the findings of their research show that the utilization of a food additive in the shape of an oral postbiotic or heat-inactivated probiotic lozenge has the potential to significantly augment oral immunity, impede the proliferation of oral pathogens, and elevate the abundance of advantageous oral microbiota.

In a separate study in order to assess the impact of postbiotics on oral health, a total of eight spent culture supernatants (SCSs) derived from probiotics were generated. These SCSs were then examined to determine their effects on the formation of cariogenic biofilms induced by *Streptococcus mutans*, as well as their influence on osteoclastogenesis induced by the receptor activator of the nuclear factor κB ligand (RANKL) in RAW 264.7 macrophages. The SCS derived from *L. salivarius* MG4265 showed a notable reduction of 73% in biofilm formation produced by S. mutans. Additionally, it demonstrated a considerable inhibition of tartrate-resistant acid phosphatase (TRAP) action, which serves as a biomarker for developed osteoclasts in RAW 264.7 macrophages. The inhibition of the activation of mitogen-activated protein kinases (p38, extracellular signal-regulated kinase, and c-Jun N-terminal kinase) and nuclear factor κB pathways, together with the increase in heme oxygenase-1 expression, effectively suppresses the RANKL-induced response. Inhibition of the activation triggered by RANK-L was found to minimize the expression of transcription elements, namely c-fos and nuclear factor of activated T cells cytoplasmic 1. Consequently, the expression of genes associated with osteoclastogenesis, such as matrix metalloproteinase-9, cathepsin K, and tartrate-resistant acid phosphatase-positive (TRAP) was also inhibited. Hence, the use of the SCS derived from *L. salivarius* MG4265 exhibits significant promise as a versatile oral health component, effectively impeding the production of biofilms and mitigating the detrimental alveolar bone loss often linked to periodontitis [167]. In this context, another research was conducted with the objective of evaluating the impact of postbiotic metabolites (PMs) originating from the microbiota on the development of dental caries. In pursuit of this objective, the antibacterial properties of PMs obtained from *L. curvatus* EIR/BG-2, *L. curvatus* EIR/DG-1, and *L. plantarum* EIR/IF-1 were examined using the agar diffusion technique.

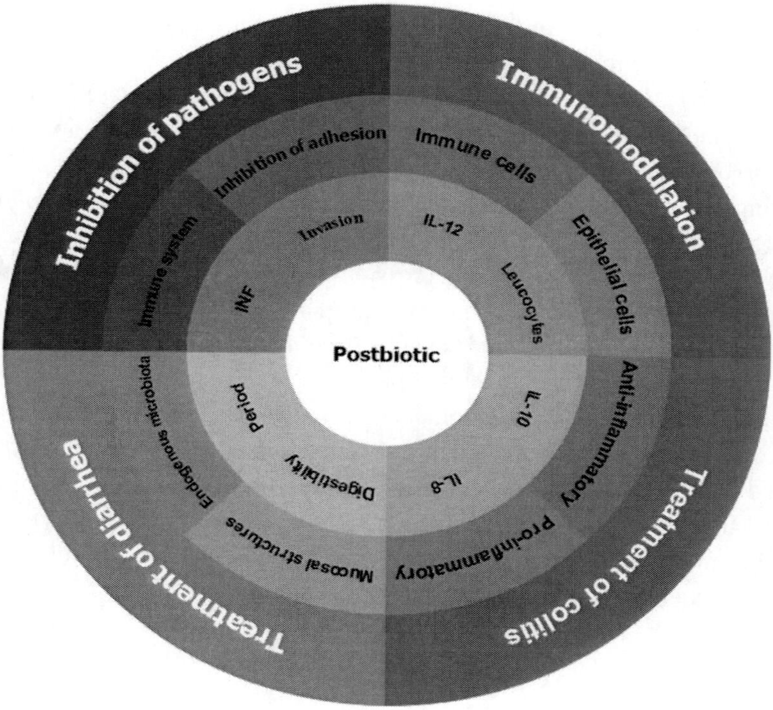

Figure 3. Main mechanisms of postbiotics regarding their biological role in the inhibition of pathogens, immunomodulation, treatment of colitis, and diarrhea. Inhibition of pathogens: in the first step, the postbiotics reduce the adherence of pathogens and promote the host's immune system; in the second step, they exert anti-bacterial and anti-viral activities through reducing the invasion of pathogens and producing INF. Immunomodulation: in the first step, postbiotics interact with immune and epithelial cells to activate innate immunity; in the second step, they stimulate the secretion of IL-12 and improve immune system functioning through increasing the phagocytic activity of leucocytes. Treatment of colitis: in the first step, postbiotics exert significant anti-inflammatory activities; in the second step, they regulate the inflammatory responses in gut epithelial cells through stimulating the production of IL-10 as an anti-inflammatory cytokine and inhibiting the production of IL-8 as a pro-inflammatory cytokine. Treatment of diarrhea: in the first step, probiotics alter the mucosal structure by increasing the villi size and fortifying the endogenous beneficial microbiota; in the second step, they reduce the symptoms of diarrhea through improving digestibility and reducing the duration of the disease.

Additionally, the antibiofilm features of these PMs were assessed using the crystal violet test. The target organism for these analyses was *S. mutans* (ATCC 25175). Based on the findings, it was observed that the strain EIR/IF-1-derived PMs, obtained from newborn feces, had the most pronounced inhibitory effect, which was shown to be dependent on pH. In addition, it was shown that the sub-minimum inhibitory concentration (sub-MIC) of all the PMs effectively eradicated the development of biofilms in both the pre-treatment and co-treatment experimental conditions. The decrease in cellular viability and significant alterations in biofilm development were further verified by the use of scanning electron microscopy and confocal laser scanning microscopy on both glass coverslips and *ex vivo* human tooth surfaces. Additionally, the sub-minimum inhibitory concentration levels of PMs were shown to decrease the expression of *comX*, *comA*, and *gtfC* without causing any notable inhibition of growth. The presence of vitamins, fatty acids, and organic acids in PMs has also been documented. In summary, the results of this study suggest that microbiota-derived PMs may have a potential preventative effect on the development of dental caries [168].

Consequently, it can be stated that postbiotic metabolites (especially those derived from oral cavity beneficial microbiota) possess significant promise as a novel host-adaptable strategy that effectively suppresses the proliferation and biofilm generation of pathogenic germs and positively stimulates the immune system (Figure 3).

Postbiotic and Halitosis

Halitosis, often known as oral malodor, is a multifactorial condition that may arise from either oral or non-oral sources [169, 170]. Halitosis is often ascribed to the presence of biofilm in the interdental gaps, the posterior region of the tongue, and chronic conditions with inflammation. The prevalence of this particular illness across various groups is believed to range from 22 to 50 percent [171]. Sulfur-containing gases, including methyl mercaptan, hydrogen sulfide, and dimethyl sulfide have a significant influence on the occurrence of halitosis. The emission of these gases occurs inside the oropharynx, namely in areas such as the gingivitis, tonsillitis, tongue coating, and periodontitis, as a result of bacterial decomposition of amino acids that include sulfur. *Porphyromonas gingivalis*, *Prevotella intermedia*, *Treponema denticola*, and *Fusobacterium nucleatum*, are among the several bacterial species that are implicated in the etiology of this particular disorder [172, 173]. Conversely, individuals with halitosis have insignificant quantities of bacterial species that constitute the predominant microbiota in the oral cavity of healthy individuals [174]. Contemporary therapeutic approaches aim to eradicate these harmful microorganisms by the use of physical or chemical antibacterial substances. Antimicrobial therapy exhibits non-selective reduction of both pathogenic bacteria and non-halitosis-causing bacteria, which likely play a role in maintaining a healthy oral microenvironment. Nevertheless, the outcome of this treatment is just a temporary reduction in malodor, since the bacteria responsible for halitosis resurface after a certain period of time [175]. Probiotics with proven efficacy in promoting periodontal health may also have the potential to address halitosis by contributing to the maintenance of a balanced microbial community on the tongue. This is particularly relevant due to the challenge of accessing specific regions of the tongue, particularly the dorsal posterior surface adjacent to the circumvallate papillae, which serves as a habitat for a substantial population of gram-negative bacteria associated with malodor [176]. However, it is widely acknowledged that the tongue is a more prominent anatomical feature compared to the periodontal grooves in terms of the species that typically inhabit them. This indicates the importance of specific adaptations to each recess, and it suggests that probiotic strains designed to colonize the periodontal grooves may not be able to effectively colonize the tongue and provide beneficial effects on oral health [177]. In their seminal study, Kang et al. (2006) [178] embarked on a scientific endeavor to identify a probiotic agent capable of mitigating or remedying halitosis. A significant reduction in hydrogen sulfide (H_2S) levels by 48.2% and methyl mercaptan (CH_3SH) levels by 59.4% has been reported in children after the use of a washing solution containing *Weissella cibaria*. Consequently, a reduction in halitosis has been noted [178, 179]. One potential contender for countering bacterial species that contribute to the elevation of sulfur-based volatile substances is *Streptococcus salivarius* since it has shown an inhibitory impact on volatile sulfur compounds. The use of chlorhexidine mouthwash, followed by the administration of lozenges containing the *S. salivarius* K12 strain, resulted in a reduction of volatile sulfur compounds in the respiratory system of the majority of participants. Furthermore, this reduction was sustained for a minimum duration of two weeks [180]. According to Meurman and Stamatova (2007) [60], this particular strain is capable of producing two lantibiotic bacteriocins that have inhibitory effects on gram-positive pathogens associated with halitosis. *S. salivarius* K12 has shown the potential to mitigate halitosis by displacing the microorganisms responsible for malodorous breath over an extended duration [181]. Previous research has shown the efficacy of this particular strain in mitigating halitosis [182, 183]. The research conducted by Iwamoto et al. (2010) [184] showed that the probiotic strain *L. salivarius* WB21 had a beneficial impact on both the organoleptic assessment results and halitosis. The use of probiotics in chewing gum has been shown to have the potential to decrease the abundance of non-sulfur odor-generating bacteria. The research conducted by Keller et al. (2012b) [185] reported a substantial reduction in organoleptic ratings after the intake of chewing gum with *L. reuteri* when matched to the placebo group. However, the study conducted by Marchetti et al. (2015) [186] revealed that the administration of *L. brevis* CD2 lozenges did not result in any significant enhancements in breath VSC levels or organoleptic ratings. Furthermore, the ingestion of milk with *L. casei* Shirota did not result in a substantial reduction in breath volatile sulfur compound content or organoleptic ratings [187]. Pre-clinical investigations have shown the occurrence of anti-volatile sulfur compound effects caused by non-oral bacteria, including *W. cibaria*, *E. faecium*, and *S. thermophilus* [188, 189].

Research was conducted that included randomized controlled trials (RCTs) to evaluate the impact of Lactobacillus paracasei ET-22 in both live and heat-inactivated forms on halitosis and the associated oral microbiota. The participants with halitosis were allocated into three groups: placebo, ET-22 live (ET-22.L), and ET-22 heat-inactivated (ET-22.HI). Participants were administered various lozenges on three separate occasions, daily, over a period of four weeks. Saliva samples were collected, and the levels of breath volatile sulfur compounds were assessed at the commencement and conclusion of the intervention. The measurement of salivary VOC was conducted using the HS-SPME-GC/MS technique, while the characterization of the microbiome profile was achieved using 16S rRNA gene amplicon sequencing. After a period of 4 weeks, a significant reduction in breath VSC concentrations was found in both the ET-22.L and ET-22.HI groups. However, the reduction was more pronounced in the ET-22.L group ($P = 0.0148$). In addition, the intervention of ET-22.L and ET-22.HI had a significant impact on the composition of both aroma-active VOCs and total salivary VOCs . A notable decrease was seen in the concentrations of many important volatile organic compounds, including benzothiazole, indole, nonanoic acid, pyridine, and valeric acid. Simultaneously, the presence of ET-22.L or ET-22.HI resulted in modifications to the taxonomic makeup of the salivary microbial ecosystem. The presence of halitosis-causing pathogens, namely *Streptococcus*, and *Rothia* exhibited a notable decrease in the ET-22.HI group. Similarly, the pathogenic microorganisms *Peptostreptococcus* and *Solobacterium* saw considerable inhibition in the ET-22.L group. This research together indicates that both ET-22.L and ET-22.HI have the potential to effectively suppress the generation of malodorous chemicals in individuals suffering from halitosis. This effect is likely attributed to alterations in the oral microbiota [190].

Postbiotic and Periodontal Diseases

One of the most prevalent chronic infectious dental disorders is periodontal disease. Antibiotics and chemical agents are typically used to treat many dental diseases, which have several unfavorable effects [191]. Multidrug-resistant bacteria are frequently produced as a result of the continued use of antibiotics to treat dental diseases, which can have long-term negative effects on public health. In addition, the World Health Organization listed antibiotic resistance as one of the top ten global health issues facing people [192]. Some antibiotics also do not penetrate the bacterial biofilm, which is another drawback. Antibiotic resistance in bacteria today is primarily due to bacterial biofilms, which are more resistant to antibiotics than planktonic bacteria [193, 194].

Butrungrod et al. (2023) investigated the efficiency of a postbiotic metabolite of *L. plantarum* PD18 isolated from fermented food that has antimicrobial activity against *P. gingivalis*, *S. mutans*, *T. forsythia*, and *P. loescheii.* It also has anti-biofilm activity against two representative oral biofilm formation strains, *P. gingivalis* and *S. mutans,* on both glass cover slips and molar typodont teeth. The results revealed that the postbiotic metabolites of *L. plantarum* PD18 showed promise as a natural adjunctive agent that could be applied in a variety of oral care formulations to inhibit periodontal pathogens and their biofilms. However, additional research is required to thoroughly assess the anti-periodontitis pathogens' mechanisms and the main active substances involved [195].

Some researchers reported the effect of postbiotics (postbiotics with whey bioconversion products produced by *Enterococcus faecalis* M157 KACC 81148BP and mixed whey bioconversion products produced by *E. faecalis* M157 KACC 81148BP and *Lactococcus lactis* ssp. *lactis* CAU2013 KACC 81152BP) for the improvement of gut health and the treatment of periodontal disease. The products were administered orally to PD-induced rats for 8 weeks. Results showed that periodontal lesions decreased in the case of previous treatment with postbiotics in comparison to the control treatment. The cytokine levels and bone loss volumes were lower as well. They concluded that the whey bioconversion product produced by *E. faecalis* M157 KACC 81148BP and mixed whey bioconversion products produced by *L. lactis* CAU2013 KACC 81152BP and *E. faecalis* M157 KACC 81148BP were effective in improving gut health and relieving periodontitis [196].

In dentistry, chlorhexidine (CHX) is one of the most widely used antiseptics. It is regarded as an adjuvant tool for mechanical oral hygiene procedures and is available in a variety of forms, including gel, mouthwash, aerosol, disks, and spray. It has broad-spectrum antibacterial activity and is able to reduce plaque, bleeding and gingival inflammation [197]. Chlorhexidine has a number of drawbacks, including dysgeusia and tooth discoloration, despite its effectiveness. Additionally, there is a high likelihood of bacterial recolonization. According to the findings of studies, postbiotics are at least as effective as regular chlorhexidine because of their antioxidant effect. Scientists recently published an in vitro study which examined free pH-neutralized supernatants (CFS) of *Lactobacillus rhamnosus* Lr32, *Lactobacillus acidophilus* LA5, *L. rhamnosus* HN001 and *L. acidophilus* NCFM against a fimbriated clinical isolate of the Aa JP2 genotype on biofilm formation for 24 h and early and mature preformed biofilms. The results showed that postbiotics derived from *lactobacilli*, particularly LA5, were able to decrease the levels of Aa colonization and to modulate the expression of virulence factors involved in the evasion of host defenses [198].

The effectiveness of both postbiotics and chlorhexidine can be explained by the fact that the latter can act as an antiseptic agent while also acting as an antioxidant, immunomodulator, and even having an anti-inflammatory effect on the periodontal tissues. The former, meanwhile, is an antiseptic agent that reduces the number of bacteria. Therefore, compared to the standard chlorhexidine-based gel used as the control, it might be assumed that using Biorepair Parodontgel Intensive can result in a prolonged effect. In contrast to postbiotics, chlorhexidine should only be used for a maximum of 15 days (with a worsening of periodontal indices at the end of the period). It is noteworthy that Biorepair Parodontgel Intensive contains biomimetic Zn-Carbonate Hydroxyapatite, which is known for its significant impact on tooth remineralization in addition to its effect on soft tissues [199, 200].

Due to the absence of analog studies, no direct comparisons can be done for the results obtained in the current study, aimed at evaluating the efficacy of antioxidant postbiotics contained in a gel formulation [201-203]. Anyway, the efficacy of both chlorhexidine and postbiotics can be justified by the fact that the former is an antiseptic agent reducing the bacterial amount, whereas postbiotics can act as antiseptics as well but also as antioxidant and immunomodulant-promoting, even having an anti-inflammatory effect on the periodontal tissues. Therefore, it might be assumed that the use of Biorepair Parodontgel Intensive is able to lead to a prolonged effect with respect to the conventional chlorhexidine-based gel considered as the control. It is also important to notice that chlorhexidine should be used for a maximum of 15 days (with a worsening of periodontal indexes at the end of the period), differently from postbiotics. In addition to the effect on soft tissues, it is also remarkable that Biorepair Parodontgel Intensive contains biomimetic Zn-Carbonate Hydroxyapatite, which is recognized for its significant effect on tooth remineralization [199]. Therefore, while chlorhexidine has acted only as an antimicrobial agent, the experimental product here considered might have caused multiple effects on both soft and hard tissues. In fact, the presence of biomimetic Zn-Carbonate Hydroxyapatite might have induced a remineralization of the radicular surface of the teeth; in addition to that, antioxidant postbiotics are likely to have induced an anti-inflammatory and regenerative effect on periodontal tissues, with a repositioning of the junctional epithelium on a remineralized radicular surface [204].

On the basis of some considerations and the absence of similar studies, no final conclusions can be drawn about the use of postbiotics in periodontology. Additional studies are needed, and, in particular, the impact of postbiotics and chlorhexidine should be investigated not only on the marketed product (due to the presence of other ingredients that could bias the results) but, especially, on the specific singular chemical compounds in order to enable a direct comparison with no confounding variables [204, 205].

Postbiotic and Oral Cancer

Oral cancer ranks as the 16th most prevalent form of cancer globally, with a greater occurrence and fatality rate among males in comparison to females. The continent of Asia accounts for the largest proportion of global incidences (65.8%) and mortalities (74%) related to lips and oral cancer, with Europe and North America following suit. According to the GLOBOCAN 2020 study, there were a cumulative 377,713 incidences of newly diagnosed lip and mouth cancer cases, resulting in 177,757 recorded deaths [206, 207]. Alcohol intake, tobacco smoking, the consumption of areca nuts (betel quid), and the presence of infections caused by microbes such as *Candida albicans* and Human Papilloma Virus are recognized as significant variables that contribute to the development of oral carcinogenesis [208]. Kleinstein et al. conducted a study proposing a novel approach to prevent and treat the effects of oral conditions. Their research focused on manipulating the oral microbiome by providing proresolving tiny lipid compounds that specifically target immunemicrobial indicators [209]. A separate research has shown that maintaining a well-balanced oral microbiome might potentially address oral disorders resulting from dysbiosis. This, in turn, may lead to a decrease in the reliance on antimicrobial medicines, which have posed ongoing challenges in the treatment of oral cancer patients owing to the emergence of antibiotic resistance [210]. Dysbiosis is characterized by an imbalance in the composition of the oral microbiome, resulting in a disruption of its normal equilibrium. The aforementioned state induces alterations in both the arrangement and functional composition of the oral microbiome, potentially leading to the activation of pathogenic properties in opportunistic bacteria, including *C. albicans* [211]. Persistent dysbiosis might potentially result in the establishment of microbial-mediated inflammation, such as *C. albicans*, which has been shown to contribute to the development of oral carcinogenesis [212]. In addition, it has been shown that some infections, such as *Helicobacter* spp., have the ability to generate genotoxins and other metabolites that are known to cause cancer. These substances have been found to initiate the development of tumors [213]. The relationship between dysbiosis and carcinogenesis in mouth cancer is not yet fully understood. While oral cancer is often linked to the use of alcohol and cigarettes, research has shown that inadequate oral hygiene is a significant risk factor for those who do not engage in smoking or drinking behaviors [214]. Therefore, it is hypothesized that dysbiosis may potentially be linked to the development of oral cancer. Chronic inflammation is recognized as a significant factor in the pathogenesis of cancer [215]. Periodontitis has been identified as a contributing factor in the development of oral squamous cell carcinoma (OSCC), a prevalent form of oral cancer. This association arises from the recognition of periodontitis as a frequently occurring inflammatory condition that affects the oral cavity [216]. Chronic periodontal inflammation has been identified as a well-established risk factor for oral cancer. Research has shown that persons with chronic inflammation have a significantly elevated chance of acquiring malignancy in comparison to those who have a healthy oral status [217]. Moreover, La Rosa et al. showed that the activation of microorganisms in the context of chronic inflammation leads to an upregulation of inflammatory cytokines and mediators. Consequently, these processes would promote mutagenesis, angiogenesis, and unregulated cellular proliferation, ultimately resulting in the development of mouth cancer [218]. Chronic inflammation linked to periodontal inflammation is often attributed to anaerobic bacteria, including *Prevotella*, *Porphyromonas*, and *Fusobacterium*. These bacteria secrete an inflammatory mediator that engages with several kinds of tissues, hence initiating inflammation. The bacteria further induce the secretion of pro-inflammatory cytokines, including IL-23, IL-17, IL-6, IL-1, tumor necrosis factor-alpha (TNF-α), and proteinases that possess the ability to degrade the extracellular matrix. Certain bacteria, including *Pseudomonas aeruginosa*, *Porphyromonas gingivalis*, and *Mycoplasma salivarium* have the ability to modulate cell proliferation by activating NF-κB and suppressing apoptosis [218, 219]. According to a research conducted by Hanahan, it was shown that the oral microbiome has the capacity to influence cancer via processes such as immunomodulation, toxin production leading to DNA damage, and adherence to epithelial receptors that promote cell proliferation [220]. Moreover, in situations where there is a disruption of the intestinal barrier caused by dysbiosis, the pathogen has the ability to generate butyrate. This substance exhibits diverse and contradictory effects on specialized cells within the epithelium, impacting cellular energy production and metabolism, modifications of histones, progression of the cell cycle, and the promotion of inflammation (which can contribute to tumor development) while simultaneously suppressing the adaptive immune response [221].

The *Lactobacilli* spp. are recognized for their production of postbiotics, which are abundant in a bacteriostatic compound known as bacteriocin [222]. The bacterium *L. reuteri* produces a chemical known as reuterin, which is generated from glycerol. Reuterin has shown significant antimicrobial properties, since it is capable of effectively inhibiting a wide range of microbes. Reuterin functions to preserve the integrity of the intestinal gut mucosa by preventing the excessive proliferation of both harmful and commensal bacteria. This system may be used in the mucosa of the mouth [223]. *L. reuteri* has been shown to have significant efficacy in mitigating the severity of gingivitis, indicating the potential of its postbiotic to possess similar properties. The inhibitory effects of postbiotics derived from the culture supernatant of *L. rhamnosus* GG have been shown to effectively suppress the development of *Candida albicans*, *Streptococcus mutans*, and *Porphyromonas gingivalis* [224]. The spent-culture supernatant (SCS) derived from *L. salivarius* MG4265, and *Lactococcus lactis* MG5125 showed inhibitory effects on the proliferation and biofilm formation of *S. mutans*. This suggests that these strains produce extracellular components and metabolites that contain anticarcinogenic properties [167].

Secretion of Anticancer Agent

Postbiotics containing anticancer drugs provide a potential alternative to traditional chemotherapy, which is often associated with significant adverse effects including hypertension, hemorrhage, and renal impairment [225]. The constituents of postbiotics include several elements such as extracellular polymeric substances (EPS), short-chain fatty acids (SCFA), functional proteins, microbial cell fractions, metabolites, cell lysates, and polysaccharides [226]. Polysaccharides had the most prominent anticancer activity among the many compounds often present in postbiotics [225]. The postbiotics derived from *B. longum*, *L. casei*, and *L. acidophilus* had a notable anticancer effect when tested against both an implanted tumor model and a chemically produced tumor model. In a research conducted *in vivo*, the treatment of the cytoplasmic compound of Lactic acid bacteria (LAB) was shown to enhance specific antitumor activity through modulating cellular immunity. There were no recorded instances of immediate tumor eradication [227]. The inclusion of *Propionibacterium freudenreichii* in fermented milk was shown to enhance the cytotoxic effects of camptothecin, a chemotherapeutic drug often used in the treatment of stomach cancer. The protective effects of beetroot juice fermentation by *L. paracasei* and *L. brevis* against the development of aberrant crypt foci (ACF) in N-nitroso-N-methylurea-induced tumor regression in advanced cancer have been seen during treatment with sterile filtrates derived from *Clostridium histolyticum* [228]. While the research mentioned does not specifically focus on oral cancer, they suggest that probiotics may have potential as an adjunctive treatment for mouth-related disorders, including various forms of tumors. While the anticancer properties of postbiotics may not exhibit the same level of efficacy as conventional chemotherapy, their mechanism mostly includes the indirect eradication of tumor cells through immunomodulatory actions. However, it has the potential to serve as an adjunctive treatment for cancer, therefore mitigating the adverse effects associated with chemotherapy. However, more research is required to substantiate the concept.

Anti-Metastasis Activity

Metastasis, the process by which cancer spreads from the original tumor to other parts of the body, has been shown to occur many years beyond the initial diagnosis of the primary tumor. In fact, it has been identified as the leading cause of mortality in over 90% of individuals diagnosed with cancer [229]. Metastasis refers to the process through which cancer cells disseminate from the original tumor to adjacent tissues and distant organs [230]. The principal factor contributing to the development of metastasis is the process known as epithelial-mesenchymal transition (EMT) in cancer cells [231]. Epithelial-mesenchymal transition is a biological process in which epithelial cells undergo a transformation, acquiring the physiological and morphological traits often associated with mesenchymal cells [232]. While it is crucial to focus on preventing the initial spread of cancer cells to other parts of the body, it is equally critical to block the development of further metastases in patients who already have existing metastases. This is necessary in order to enhance their overall prognosis [233]. *L. delbrueckii* subsp. *Lactis* demonstrated a noteworthy increase in the expression of E-cadherin in cell lines derived from human cancer of the uterine cervix (HeLa cells). E-cadherin is considered the principal protein responsible for mediating cell-to-cell adhesion. Therefore, the enhanced reaction of E-cadherin impeded the migration of cancer cells [234]. In addition, it has been shown that the administration of *L. paracasei* GMNL-133 and *L. reuteri* GMNL-89 effectively reduces the expression of epithelial-mesenchymal transition-related markers in mice models of pancreatic cancer, hence mitigating the likelihood of metastatic spread] 235]. The concentrations of matrix metalloproteinase-9 (MMP-9) were reduced and the concentrations of tight junction protein ZO-1 were elevated by the postbiotics derived from *L. rhamnosus* GG, and *L. casei* specifically in the form of cell-free supernatants. As a consequence, there was a decrease in the occurrence of colon cancer, leading to a subsequent reduction in its metastatic consequences [236]. The use of kefir water, a grain-free supernatant, in the management of murine breast cancer cells has shown notable anti-angiogenic and anti-metastatic effects. These results were attributed to its capacity to stimulate the upregulation of tissue-specific inhibitors of matrix metalloproteinases (TIMPs) [237]. The metastasis of colon cancer cells was prevented by the cell-free supernatant of *L. plantarum* YYC-3 via the suppression of the vascular endothelial growth factor (VEGF)- MMP2/9 signaling pathway [238]. The first stage of metastasis involves the deterioration of the basement membrane, which may be impeded by the suppression of the VEGF-MMP2/9 signaling pathway. The reason for this phenomenon may be attributed to the role of the Vascular Endothelial Growth Factor as a signalling protein that facilitates the proliferation of nascent blood vessels, juxtaposed with the function of matrix metalloproteinases in the degradation of the extracellular matrix. Therefore, the use of postbiotic therapy effectively inhibited the signaling pathway of vascular endothelial growth factor-matrix metalloproteinase 2/9 (MMP2/9), thereby mitigating the potential for metastasis in colon cancer cells [239, 240]. The aforementioned studies demonstrate the efficacy of probiotics and postbiotics in their anti-metastatic properties against several cancer cell types. However, more work is required to explore their efficacy in inhibiting oral cancer via the prevention of metastasis.

Conclusion

The investigation of probiotics and their potential therapeutic benefits in the prevention, treatment, and management of many illnesses has garnered significant interest over an extended period of time. Hence, there is a growing inclination among individuals to utilize probiotic dietary and pharmaceutical goods. The demand for probiotic byproducts and secretions, particularly postbiotics, has grown due to the challenges associated with the viability of probiotics in food items until the point of utilization, as well as under unfavorable ambient and gastrointestinal circumstances. Due to the absence of a survival imperative for probiotics and their ability to remain stable over extended periods, as well as their ease of incorporation into various food formulations, postbiotics may serve as a viable substitute for live probiotics. One emerging subject of study is the utilization of postbiotics for the purpose of preserving and enhancing oral cavity health. Numerous studies have shown that the incorporation of probiotics into the oral cavity yields notable outcomes in the mitigation of anomalies, including tooth decay, oral cavity fungus, infection, and inflammation of the gums and palate. The use of postbiotics as an alternative to probiotics seems to provide comparable outcomes and demonstrates efficacy in both the prevention and treatment of numerous oral and dental infectious disorders attributed to the presence of pathogens like *S. mutans*. The results obtained from recent studies provide support for the previously described impact. Nevertheless, there are some obstacles regarding the durability of postbiotics in comparison to probiotics. In order to substantiate the preventative and therapeutic benefits of postbiotics derived from various kinds and species of probiotics, it is essential to conduct several animal and human clinical trials. These investigations are crucial for establishing the ultimate efficacy of such interventions. Given that probiotics share acidogenic properties with cariogenic bacteria like *S. mutans*, it would be beneficial for future research to investigate the distinctions in both the quantity and kind of acids generated by probiotic and pathogenic bacteria. The findings of these investigations may provide more conclusive data and rationales about the potential disparity in carcinogenicity between these acids and the respective bacterial strains responsible for their production.

Disclaimer

None.

References

[1] Bernabe E, Marcenes W, Hernandez CR, Bailey J, Abreu LG, Alipour V, Amini S, Arabloo J, Arefi Z, Arora A, Ayanore MA, Bärnighausen TW, Bijani A, Cho DY, Chu DT, Crowe CS, Demoz GT, Demsie DG, Dibaji Forooshani ZS, Du M, El Tantawi M, Fischer F, Folayan MO, Futran ND, Geramo YCD, Haj-Mirzaian A, Hariyani N, Hasanzadeh A, Hassanipour S, Hay SI, Hole MK, Hostiuc S, Ilic MD, James SL, Kalhor R, Kemmer L, Keramati M, Khader YS, Kisa S, Kisa A, Koyanagi A, Lalloo R, Le Nguyen Q, London SD, Manohar ND, Massenburg BB, Mathur MR, Meles HG, Mestrovic T, Mohammadian-Hafshejani A, Mohammadpourhodki R, Mokdad AH, Morrison SD, Nazari J, Nguyen TH, Nguyen CT, Nixon MR, Olagunju TO, Pakshir K, Pathak M, Rabiee N, Rafiei A, Ramezanzadeh K, Rios-Blancas MJ, Roro EM, Sabour S, Samy AM, Sawhney M, Schwendicke F, Shaahmadi F, Shaikh MA, Stein C, Tovani-Palone MR, Tran BX, Unnikrishnan B, Vu GT, Vukovic A, Warouw TSS, Zaidi Z, Zhang ZJ, Kassebaum NJ. Global, Regional, and National Levels and Trends in Burden of Oral Conditions from 1990 to 2017: A Systematic Analysis for the Global Burden of Disease 2017 Study. *Journal of Dental Research.* 2020;99(4):362-73.

[2] Iheozor-Ejiofor Z, Worthington HV, Walsh T, O'Malley L, Clarkson JE, Macey R, Alam R, Tugwell P, Welch V, Glenny AM. Water fluoridation for the prevention of dental caries. *Cochrane database of systematic reviews.* 2015(6).

[3] Zainab J, Raghad F, Yasameen A. Correlation between caries related microorganisms in the dental plaque and saliva with dental caries level in the upper and lower jaws in 5-9 years old children in baghdad city. *J Bagh Coll Dentistry.* 2016;28(3):132-6.

[4] Abd ST, Ali AF. The Effect of Zinc Oxide Nanoparticles on Streptococcus mutans of Human Saliva (In Vitro Study). *Journal of baghdad college of dentistry.* 2016;28(2).

[5] Ghorbani-Tajani A, Mohammadi R, Shahrooz R. Effect of Local Transplantation of Bone Marrow Derived Mast Cells (BMMCs) Combined with Chitosan Biofilm on Excisional and Incisional Wound Healing: A Novel Preliminary Animal Study on Lamb. *Iranian Journal of Veterinary Surgery.* 2019;14(1):34-43.

[6] Tanzer JM, Livingston J, Thompson AM. The microbiology of primary dental caries in humans. *Journal of dental education.* 2001;65(10):1028-37.

[7] Renuka P, Pushpanjali K, Sangeetha R. Review on "Influence of host genes on dental caries." *IOSR J Dent Med Sci.* 2013;4(3):86-92.

[8] Gruner D, Paris S, Schwendicke F. Probiotics for managing caries and periodontitis: systematic review and meta-analysis. *Journal of Dentistry.* 2016;48:16-25.

[9] Burton JP, Wescombe PA, Macklaim JM, Chai MH, MacDonald K, Hale JD, Tagg J, Reid G, Gloor GB, Cadieux PA. Persistence of the oral probiotic Streptococcus salivarius M18 is dose dependent and megaplasmid transfer can augment their bacteriocin production and adhesion characteristics. *PloS One.* 2013;8(6):e65991.

[10] Walker R, Buckley M. *Probiotic microbes: the scientific basis.* 2006.

[11] Lee S-H, Kim Y-J. A comparative study of the effect of probiotics on cariogenic biofilm model for preventing dental caries. *Archives of microbiology.* 2014;196:601-9.

[12] Han N, Jia L, Su Y, Du J, Guo L, Luo Z, Liu Y. Lactobacillus reuteri extracts promoted wound healing via PI3K/AKT/β-catenin/TGFβ1 pathway. *Stem cell research & therapy.* 2019 Dec;10:1-1.

[13] Jayaram P, Chatterjee A, Raghunathan V. Probiotics in the treatment of periodontal disease: a systematic review. *Journal of Indian Society of Periodontology.* 2016;20(5):488.

[14] Meurman JH. Probiotics: do they have a role in oral medicine and dentistry? *European journal of oral sciences.* 2005;113(3):188-96.

[15] Cheng Y, Liu J, Ling Z. Short-chain fatty acids-producing probiotics: A novel source of psychobiotics. *Critical reviews in food science and nutrition.* 2022;62(28):7929-59.

[16] Ghorbani Tajani A, Bisha B. Effect of Food Matrix and Treatment Time on the Effectiveness of Grape Seed Extract as an Antilisterial Treatment in Fresh Produce. *Microorganisms.* 2023;11(4):1029.

[17] Rad AH, Aghebati-Maleki L, Kafil HS, Gilani N, Abbasi A, Khani N. Postbiotics, as dynamic biomolecules, and their promising role in promoting food safety. *Biointerface Res Appl Chem.* 2021;11(6):14529-44.

[18] Sartor R. the potential mechanisms of action of rifaximin in the management of inflammatory bowel diseases. *Alimentary pharmacology & therapeutics.* 2016;43:27-36.

[19] Mathur S, Singh R. Antibiotic resistance in food lactic acid bacteria—a review. *International journal of food microbiology.* 2005;105(3):281-95.

[20] Sawada D, Sugawara T, Ishida Y, Aihara K, Aoki Y, Takehara I, Takano K, Fujiwara S. Effect of continuous ingestion of a beverage prepared with Lactobacillus gasseri CP2305 inactivated by heat treatment on the regulation of intestinal function. *Food Research International.* 2016 Jan 1;79:33-9.

[21] Verma D, Garg PK, Dubey AK. Insights into the human oral microbiome. *Archives of Microbiology.* 2018;200(4):525-40.

[22] Wang S, Song F, Wang Y, Huang Y, Xie B, Luo H. High resolution melting analysis (HRM) based on 16SrRNA as a tool for personal identification with the

human oral microbiome. *Forensic Science International: Genetics Supplement Series.* 2019;7(1):161-3.
[23] Abeles SR, Pride DT. Molecular Bases and Role of Viruses in the Human Microbiome. *Journal of Molecular Biology.* 2014;426(23):3892-906.
[24] Baker JL, Bor B, Agnello M, Shi W, He X. Ecology of the oral microbiome: beyond bacteria. *Trends in microbiology.* 2017;25(5):362-74.
[25] Pride DT, Salzman J, Haynes M, Rohwer F, Davis-Long C, White RA, Loomer P, Armitage GC, Relman DA. Evidence of a robust resident bacteriophage population revealed through analysis of the human salivary virome. *The ISME journal.* 2012 May;6(5):915-26.
[26] Gruffaz M, Zhang T, Marshall V, Gonçalves P, Ramaswami R, Labo N, Whitby D, Uldrick TS, Yarchoan R, Huang Y, Gao SJ. Signatures of oral microbiome in HIV-infected individuals with oral Kaposi's sarcoma and cell-associated KSHV DNA. *PLoS pathogens.* 2020 Jan 17;16(1):e1008114.
[27] Hayes RB, Ahn J, Fan X, Peters BA, Ma Y, Yang L, Agalliu I, Burk RD, Ganly I, Purdue MP, Freedman ND. Association of oral microbiome with risk for incident head and neck squamous cell cancer. *JAMA oncology.* 2018 Mar 1;4(3):358-65.
[28] Gomez A, Espinoza JL, Harkins DM, Leong P, Saffery R, Bockmann M, Torralba M, Kuelbs C, Kodukula R, Inman J, Hughes T, Craig JM, Highlander SK, Jones MB, Dupont CL, Nelson KE. Host genetic control of the oral microbiome in health and disease. *Cell host & microbe.* 2017;22(3):269-78. e3.
[29] Wade WG. The oral microbiome in health and disease. *Pharmacological Research.* 2013;69(1):137-43.
[30] Matarazzo F, Ribeiro AC, Feres M, Faveri M, Mayer MPA. Diversity and quantitative analysis of Archaea in aggressive periodontitis and periodontally healthy subjects. *Journal of clinical periodontology.* 2011;38(7):621-7.
[31] Liu NN, Jiao N, Tan JC, Wang Z, Wu D, Wang AJ, Chen J, Tao L, Zhou C, Fang W, Cheong IH. Multi-kingdom microbiota analyses identify bacterial–fungal interactions and biomarkers of colorectal cancer across cohorts. *Nature Microbiology.* 2022 Feb;7(2):238-50.
[32] Ghannoum MA, Jurevic RJ, Mukherjee PK, Cui F, Sikaroodi M, Naqvi A, Gillevet PM. Characterization of the oral fungal microbiome (mycobiome) in healthy individuals. *PLoS pathogens.* 2010 Jan 8;6(1):e1000713.
[33] Cheung MK, Chan JY, Wong MC, Wong PY, Lei P, Cai L, Lan L, Ho WC, Yeung AC, Chan PK, Chen Z. Determinants and interactions of oral bacterial and fungal microbiota in healthy Chinese adults. *Microbiology Spectrum.* 2022 Feb 23;10(1):e02410-21.
[34] Sultan AS, Kong EF, Rizk AM, Jabra-Rizk MA. The oral microbiome: A Lesson in coexistence. *PLoS pathogens.* 2018;14(1):e1006719.
[35] Burgain A, Pic É, Markey L, Tebbji F, Kumamoto CA, Sellam A. A novel genetic circuitry governing hypoxic metabolic flexibility, commensalism and virulence in the fungal pathogen Candida albicans. *PLoS pathogens.* 2019;15(12):e1007823.
[36] Vylkova S, Lorenz MC. Phagosomal Neutralization by the Fungal Pathogen Candida albicans Induces Macrophage Pyroptosis. *Infection and Immunity.* 2017;85(2):10.1128/iai.00832-16.

[37] Metwalli KH, Khan SA, Krom BP, Jabra-Rizk MA. Streptococcus mutans, Candida albicans, and the human mouth: a sticky situation. *PLoS Pathog.* 2013;9(10):e1003616.

[38] Krom BP, Kidwai S, ten Cate JM. Candida and Other Fungal Species:Forgotten Players of Healthy Oral Microbiota. *Journal of Dental Research.* 2014;93(5):445-51.

[39] Morse DJ, Wilson MJ, Wei X, Bradshaw DJ, Lewis MAO, Williams DW. Modulation of Candida albicans virulence in in vitro biofilms by oral bacteria. *Letters in applied microbiology.* 2019;68(4):337-43.

[40] Ishijima SA, Hayama K, Burton JP, Reid G, Okada M, Matsushita Y, Abe S. Effect of Streptococcus salivarius K12 on the in vitro growth of Candida albicans and its protective effect in an oral candidiasis model. *Applied and environmental microbiology.* 2012 Apr 1;78(7):2190-9.

[41] Verma A, Gaffen SL, Swidergall M. Innate Immunity to Mucosal Candida Infections. *Journal of Fungi.* 2017;3(4):60.

[42] Nasidze I, Li J, Quinque D, Tang K, Stoneking M. Global diversity in the human salivary microbiome. *Genome research.* 2009;19(4):636-43.

[43] Benn A, Heng N, Broadbent J, Thomson W. Studying the human oral microbiome: challenges and the evolution of solutions. *Australian dental journal.* 2018;63(1):14-24.

[44] Dewhirst FE, Chen T, Izard J, Paster BJ, Tanner ACR, Yu W-H, Lakshmanan A, Wade WG. The Human Oral Microbiome. *Journal of Bacteriology.* 2010;192(19):5002-17.

[45] Perera M, Al-Hebshi NN, Speicher DJ, Perera I, Johnson NW. Emerging role of bacteria in oral carcinogenesis: a review with special reference to perio-pathogenic bacteria. *Journal of oral microbiology.* 2016;8(1):32762.

[46] Pushalkar S, Paul B, Li Q, Yang J, Vasconcelos R, Makwana S, González JM, Shah S, Xie C, Janal MN, Queiroz E. Electronic cigarette aerosol modulates the oral microbiome and increases risk of infection. *Iscience.* 2020 Mar 27;23(3).

[47] Ibrahim M, Subramanian A, Anishetty S. Comparative pan genome analysis of oral Prevotella species implicated in periodontitis. *Functional & integrative genomics.* 2017;17(5):513-36.

[48] Eribe ERK, Olsen I. Leptotrichia species in human infections II. *Journal of Oral Microbiology.* 2017;9(1):1368848.

[49] Hasslöf P, Stecksén-Blicks C. Probiotic bacteria and dental caries. *The Impact of Nutrition and Diet on Oral Health.* 2020;28:99-107.

[50] Deepti A, Jeevarathan J, Muthu M. Effect of fluoride varnish on Streptococcus mutans count in saliva of caries free children using Dentocult SM Strip mutans test: a randomized controlled triple blind study. *International Journal of Clinical Pediatric Dentistry.* 2008;1(1):1.

[51] Klock B, Krasse B. A comparison between different methods for prediction of caries activity. *European Journal of Oral Sciences.* 1979;87(2):129-39.

[52] Ghasemi E, Mazaheri R, Tahmourespour A. Effect of probiotic yogurt and xylitol-containing chewing gums on salivary S mutans count. *Journal of Clinical Pediatric Dentistry.* 2017;41(4):257-63.

[53] Bafna HP, Ajithkrishnan CG, Kalantharakath T, Singh RP, Kalyan P, Vathar JB, Patel HR. Effect of short-term consumption of amul probiotic yogurt containing Lactobacillus acidophilus La5 and Bifidobacterium lactis Bb12 on salivary Streptococcus mutans count in high caries risk individuals. *International Journal of applied and basic medical research.* 2018 Apr;8(2):111.

[54] Teughels W, Kinder Haake S, Sliepen I, Pauwels M, Van Eldere J, Cassiman JJ, Quirynen M. Bacteria interfere with A. actinomycetemcomitans colonization. *Journal of dental research.* 2007 Jul;86(7):611-7.

[55] Morales A, Carvajal P, Silva N, Hernandez M, Godoy C, Rodriguez G, Cabello R, Garcia-Sesnich J, Hoare A, Diaz PI, Gamonal J. Clinical effects of Lactobacillus rhamnosus in non-surgical treatment of chronic periodontitis: a randomized placebo-controlled trial with 1-year follow-up. *Journal of periodontology.* 2016 Aug;87(8):944-52.

[56] Wattanarat O, Makeudom A, Sastraruji T, Piwat S, Tianviwat S, Teanpaisan R, Krisanaprakornkit S. Enhancement of salivary human neutrophil peptide 1–3 levels by probiotic supplementation. *BMC Oral Health.* 2015 Dec;15:1-1.

[57] Jindal G, Pandey R, Agarwal J, Singh M. A comparative evaluation of probiotics on salivary mutans streptococci counts in Indian children. *European Archives of Paediatric Dentistry.* 2011;12:211-5.

[58] Nadelman P, Magno MB, Masterson D, da Cruz AG, Maia LC. Are dairy products containing probiotics beneficial for oral health? A systematic review and meta-analysis. *Clinical oral investigations.* 2018;22:2763-85.

[59] Laleman I, Detailleur V, Slot DE, Slomka V, Quirynen M, Teughels W. Probiotics reduce mutans streptococci counts in humans: a systematic review and meta-analysis. *Clinical oral investigations.* 2014;18:1539-52.

[60] Meurman JH, Stamatova I. Probiotics: contributions to oral health. *Oral diseases.* 2007;13(5):443-51.

[61] Kõll-Klais P, Mändar R, Leibur E, Marcotte H, Hammarström L, Mikelsaar M. Oral lactobacilli in chronic periodontitis and periodontal health: species composition and antimicrobial activity. *Oral microbiology and immunology.* 2005;20(6):354-61.

[62] Strahinic I, Busarcevic M, Pavlica D, Milasin J, Golic N, Topisirovic L. Molecular and biochemical characterizations of human oral lactobacilli as putative probiotic candidates. *Oral microbiology and immunology.* 2007;22(2):111-7.

[63] Ishikawa H, Aiba Y, Nakanishi M, Oh-hashi Y, Koga Y. Suppression of periodontal pathogenic bacteria in the saliva of humans by the administration of Lactobacillus salivarius TI 2711. Nihon Shishubyo Gakkai *Kaishi (Journal of the Japanese Society of Periodontology).* 2003;45(1):105-12.

[64] Sookkhee S, Chulasiri M, Prachyabrued W. Lactic acid bacteria from healthy oral cavity of Thai volunteers: inhibition of oral pathogens. *Journal of applied microbiology.* 2001;90(2):172-9.

[65] Meurman J, Antila H, Korhonen A, Salminen S. Effect of Lactobacillus rhamnosus strain GG (ATCC 53103) on the growth of Streptococcus sobrinus in vitro. *European journal of oral sciences.* 1995;103(4):253-8.

[66] Stamatova I, Meurman JH. Probiotics: health benefits in the mouth. *American Journal of Dentistry.* 2009;22(6):329.

[67] Haukioja A, Yli-Knuuttila H, Loimaranta V, Kari K, Ouwehand AC, Meurman JH, Tenovuo J. Oral adhesion and survival of probiotic and other lactobacilli and bifidobacteria in vitro. *Oral microbiology and immunology.* 2006 Oct;21(5):326-32.

[68] Comelli EM, Guggenheim B, Stingele F, Neeser JR. Selection of dairy bacterial strains as probiotics for oral health. *European journal of oral sciences.* 2002;110(3):218-24.

[69] Sidhu GK, Mantha S, Murthi S, Sura H, Kadaru P, Jangra JK. Evaluation of Lactobacillus and Streptococcus mutans by Addition of Probiotics in the form of Curd in the Diet. *Journal of international oral health: JIOH.* 2015;7(7):85.

[70] Huang X, Schulte RM, Burne RA, Nascimento MM. Characterization of the arginolytic microflora provides insights into pH homeostasis in human oral biofilms. *Caries research.* 2015;49(2):165-76.

[71] Shimada A, Noda M, Matoba Y, Kumagai T, Kozai K, Sugiyama M. Oral lactic acid bacteria related to the occurrence and/or progression of dental caries in Japanese preschool children. *Bioscience of microbiota, food and health.* 2015;34(2):29-36.

[72] Caufield P, Schön C, Saraithong P, Li Y, Argimón S. Oral lactobacilli and dental caries: a model for niche adaptation in humans. *Journal of dental research.* 2015;94(9_suppl):110S-8S.

[73] Karpiński TM, Szkaradkiewicz AK. Microbiology of dental caries. *J Biol Earth Sci.* 2013;3(1):M21-4.

[74] Mortazavi S, Akhlaghi N. Salivary Streptococcus mutans and Lactobacilli levels following probiotic cheese consumption in adults: A double blind randomized clinical trial. *Journal of research in medical sciences: the official journal of Isfahan University of Medical Sciences.* 2012;17(1):57.

[75] Cogulu D, Topaloglu-Ak A, Caglar E, Sandalli N, Karagozlu C, Ersin N, Yerlikaya O. Potential effects of a multistrain probiotic-kefir on salivary Streptococcus mutans and Lactobacillus spp. *Journal of Dental Sciences.* 2010 Sep 1;5(3):144-9.

[76] Keller MK, Twetman S. Acid production in dental plaque after exposure to probiotic bacteria. *BMC oral health.* 2012;12(1):1-6.

[77] Aminabadi N, Erfanparast L, Ebrahimi A, Oskouei S. Effect of chlorhexidine pretreatment on the stability of salivary lactobacilli probiotic in six-to twelve-year-old children: a randomized controlled trial. *Caries research.* 2011;45(2):148-54.

[78] Reddy RS, Swapna L, Ramesh T, Singh TR, Vijayalaxmi N, Lavanya R. Bacteria in oral health-probiotics and prebiotics a review. *Int J Biol Med Res.* 2011;2(4):1226-33.

[79] Nozari A, Motamedifar M, Seifi N, Hatamizargaran Z, Ranjbar MA. The effect of Iranian customary used probiotic yogurt on the children's salivary cariogenic microflora. *Journal of Dentistry.* 2015;16(2):81.

[80] Pinto G, Cenci M, Azevedo M, Epifanio M, Jones M. Effect of yogurt containing bifidobacteriumanimalis subsp. lactis DN-173010 probiotic on dental plaque and saliva in orthodontic patients. *Caries research.* 2014;48(1):63-8.

[81] Srivastava S, Saha S, Kumari M, Mohd S. Effect of probiotic curd on salivary pH and Streptococcus mutans: a double blind parallel randomized controlled trial. *Journal of clinical and diagnostic research: JCDR*. 2016;10(2):ZC13.

[82] Zare Javid A, Amerian E, Basir L, Ekrami A, Haghighizadeh MH, Maghsoumi-Norouzabad L. Effects of the consumption of probiotic yogurt containing bifidobacterium lactis Bb12 on the levels of streptococcus mutans and lactobacilli in saliva of students with initial stages of dental caries: A double-blind randomized controlled trial. *Caries research*. 2020;54(1):68-74.

[83] Nagarajappa R, Daryani H, Sharda AJ, Asawa K, Batra M, Sanadhya S, Ramesh G. Effect of chocobar ice cream containing Bifidobacterium on salivary Streptococcus mutans and Lactobacilli: A randomised controlled trial. *Oral Health Prev Dent*. 2015 Jan 1;13(3):213-8.

[84] Jäsberg H, Söderling E, Endo A, Beighton D, Haukioja A. Bifidobacteria inhibit the growth of Porphyromonas gingivalis but not of Streptococcus mutans in an in vitro biofilm model. *European journal of oral sciences*. 2016;124(3):251-8.

[85] Valdez RM, Dos Santos VR, Caiaffa KS, Danelon M, Arthur RA, de Cássia Negrini T, Delbem AC, Duque C. Comparative in vitro investigation of the cariogenic potential of bifidobacteria. *Archives of Oral Biology*. 2016 Nov 1;71:97-103.

[86] Haukioja A, Söderling E, Tenovuo J. Acid production from sugars and sugar alcohols by probiotic lactobacilli and bifidobacteria in vitro. *Caries research*. 2008;42(6):449-53.

[87] de Matos BM, Brighenti FL, Do T, Beighton D, Koga-Ito CY. Acidogenicity of dual-species biofilms of bifidobacteria and Streptococcus mutans. *Clinical Oral Investigations*. 2017;21:1769-76.

[88] Zhai J-J, Zou J, Lu L-Y. Distribution of Bifidobacterium in oral cavities of children and the relations with caries. *Hua xi kou Qiang yi xue za zhi= Huaxi Kouqiang Yixue Zazhi= West China Journal of Stomatology*. 2009;27(6):618-21.

[89] Eribe ERK, Olsen I. Leptotrichia species in human infections. *Anaerobe*. 2008;14(3):131-7.

[90] Langfeldt D, Neulinger SC, Stiesch M, Stumpp N, Bang C, Schmitz RA, Eberhard J. Health-and disease-associated species clusters in complex natural biofilms determine the innate immune response in oral epithelial cells during biofilm maturation. *FEMS Microbiology Letters*. 2014 Nov 1;360(2):137-43.

[91] Randis TM, Ratner AJ. Gardnerella and Prevotella: Co-conspirators in the Pathogenesis of Bacterial Vaginosis. *The Journal of Infectious Diseases*. 2019;220(7):1085-8.

[92] Lukens JR, Gurung P, Vogel P, Johnson GR, Carter RA, McGoldrick DJ, Bandi SR, Calabrese CR, Walle LV, Lamkanfi M, Kanneganti TD. Dietary modulation of the microbiome affects autoinflammatory disease. *Nature*. 2014 Dec 11;516(7530):246-9.

[93] de Brito BB, da Silva FA, Soares AS, Pereira VA, Santos ML, Sampaio MM, Neves PH, de Melo FF. Pathogenesis and clinical management of Helicobacter pylori gastric infection. *World journal of gastroenterology*. 2019 Oct 10;25(37):5578.

[94] Yee JKC. Are the view of Helicobacter pylori colonized in the oral cavity an illusion? *Experimental & Molecular Medicine*. 2017;49(11):e397-e.

[95] Abbasi A, Bazzaz S, A. Ibrahim S, Hekmatdoost A, Hosseini H, Sabahi S, Sheykhsaran E, Rahbar Saadat Y, Asghari Ozma M, Lahouty M. A Critical Review on the Gluten-Induced Enteropathy/Celiac Disease: Gluten-Targeted Dietary and Non-Dietary Therapeutic Approaches. *Food Reviews International.* 2023 Apr 15:1-41.

[96] Brown LM. Helicobacter Pylori : Epidemiology and Routes of Transmission. *Epidemiologic Reviews.* 2000;22(2):283-97.

[97] Loster BW, Majewski SW, Cześnikiewicz-Guzik M, Bielanski W, Pierzchalski P, Konturek SJ. The relationship between the presence of Helicobacter pylori in the oral cavity and gastric in the stomach. *Journal of physiology and pharmacology : an official journal of the Polish Physiological Society.* 2006;57 Suppl 3:91-100.

[98] Namiot DB, Namiot Z, Kemona A, Bucki R, Gotębiewska M. Oral health status and oral hygiene practices of patients with peptic ulcer and how these affect Helicobacter pylori eradication from the stomach. *Helicobacter.* 2007;12(1):63-7.

[99] Regis W, Reis A, Rocha F, Guedes S, Maia D, Rodrigues L. The Role of Candida Albicans and Streptococcus Mutans Spent Culture Supernatant in Single and Dual-Species Biofilm. *J Sci Tech Res.* 2019;14:1-3.

[100] Falsetta ML, Klein MI, Colonne PM, Scott-Anne K, Gregoire S, Pai CH, Gonzalez-Begne M, Watson G, Krysan DJ, Bowen WH, Koo H. Symbiotic relationship between Streptococcus mutans and Candida albicans synergizes virulence of plaque biofilms in vivo. *Infection and immunity.* 2014 May;82(5):1968-81.

[101] Dashper SG, Mitchell HL, Lê Cao KA, Carpenter L, Gussy MG, Calache H, Gladman SL, Bulach DM, Hoffmann B, Catmull DV, Pruilh S. Temporal development of the oral microbiome and prediction of early childhood caries. *Scientific reports.* 2019 Dec 24;9(1):19732.

[102] Baker JL, He X, Shi W. Precision Reengineering of the Oral Microbiome for Caries Management. *Advances in Dental Research.* 2019;30(2):34-9.

[103] Krzyściak W, Kościelniak D, Papież M, Vyhouskaya P, Zagórska-Świeży K, Kołodziej I, Bystrowska B, Jurczak A. Effect of a Lactobacillus salivarius probiotic on a double-species Streptococcus mutans and Candida albicans caries biofilm. *Nutrients.* 2017 Nov 14;9(11):1242.

[104] Teodorescu AC, Teslaru S, Solomon SM, Zetu L, Luchian I, Sioustis IA, Martu MA, Vasiliu B, Martu S. Assessment of Bacterial Associations Involved in Periodontal Disease Using Crevicular Fluid. *Rev. Chim.* 2019 Jun 1;70:2145-9.

[105] Olsen I, Lambris JD, Hajishengallis G. Porphyromonas gingivalis disturbs host-commensal homeostasis by changing complement function. *J Oral Microbiol.* 2017;9(1):1340085.

[106] Irshad M, van der Reijden WA, Crielaard W, Laine ML. In vitro invasion and survival of Porphyromonas gingivalis in gingival fibroblasts; role of the capsule. *Archivum immunologiae et therapiae experimentalis.* 2012;60(6):469-76.

[107] How KY, Song KP, Chan KG. Porphyromonas gingivalis: An Overview of Periodontopathic Pathogen below the Gum Line. *Frontiers in Microbiology.* 2016;7.

[108] Amano A. Bacterial adhesins to host components in periodontitis. *Periodontology 2000.* 2010;52:12-37.

[109] Xiao L, Zhang Q, Peng Y, Wang D, Liu Y. The effect of periodontal bacteria infection on incidence and prognosis of cancer: A systematic review and meta-analysis. *Medicine.* 2020;99(15):e19698.

[110] Olsen I, Yilmaz Ö. Possible role of Porphyromonas gingivalis in orodigestive cancers. *J Oral Microbiol.* 2019; 11(1): 1563410.

[111] Surdu AE, Popa C, Luchian I. Identification of bacteria involved in periodontal disease using molecular biology techniques. *Rev Chim.* 2017;68:2407-12.

[112] Loozen G, Ozcelik O, Boon N, De Mol A, Schoen C, Quirynen M, Teughels W. Inter-bacterial correlations in subgingival biofilms: a large-scale survey. *Journal of clinical periodontology.* 2014 Jan;41(1):1-0.

[113] Cao P, Chen Y, Guo X, Chen Y, Su W, Zhan N, Dong W. Fusobacterium nucleatum activates endoplasmic reticulum stress to promote Crohn's disease development via the upregulation of CARD3 expression. *Frontiers in pharmacology.* 2020 Feb 21;11:106.

[114] Hattori T, Yuasa N, Ikegami S, Nishiyama H, Takeuchi E, Miyake H, Kuno R, Miyata K, Fujino M, Minami M. Culture-based bacterial evaluation of the appendix lumen in patients with and without acute appendicitis. *Journal of Infection and Chemotherapy.* 2019 Sep 1;25(9):708-13.

[115] Han YW, Wang X. Mobile Microbiome:Oral Bacteria in Extra-oral Infections and Inflammation. *Journal of Dental Research.* 2013;92(6):485-91.

[116] Han YW. Fusobacterium nucleatum: a commensal-turned pathogen. *Current Opinion in Microbiology.* 2015;23:141-7.

[117] Amer A, Galvin S, Healy CM, Moran GP. The microbiome of potentially malignant oral leukoplakia exhibits enrichment for Fusobacterium, Leptotrichia, Campylobacter, and Rothia species. *Frontiers in microbiology.* 2017;8:2391.

[118] Brennan CA, Garrett WS. Fusobacterium nucleatum — symbiont, opportunist and oncobacterium. *Nature Reviews Microbiology.* 2019;17(3):156-66.

[119] Coppenhagen-Glazer S, Sol A, Abed J, Naor R, Zhang X, Han YW, Bachrach G. Fap2 of Fusobacterium nucleatum is a galactose-inhibitable adhesin involved in coaggregation, cell adhesion, and preterm birth. *Infection and immunity.* 2015 Mar;83(3):1104-13.

[120] Park SR, Kim DJ, Han SH, Kang MJ, Lee JY, Jeong YJ, Lee SJ, Kim TH, Ahn SG, Yoon JH, Park JH. Diverse Toll-like receptors mediate cytokine production by Fusobacterium nucleatum and Aggregatibacter actinomycetemcomitans in macrophages. *Infection and immunity.* 2014 May;82(5):1914-20.

[121] Chaushu S, Wilensky A, Gur C, Shapira L, Elboim M, Halftek G, Polak D, Achdout H, Bachrach G, Mandelboim O. Direct recognition of Fusobacterium nucleatum by the NK cell natural cytotoxicity receptor NKp46 aggravates periodontal disease. *PLoS pathogens.* 2012 Mar 22;8(3):e1002601.

[122] Feng X, Zhang L, Xu L, Meng H, Lu R, Chen Z, Shi D, Wang X. Detection of eight periodontal microorganisms and distribution of Porphyromonas gingivalis fimA genotypes in Chinese patients with aggressive periodontitis. *Journal of periodontology.* 2014 Jan;85(1):150-9.

[123] Li Q, Tan L, Wang H, Kou Y, Shi X, Zhang S, Pan Y. Fusobacterium nucleatum interaction with Pseudomonas aeruginosa induces biofilm-associated antibiotic

tolerance via Fusobacterium adhesin A. *ACS Infectious Diseases.* 2020 Apr 22;6(7):1686-96.

[124] Yu T, Guo F, Yu Y, Sun T, Ma D, Han J, Qian Y, Kryczek I, Sun D, Nagarsheth N, Chen Y. Fusobacterium nucleatum promotes chemoresistance to colorectal cancer by modulating autophagy. *Cell.* 2017 Jul 27;170(3):548-63.

[125] Gallimidi AB, Fischman S, Revach B, Bulvik R, Maliutina A, Rubinstein AM, Nussbaum G, Elkin M. Periodontal pathogens Porphyromonas gingivalis and Fusobacterium nucleatum promote tumor progression in an oral-specific chemical carcinogenesis model. *Oncotarget.* 2015 Sep 9;6(26):22613.

[126] Abbasi A, Sabahi S, Bazzaz S, Tajani AG, Lahouty M, Aslani R, Hosseini H. An edible coating utilizing Malva sylvestris seed polysaccharide mucilage and postbiotic from Saccharomyces cerevisiae var. boulardii for the preservation of lamb meat. *International Journal of Biological Macromolecules.* 2023 Aug 15;246:125660.

[127] Abbasi A, Sanej KD, Moradi S, Bazzaz S, Esmaeili A, Ghafourian K, Sabahi S, Lahouty M, Akrami S, Aslani R, Hosseini H. Bioactive Compounds and Biological Activities of Allium sativum L. In *Bioactive Compounds in the Storage Organs of Plants* 2023 Jul 15 (pp. 1-40). Cham: Springer Nature Switzerland.

[128] Salminen S, Collado MC, Endo A, Hill C, Lebeer S, Quigley EM, Sanders ME, Shamir R, Swann JR, Szajewska H, Vinderola G. The International Scientific Association of Probiotics and Prebiotics (ISAPP) consensus statement on the definition and scope of postbiotics. *Nature Reviews Gastroenterology & Hepatology.* 2021 Sep;18(9):649-67.

[129] Abbasi A, Bazzaz S, Da Cruz AG, Khorshidian N, Saadat YR, Sabahi S, Ozma MA, Lahouty M, Aslani R, Mortazavian AM. A Critical Review on Akkermansia muciniphila: Functional Mechanisms, Technological Challenges, and Safety Issues. *Probiotics and Antimicrobial Proteins.* 2023 Jul 11:1-23.

[130] Carmen CM, Seppo S, Vinderola G. Postbiotics: defining the impact of inactivated microbes and their metabolites on promotion of health. *The Human Microbiome in Early Life:* Elsevier; 2021. p. 257-68.

[131] Hosseini H, Abbasi A, Sabahi S, Akrami S, Yousefi-Avarvand A. Assessing the Potential Biological Activities of Postbiotics Derived from Saccharomyces cerevisiae: An In Vitro Study. *Probiotics and Antimicrobial Proteins.* 2023:1-17.

[132] Nataraj BH, Ali SA, Behare PV, Yadav H. Postbiotics-parabiotics: the new horizons in microbial biotherapy and functional foods. *Microbial Cell Factories.* 2020;19(1):168.

[133] Rooks MG, Garrett WS. Gut microbiota, metabolites and host immunity. *Nature Reviews Immunology.* 2016;16(6):341-52.

[134] Breyner NM, Michon C, de Sousa CS, Vilas Boas PB, Chain F, Azevedo VA, Langella P, Chatel JM. Microbial anti-inflammatory molecule (MAM) from Faecalibacterium prausnitzii shows a protective effect on DNBS and DSS-induced colitis model in mice through inhibition of NF-κB pathway. *Frontiers in microbiology.* 2017 Feb 1;8:114.

[135] He X, Zhao S, Li Y. Faecalibacterium prausnitzii: A next-generation probiotic in gut disease improvement. *Canadian Journal of Infectious Diseases and Medical Microbiology.* 2021;2021:1-10.

[136] Wieërs G, Belkhir L, Enaud R, Leclercq S, Philippart de Foy JM, Dequenne I, de Timary P, Cani PD. How probiotics affect the microbiota. *Frontiers in cellular and infection microbiology.* 2020 Jan 15;9:454.

[137] Eisenstein M. The hunt for a healthy microbiome. *Nature.* 2020;577(7792):S6-S.

[138] Tian L, Wang XW, Wu AK, Fan Y, Friedman J, Dahlin A, Waldor MK, Weinstock GM, Weiss ST, Liu YY. Deciphering functional redundancy in the human microbiome. *Nature communications.* 2020 Dec 4;11(1):6217.

[139] de Almada CN, Almada CN, Martinez RCR, Sant'Ana AS. Paraprobiotics: Evidences on their ability to modify biological responses, inactivation methods and perspectives on their application in foods. *Trends in Food Science & Technology.* 2016;58:96-114.

[140] Baird B, Lucia L, Acuff G, Harris K, Savell J. Beef hide antimicrobial interventions as a means of reducing bacterial contamination. *Meat science.* 2006;73(2):245-8.

[141] Šušković J, Kos B, Beganović J, Leboš Pavunc A, Habjanič K, Matošić S. Antimicrobial activity–the most important property of probiotic and starter lactic acid bacteria. *Food Technology and Biotechnology.* 2010;48(3):296-307.

[142] Yoon BK, Jackman JA, Valle-González ER, Cho N-J. Antibacterial free fatty acids and monoglycerides: biological activities, experimental testing, and therapeutic applications. *International journal of molecular sciences.* 2018;19(4):1114.

[143] Abbasi A, Rad AH, Maleki LA, Kafil HS, Baghbanzadeh A. Antigenotoxicity and Cytotoxic Potentials of Cell-Free Supernatants Derived from Saccharomyces cerevisiae var. boulardii on HT-29 Human Colon Cancer Cell Lines. *Probiotics and Antimicrobial Proteins.* 2023:1-13.

[144] Osborn H, Akoh C. Structured lipids-novel fats with medical, nutraceutical, and food applications. *Comprehensive reviews in food science and food safety.* 2002;1(3):110-20.

[145] Twetman L, Larsen U, Fiehn N-E, Stecksén-Blicks C, Twetman S. Coaggregation between probiotic bacteria and caries-associated strains: an in vitro study. *Acta Odontologica Scandinavica.* 2009;67(5):284-8.

[146] Abbasi A, Saadat TR, Saadat YR. Microbial exopolysaccharides–β-glucans–as promising postbiotic candidates in vaccine adjuvants. *International Journal of Biological Macromolecules.* 2022.

[147] Talarico T, Casas I, Chung TC, Dobrogosz W. Production and isolation of reuterin, a growth inhibitor produced by Lactobacillus reuteri. *Antimicrobial agents and chemotherapy.* 1988;32(12):1854-8.

[148] Ganzle MG, Höltzel A, Walter J, Jung Gn, Hammes WP. Characterization of reutericyclin produced by Lactobacillus reuteri LTH2584. *Applied and environmental microbiology.* 2000;66(10):4325-33.

[149] El-Ziney M, Debevere J. The Effect of Reuterin on Listeria monocytogenes and Escherichia coliO157: H7 in Milk and Cottage Cheese. *Journal of Food Protection.* 1998;61(10):1275-80.

[150] López-López A, Camelo-Castillo A, Ferrer MD, Simon-Soro Á, Mira A. Health-associated niche inhabitants as oral probiotics: the case of Streptococcus dentisani. *Frontiers in microbiology*. 2017;8:379.

[151] Di Pierro F, Zanvit A, Nobili P, Risso P, Fornaini C. Cariogram outcome after 90 days of oral treatment with Streptococcus salivarius M18 in children at high risk for dental caries: results of a randomized, controlled study. *Clinical, cosmetic and investigational dentistry*. 2015:107-13.

[152] Abbasi A, Aghebati-Maleki L, Homayouni-Rad A. The promising biological role of postbiotics derived from probiotic Lactobacillus species in reproductive health. *Critical Reviews in Food Science and Nutrition*. 2022;62(32):8829-41.

[153] Trüper HG, De'Clari L. Taxonomic note: necessary correction of specific epithets formed as substantives (nouns) "in apposition." *International Journal of Systematic Bacteriology*. 1997;47(3):908-9.

[154] Nørskov-Lauritsen N, Kilian M. Reclassification of Actinobacillus actinomycetemcomitans, Haemophilus aphrophilus, Haemophilus paraphrophilus and Haemophilus segnis as Aggregatibacter actinomycetemcomitans gen. nov., comb. nov., Aggregatibacter aphrophilus comb. nov. and Aggregatibacter segnis comb. nov., and emended description of Aggregatibacter aphrophilus to include V factor-dependent and V factor-independent isolates. *International journal of systematic and evolutionary microbiology*. 2006;56(9):2135-46.

[155] Hillman J, Socransky S, Shivers M. The relationships between streptococcal species and periodontopathic bacteria in human dental plaque. *Archives of Oral Biology*. 1985;30(11-12):791-5.

[156] Hillman J, Shivers M. Interaction between wild-type, mutant and revertant forms of the bacterium Streptococcus sanguis and the bacterium Actinobacillus actinomycetemcomitans in vitro and in the gnotobiotic rat. *Archives of oral biology*. 1988;33(6):395-401.

[157] Kidd E, Fejerskov O. What constitutes dental caries? Histopathology of carious enamel and dentin related to the action of cariogenic biofilms. *Journal of dental research*. 2004;83(1_suppl):35-8.

[158] Conrads G, de Soet JJ, Song L, Henne K, Sztajer H, Wagner-Döbler I, Zeng AP. Comparing the cariogenic species Streptococcus sobrinus and S. mutans on whole genome level. *Journal of oral microbiology*. 2014 Jan 1;6(1):26189.

[159] Shakovetz N, Borutta A, Kneist S. Probiotica in caries prevention for preschool children. *Oralprophylaxe und Kinderzahnheilkunde*. 2013;35(3):120-6.

[160] Sabahi S, Abbasi A, Mortazavi SA. Characterization of cinnamon essential oil and its application in Malva sylvestris seed mucilage edible coating to the enhancement of the microbiological, physicochemical and sensory properties of lamb meat during storage. *Journal of Applied Microbiology*. 2022;133(2):488-502.

[161] Abbasi A, Rad AH, Ghasempour Z, Sabahi S, Kafil HS, Hasannezhad P, Rahbar Saadat Y, Shahbazi N. The biological activities of postbiotics in gastrointestinal disorders. *Critical Reviews in Food Science and Nutrition*. 2022 Jul 23;62(22):5983-6004.

[162] Hillman J, Brooks T, Michalek S, Harmon C, Snoep J, van Der Weijden C. Construction and characterization of an effector strain of Streptococcus mutans for replacement therapy of dental caries. *Infection and immunity.* 2000;68(2):543-9.
[163] Garcia-Varela R, Garcia H, Mata-Haro V, Vallejo-Cordoba B. Postbiotics: An evolving term within the functional foods field. *Trends in food science & technology.* 2018.
[164] Patel RM, Denning PW. Therapeutic use of prebiotics, probiotics, and postbiotics to prevent necrotizing enterocolitis: what is the current evidence? *Clinics in perinatology.* 2013;40(1):11-25.
[165] Dinić M, Lukić J, Djokić J, Milenković M, Strahinić I, Golić N, Begović J. Lactobacillus fermentum postbiotic-induced autophagy as potential approach for treatment of acetaminophen hepatotoxicity. *Frontiers in microbiology.* 2017 Apr 6;8:594.
[166] Abbasi A, Hajipour N, Hasannezhad P, Baghbanzadeh A, Aghebati-Maleki L. Potential in vivo delivery routes of postbiotics. *Critical Reviews in Food Science and Nutrition.* 2022;62(12):3345-69.
[167] Jung JI, Baek SM, Nguyen TH, Kim JW, Kang CH, Kim S, Imm JY. Effects of probiotic culture supernatant on cariogenic biofilm formation and RANKL-induced osteoclastogenesis in RAW 264.7 macrophages. *Molecules.* 2021 Jan 31;26(3):733.
[168] OmerOglou E, Karaca B, Kibar H, Haliscelik O, Kiran F. The role of microbiota-derived postbiotic mediators on biofilm formation and quorum sensing-mediated virulence of Streptococcus mutans: A perspective on preventing dental caries. *Microbial Pathogenesis.* 2022;164:105390.
[169] Dubar M, Decock A-C, Petit J, Delcourt-Debruyne E, Blaizot A, Agossa K. How effective are essential oils and essential oil constituents in the management of intra-oral halitosis: A systematic review. *Journal of Herbal Medicine.* 2023;39:100663.
[170] Sabahi S, Homayouni Rad A, Aghebati-Maleki L, Sangtarash N, Ozma MA, Karimi A, Hosseini H, Abbasi A. Postbiotics as the new frontier in food and pharmaceutical research. *Critical Reviews in Food Science and Nutrition.* 2022 Mar 22:1-28.
[171] Akaji EA, Folaranmi N, Ashiwaju O. Halitosis: a review of the literature on its prevalence, impact and control. *Oral Health Prev Dent.* 2014;12(4):297-304.
[172] Cabanillas-Lazo M, Pascual-Guevara M, Hilario-Gomez MM, Salazar-Alarcón JL, León-Figueroa DA, Caballero-Alvarado JA, Barboza JJ. Effects of probiotic, prebiotic or synbiotic supplementation after Roux-en-Y gastric bypass: a systematic review with meta-analysis.
[173] Ozma MA, Abbasi A, Sabahi S. Characterization of postbiotics derived from Lactobacillus paracasei ATCC 55544 and its application in Malva sylvestris seed mucilage edible coating to the improvement of the microbiological, and sensory properties of lamb meat during storage. *Biointerface Res Appl Chem.* 2022;13.
[174] Kazor CE, Mitchell PM, Lee AM, Stokes LN, Loesche WJ, Dewhirst FE, Paster BJ. Diversity of bacterial populations on the tongue dorsa of patients with halitosis and healthy patients. *Journal of clinical microbiology.* 2003 Feb;41(2):558-63.

[175] Burton JP, Chilcott CN, Tagg JR. The rationale and potential for the reduction of oral malodour using Streptococcus salivarius probiotics. *Oral Dis.* 2005;11 Suppl 1:29-31.

[176] Allaker RP, Waite RD, Hickling J, North M, McNab R, Bosma MP. Topographic distribution of bacteria associated with oral malodour on the tongue. *Archives of oral biology.* 2008 Apr 1;53:S8-12.

[177] Eren AM, Borisy GG, Huse SM, Mark Welch JL. Oligotyping analysis of the human oral microbiome. *Proceedings of the National Academy of Sciences.* 2014;111(28):E2875-E84.

[178] Kang MS, Kim BG, Chung J, Lee HC, Oh JS. Inhibitory effect of Weissella cibaria isolates on the production of volatile sulphur compounds. *Journal of clinical periodontology.* 2006;33(3):226-32.

[179] Lima LM, Motisuki C, D Spolidorio MP, Santos-Pinto L. In vitro evaluation of probiotics microorganisms adhesion to an artificial caries model. *European journal of clinical nutrition.* 2005;59(7):884-6.

[180] Sullivan Å, Nord C. Probiotics and gastrointestinal diseases. *Journal of internal Medicine.* 2005;257(1):78-92.

[181] Burton J, Chilcott C, Moore C, Speiser G, Tagg J. A preliminary study of the effect of probiotic Streptococcus salivarius K12 on oral malodour parameters. *Journal of applied microbiology.* 2006;100(4):754-64.

[182] Wescombe PA, Heng NC, Burton JP, Tagg JR. Something old and something new: an update on the amazing repertoire of bacteriocins produced by Streptococcus salivarius. *Probiotics and antimicrobial proteins.* 2010;2:37-45.

[183] Masdea L, Kulik EM, Hauser-Gerspach I, Ramseier AM, Filippi A, Waltimo T. Antimicrobial activity of Streptococcus salivarius K12 on bacteria involved in oral malodour. *Archives of Oral Biology.* 2012;57(8):1041-7.

[184] Iwamoto T, Suzuki N, Tanabe K, Takeshita T, Hirofuji T. Effects of probiotic Lactobacillus salivarius WB21 on halitosis and oral health: an open-label pilot trial. *Oral Surgery, Oral Medicine, Oral Pathology, Oral Radiology, and Endodontology.* 2010;110(2):201-8.

[185] Keller MK, Bardow A, Jensdottir T, Lykkeaa J, Twetman S. Effect of chewing gums containing the probiotic bacterium Lactobacillus reuteri on oral malodour. *Acta Odontologica Scandinavica.* 2012;70(3):246-50.

[186] Marchetti E, Tecco S, Santonico M, Vernile C, Ciciarelli D, Tarantino E, Marzo G, Pennazza G. Multi-sensor approach for the monitoring of halitosis treatment via Lactobacillus brevis (CD2)—containing lozenges—a randomized, double-blind placebo-controlled clinical trial. *Sensors.* 2015 Aug 10;15(8):19583-96.

[187] Sutula J, Coulthwaite LA, Thomas LV, Verran J. The effect of a commercial probiotic drink containing Lactobacillus casei strain Shirota on oral health in healthy dentate people. *Microbial ecology in health and disease.* 2013;24(1):21003.

[188] Lee S-H, Baek D-H. Effects of Streptococcus thermophilus on volatile sulfur compounds produced by Porphyromonas gingivalis. *Archives of Oral Biology.* 2014;59(11):1205-10.

[189] Suzuki N, Higuchi T, Nakajima M, Fujimoto A, Morita H, Yoneda M, Hanioka T, Hirofuji T. Inhibitory effect of Enterococcus faecium WB2000 on volatile sulfur compound production by Porphyromonas gingivalis. *International Journal of Dentistry.* 2016 Oct 9;2016.

[190] Wuri G, Liu F, Sun Z, Fang B, Zhao W, Hung WL, Liu WH, Zhang X, Wang R, Wu F, Zhao L. Lactobacillus paracasei ET-22 and derived postbiotics reduce halitosis and modulate oral microbiome dysregulation–a randomized, double-blind placebo-controlled clinical trial. *Food & Function.* 2023;14(16):7335-46.

[191] Ozma MA, Abbasi A, Akrami S, Lahouty M, Shahbazi N, Ganbarov K, Pagliano P, Sabahi S, Köse Ş, Yousefi M, Dao S. Postbiotics as the key mediators of the gut microbiota-host interactions. Le infezioni in medicina. 2022;30(2):180.

[192] Haque M, Sartelli M, Haque SZ. Dental infection and resistance—global health consequences. *Dentistry journal.* 2019;7(1):22.

[193] Lin X, Xu J, Shi Z, Xu Y, Fu T, Zhang L, He F. Evaluation of the antibacterial effects and mechanism of Plantaricin 149 from Lactobacillus plantarum NRIC 149 on the peri-implantitis pathogens. *Scientific Reports.* 2021 Oct 25;11(1):21022.

[194] Homayouni-rad A, Aghebati-Maleki L, Samadi-Kafil H, Abbasi A, Khani N. Postbiotics as a safe alternative to live probiotic bacteria in the food and pharmaceutical industries. *HBI_Journals.* 2021;26:132-57.

[195] Butrungrod W, Chaiyasut C, Makhamrueang N, Peerajan S, Chaiyana W, Sirilun S. Postbiotic Metabolite of Lactiplantibacillus plantarum PD18 against Periodontal Pathogens and Their Virulence Markers in Biofilm Formation. *Pharmaceutics.* 2023;15(5):1419.

[196] Park E, Ha J, Lim S, Kim G, Yoon Y. Development of postbiotics by whey bioconversion with Enterococcus faecalis M157 KACC81148BP and Lactococcus lactis CAU2013 KACC81152BP for treating periodontal disease and improving gut health. *Journal of Dairy Science.* 2021;104(12):12321-31.

[197] Varoni E, Tarce M, Lodi G, Carrassi A. Chlorhexidine (CHX) in dentistry: state of the art. *Minerva Stomatol.* 2012;61(9):399-419.

[198] Ishikawa KH, Bueno MR, Kawamoto D, Simionato MR, Mayer MP. Lactobacilli postbiotics reduce biofilm formation and alter transcription of virulence genes of Aggregatibacter actinomycetemcomitans. *Molecular Oral Microbiology.* 2021;36(1):92-102.

[199] Butera A, Pascadopoli M, Gallo S, Lelli M, Tarterini F, Giglia F, Scribante A. SEM/EDS evaluation of the mineral deposition on a polymeric composite resin of a toothpaste containing biomimetic Zn-carbonate hydroxyapatite (microRepair®) in oral environment: a randomized clinical trial. *Polymers.* 2021 Aug 16;13(16):2740.

[200] Rad AH, Aghebati-Maleki L, Kafil HS, Abbasi A. Molecular mechanisms of postbiotics in colorectal cancer prevention and treatment. *Critical reviews in food science and nutrition.* 2021;61(11):1787-803.

[201] Abbasi A, Sheykhsaran E, Kafil HS. *Postbiotics: science, technology and applications:* Bentham Science Publishers; 2021.

[202] Homayouni Rad A, Aghebati Maleki L, Samadi Kafil H, Abbasi A. Postbiotics: A novel strategy in food allergy treatment. *Critical reviews in food science and nutrition.* 2021;61(3):492-9.

[203] Alesaeidi S, Kahrizi MS, Ghorbani Tajani A, Hajipour H, Ghorbani M. Soy protein isolate/sodium alginate hybrid hydrogel embedded with hydroxyapatite for tissue engineering. *Journal of Polymers and the Environment.* 2023;31(1):396-405.

[204] Butera A, Gallo S, Pascadopoli M, Taccardi D, Scribante A. Home oral care of periodontal patients using antimicrobial gel with postbiotics, lactoferrin, and aloe barbadensis leaf juice powder vs. conventional chlorhexidine gel: A split-mouth randomized clinical trial. *Antibiotics.* 2022;11(1):118.

[205] Abbasi A, Aghebati-Maleki A, Yousefi M, Aghebati-Maleki L. Probiotic intervention as a potential therapeutic for managing gestational disorders and improving pregnancy outcomes. *Journal of reproductive immunology.* 2021;143:103244.

[206] Bray F, Ferlay J, Soerjomataram I, Siegel RL, Torre LA, Jemal A. Global cancer statistics 2018: GLOBOCAN estimates of incidence and mortality worldwide for 36 cancers in 185 countries. *CA: a cancer journal for clinicians.* 2018;68(6):394-424.

[207] Rad AH, Abbasi A, Kafil HS, Ganbarov K. Potential pharmaceutical and food applications of postbiotics: a review. *Current pharmaceutical biotechnology.* 2020;21(15):1576-87.

[208] Peres MA, Macpherson LM, Weyant RJ, Daly B, Venturelli R, Mathur MR, Listl S, Celeste RK, Guarnizo-Herreño CC, Kearns C, Benzian H. Oral diseases: a global public health challenge. *The Lancet.* 2019 Jul 20;394(10194):249-60.

[209] Kleinstein S, Nelson K, Freire M. Inflammatory networks linking oral microbiome with systemic health and disease. *Journal of Dental Research.* 2020;99(10):1131-9.

[210] Devine DA, Marsh PD. Prospects for the development of probiotics and prebiotics for oral applications. *Journal of Oral Microbiology.* 2009;1(1):1949.

[211] DeGruttola AK, Low D, Mizoguchi A, Mizoguchi E. Current understanding of dysbiosis in disease in human and animal models. *Inflammatory bowel diseases.* 2016;22(5):1137-50.

[212] Koliarakis I, Messaritakis I, Nikolouzakis TK, Hamilos G, Souglakos J, Tsiaoussis J. Oral Bacteria and Intestinal Dysbiosis in Colorectal Cancer. *International Journal of Molecular Sciences*. 2019;20(17):4146.

[213] Sheflin AM, Whitney AK, Weir TL. Cancer-Promoting Effects of Microbial Dysbiosis. *Current Oncology Reports*. 2014;16(10):406.

[214] Shin SH, Lee YS, Shin YP, Kim B, Kim MH, Chang HR, Jang WS, Lee IH. Therapeutic efficacy of halocidin-derived peptide HG1 in a mouse model of Candida albicans oral infection. *Journal of Antimicrobial Chemotherapy.* 2013 May 1;68(5):1152-60.

[215] Hanahan D, Weinberg RA. Hallmarks of cancer: the next generation. *Cell.* 2011;144(5):646-74.

[216] Elebyary O, Barbour A, Fine N, Tenenbaum HC, Glogauer M. The crossroads of periodontitis and oral squamous cell carcinoma: immune implications and tumor promoting capacities. *Frontiers in Oral Health.* 2021;1:584705.
[217] Krüger M, Hansen T, Kasaj A, Moergel M. The correlation between chronic periodontitis and oral cancer. *Case reports in dentistry.* 2013;2013.
[218] La Rosa GRM, Gattuso G, PEduLLà E, Rapisarda E, Nicolosi D, Salmeri M. Association of oral dysbiosis with oral cancer development. *Oncology letters.* 2020;19(4):3045-58.
[219] Vyhnalova T, Danek Z, Gachova D, Linhartova PB. The Role of the Oral Microbiota in the Etiopathogenesis of Oral Squamous Cell Carcinoma. *Microorganisms.* 2021;9(8):1549.
[220] Hanahan D. Hallmarks of cancer: new dimensions. *Cancer discovery.* 2022;12(1):31-46.
[221] Salvi PS, Cowles RA. Butyrate and the intestinal epithelium: modulation of proliferation and inflammation in homeostasis and disease. *Cells.* 2021;10(7):1775.
[222] Fayol-Messaoudi D, Berger CN, Coconnier-Polter M-H, Lievin-Le Moal V, Servin AL. pH-, Lactic acid-, and non-lactic acid-dependent activities of probiotic Lactobacilli against Salmonella enterica Serovar Typhimurium. *Applied and environmental microbiology.* 2005;71(10):6008-13.
[223] Jones SE, Versalovic J. Probiotic Lactobacillus reuteribiofilms produce antimicrobial and anti-inflammatory factors. *BMC microbiology.* 2009;9(1):1-9.
[224] Kojima Y, Ohshima T, Seneviratne CJ, Maeda N. Combining prebiotics and probiotics to develop novel synbiotics that suppress oral pathogens. *Journal of Oral Biosciences.* 2016;58(1):27-32.
[225] Khan T, Date A, Chawda H, Patel K. Polysaccharides as potential anticancer agents—A review of their progress. *Carbohydrate polymers.* 2019;210:412-28.
[226] Wegh CA, Geerlings SY, Knol J, Roeselers G, Belzer C. Postbiotics and their potential applications in early life nutrition and beyond. *International journal of molecular sciences.* 2019;20(19):4673.
[227] Lee JW, Shin JG, Kim EH, Kang HE, Yim IB, Kim JY, Joo HG, Woo HJ. Immunomodulatory and antitumor effects in vivo by the cytoplasmic fraction of Lactobacillus casei and Bifidobacterium longum. *Journal of veterinary science.* 2004 Mar 1;5(1):41-8.
[228] Cousin FJ, Jouan-Lanhouet S, Dimanche-Boitrel M-T, Corcos L, Jan G. Milk fermented by Propionibacterium freudenreichii induces apoptosis of HGT-1 human gastric cancer cells. *PloS one.* 2012;7(3):e31892.
[229] Dillekås H, Rogers MS, Straume O. Are 90% of deaths from cancer caused by metastases? *Cancer medicine.* 2019;8(12):5574-6.
[230] Seyfried TN, Huysentruyt LC. On the origin of cancer metastasis. *Critical Reviews™ in Oncogenesis.* 2013;18(1-2).
[231] Ribatti D, Tamma R, Annese T. Epithelial-mesenchymal transition in cancer: a historical overview. *Translational oncology.* 2020;13(6):100773.
[232] Bukhari SZ, Zeth K, Iftikhar M, Rehman M, Munir MU, Khan WS, Ihsan A. Supramolecular lipid nanoparticles as delivery carriers for non-invasive cancer

theranostics. *Current Research in Pharmacology and Drug Discovery.* 2021 Jan 1;2:100067.
[233] Steeg PS. Targeting metastasis. *Nature reviews cancer.* 2016;16(4):201-18.
[234] Li X, Wang H, Du X, Yu W, Jiang J, Geng Y, Guo X, Fan X, Ma C. Lactobacilli inhibit cervical cancer cell migration in vitro and reduce tumor burden in vivo through upregulation of E-cadherin. *Oncology Reports.* 2017 Sep 1;38(3):1561-8.
[235] Chen SM, Hsu LJ, Lee HL, Lin CP, Huang SW, Lai CJ, Lin CW, Chen WT, Chen YJ, Lin YC, Yang CC. Lactobacillus attenuate the progression of pancreatic cancer promoted by Porphyromonas gingivalis in K-rasG12D transgenic mice. *Cancers.* 2020 Nov 26;12(12):3522.
[236] Escamilla J, Lane MA, Maitin V. Cell-free supernatants from probiotic Lactobacillus casei and Lactobacillus rhamnosus GG decrease colon cancer cell invasion in vitro. *Nutrition and cancer.* 2012;64(6):871-8.
[237] Zamberi NR, Abu N, Mohamed NE, Nordin N, Keong YS, Beh BK, Zakaria ZA, Nik Abdul Rahman NM, Alitheen NB. The antimetastatic and antiangiogenesis effects of kefir water on murine breast cancer cells. *Integrative cancer therapies.* 2016 Dec;15(4):NP53-66.
[238] Yue YC, Yang BY, Lu J, Zhang SW, Liu L, Nassar K, Xu XX, Pang XY, Lv JP. Metabolite secretions of Lactobacillus plantarum YYC-3 may inhibit colon cancer cell metastasis by suppressing the VEGF-MMP2/9 signaling pathway. *Microbial cell factories.* 2020 Dec;19:1-2.
[239] Sankarapandian V, Venmathi Maran BA. An Update on the Effectiveness of Probiotics in the Prevention and Treatment of Cancer. 2022;12(1).
[240] Abbasi A, Sanej KD, Mohammadi A, Moradi S, Nayeri BD, Bazzaz S, Hosseini H. The Role of Postbiotics in Food Safety Promotion.

Chapter 3

Honey: A Natural Postbiotic Product

Rustem A. Ilyasov[1,*], PhD
Vener N. Sattarov[2], PhD
Valery N. Danilenko[3], PhD
and Dmitry V. Boguslavsky[1], PhD
[1]Department of Biological Sciences, Koltsov Institute of Developmental Biology, Russian Academy of Sciences, Moscow, Russia
[2]Department of Bioecology and Biological Education, Bashkir State Pedagogical University named after M. Akmulla, Ufa, Russia
[3]Department of Genetics and Biotechnology, Vavilov Institute of General Genetics, Russian Academy of Sciences, Moscow, Russia

Abstract

Since the beginning of time, people have ingested honey, the main product of beekeeping. In general, plant nectar is necessary for the production of honey. The glands in plant flowers create nectar, a tasty liquid fluid. Through enzymatic characteristics, the productive microbiota of honey bees and their own enzyme, invertase, affect nectar and honey conversion. Fermentation turns honey into a postbiotic. Bees stimulate the enzyme glucose oxidase, which changes glucose into gluconic acid and hydrogen peroxide, since honey substitutes nectar. These elements play a big part in how honey tastes and functions biologically. Depending on the process used to change the nectar, acids and other compounds may or may not be present. Because the composition of the converted nectar determines the quantity of acids and other compounds in the honey, certain honeys have stronger antibacterial effects than others. The co-fermentation of nectar and nectar

* Corresponding Author's Email: apismell@hotmail.com.

In: Exploring Microbiotics in Health and Disease
Editor: Edward L. Stillman
ISBN: 978-8-89113-410-2

modification by bee microbiota and stomach enzymes result in the production of honey. In addition to active ingredients, phytohormones, and polyphenols originating from plant nectar, such as phenolic acids, flavonoids, and other phytochemicals, honey also contains a number of compounds created by fermentation in the ventricle. Antioxidants, neuromodulation, and inflammation are all impacted. A number of ailments, such as Alzheimer's disease, Parkinson's disease, Huntington's disease, and multiple sclerosis, have been successfully treated with honey as a complementary and alternative therapy. Products known as postbiotics contain compounds that bacteria release as a result of their metabolic activities. Additionally, they could include dead bacteria that are healthy for the body. As a result, honey should be acknowledged as a natural postbiotic substance that can be used by humans to cure a range of ailments. We investigate the beneficial properties of honey as a natural postbiotic, including microbe metabolites, plant waste products, and bees.

Keywords: honey, honey bee, postbiotic, microbiome, fermentation, phytohormones, antimicrobial activity, anti-inflammatory activity, antioxidant activity, neuromodulatory activity

Introduction

The honey bee (*Apis mellifera*) produces honey from flower nectar, plant secretions, exudates produced by other insects such as aphids, or a combination of these (Rodríguez-Flores et al., 2019; Kafantaris et al., 2021). Sugars, proteins, lipids, vitamins, minerals, polyphenols, plant and bee enzymes, and microbial metabolites are just a few of the over 200 compounds found in honey (Crane, 1980; Schell et al., 2022; Bogdanov et al., 2008; Kafantaris et al., 2021).

The nectar gathered by honey bees to produce honey influences the flavor, color, and therapeutic characteristics of diverse honeys (Irish et al., 2011; Schell et al., 2022). The monosaccharides fructose and glucose account for up to 80% of honey's sugar composition, with the remaining sugars consisting of di-, tri-, oligo-, and polysaccharides. Honey also contains 15 to 20% water, proteins, organic acids (such as gluconic acid), minerals, plant phytochemicals, and vitamins (Saba et al., 2013; Miguel et al., 2017; Schell et al., 2022). Because of their floral origins, some honeys are extremely bioactive (Irish et al., 2011; Carter et al., 2016; Schell et al., 2022). Numerous in vitro, animal, and human studies have proven the impact of honey's nondigestible oligosaccharides.

Bee subspecies, intestinal microbiome fermentation, botanical and geographic origin, climatic and environmental conditions of the production area, storage method, and even harvesting technology all affect the biological properties and physicochemical composition of honey (da Silva et al., 2016; Escuredo et al., 2014; Karabagias). It was shown that honey is a nutritious natural postbiotic food that contains antibacterial and antioxidant properties (Seraglio et al., 2019). Because it has a variety of therapeutic properties, including anti-inflammatory, anti-diabetic, antimutagenic, and anticancer potential (Badolato et al., 2017; Kafantaris et al., 2021), honey is used in both traditional and modern medicine as a natural postbiotic product.

For ancient people, honey might have been a significant source of protein, fat, and energy (Crittenden 2011; Schell et al., 2022). Children who consume honey have shorter bouts of bacterial diarrhea (Haffejee, 1985; Crittenden, 2011; Schell et al., 2022), and critically ill tube-fed patients who consume honey are less likely to experience organ failure (El-Soud, 2012; Kuropatnicki, 2018; Schell et al., 2022). Those who have viral gastroenteritis benefit from honey's healing properties (Salem, 1981; Shariatpanahi et al., 2018; Schell et al., 2022). Additional studies have shown that honey shields the stomach (Al-Swayeh and Mobarok Ali, 1998; Schell et al., 2022). Due to the limited absorption of fructose in honey, consuming rather large amounts of honey (50–100 g) may also have a mild laxative effect (Bogdanov et al., 2008; Schell et al., 2022).

Among other things, honey has antibacterial, anti-inflammatory, wound-healing, and antioxidant properties (Alvarez-Suarez et al., 2010; Molan, 2001). The most thorough study on antimicrobial activity has been conducted through in vitro, in vivo, and human trials (Alvarez-Suarez et al., 2010; Carter et al., 2016; Bogdanov et al., 2008; Bogdanov, 1997; Molan, 1998; Molan, 1997; Willicks, 1992; Schell et al., 2022). Honey's continued use as a medication is a result of its broad-spectrum antibacterial properties, which have been proven effective against a variety of pathogenic organisms, including those that are multidrug-resistant. Honey has a water activity between 0.50 and 0.65. Honeys usually have an acidic pH between 3 and 5, which is due to the presence of organic acids such as gluconic acid (Olaitan et al., 2007; Balzan et al., 2020). Vegetative bacterial cells cannot thrive in honey due to its low water activity, low pH, and antimicrobial elements such as hydrogen peroxide, antioxidants, and antimicrobial peptides (Olaitan et al., 2007). The majority of the species that can tolerate the osmotic stress of honey are spore-forming bacteria and yeasts. Osmotolerant bacteria have been found in certain studies to be transferred into honey by bee pollination from flower nectar (Alvarez-Perez et al., 2012). In addition, honey's antibacterial activity is multifactorial and influenced by osmolarity, acidity, hydrogen peroxide production, and the presence of non-peroxide components (Molan, 1997). No reports of microbial resistance to honey's inhibitory effects exist, and honey cannot breed resistance (Blair et al., 2009; Cooper et al., 2010; Maddocks et al., 2013; Schell et al., 2022). This is probably because honey has a variety of antimicrobial routes (Bouzo et al., 2020). Honey prevents harmful bacteria in the intestines from growing, including *Clostridium* perfringens, Eubacterium aerofaciens, and *Listeria monocytogenes* in milk (Shin and Ustunol, 2005; Schell et al., 2022). In addition, honey also inhibits many enteropathogenic organisms such as *Salmonella* species (multidrug-resistant strains), *Shigella* species, enteropathogenic *E. coli* (including multidrug-resistant strains), *Enterobacter* spp., Yersinia entero*coli*tica, Campylobacter spp., and *Clostridium difficile* (Willix et al., 1992; Molan, 2001; AdeboLu et al., 2005; Badawy et al., 2004; Al-Waili et al., 2005; Lin et al., 2011; Lin et al., 2009; Hammond and Donkor, 2013; Schell et al., 2022). In vitro research has shown that honey, in addition to having a direct antibacterial effect, also inhibits *Salmonella* species from adhering to mucosal epithelial cells, preventing infection (Alnaqdy et al., 2005; Schell et al., 2022).

The majority of honey's antioxidant effects can be attributed to its phenolic constituents, which can provide protection to human cells and the bloodstream when taken (Schramm et al., 2003; Schell et al., 2022). Similar to its antibacterial activity, honey's antioxidant capacity varies greatly and is based on the floral source. Darker-colored honey has greater antioxidant activity than lighter-colored honey since color is also influenced by phenolic content (Schell et al., 2022). Additionally connected to its anti-inflammatory qualities are honey's phenolic components. Inflammatory mediators have been demonstrated to be interrupted and pro-inflammatory cytokine levels decreased by honey (Vallianou et al., 2014; Zhao et al., 2019; Schell et al., 2022). Therefore, the anti-inflammatory and antioxidant activities of honey are closely related. Some honeys are frequently used to treat wounds, burns, and ulcers because of their anti-inflammatory, antioxidant, antibacterial, and wound-healing properties (Molan, 2001; Molan, 2000; Molan, 1999; Molan, 2002; Schell et al., 2022); however, little is known about their systemic effects when taken orally. This chapter investigates the beneficial properties of honey as a natural postbiotic, including microbe metabolites, plant waste products, and bees.

The Postbiotic Potential of Honey

Honey contains di-, tri-, and oligosaccharides in smaller levels, but simple sugars (monosaccharides), which are readily absorbed in the small intestine, make up the majority of its chemical composition (Bogdanov et al., 2004; Sanz et al., 2004; Schell et al., 2022). Low-mass oligosaccharides and polysaccharides found in honey are anticipated to evade host enzyme degradation and reach the lower intestine, where they exert postbiotic effects (Figure 1) (Sanz et al., 2005; Schell et al., 2022).

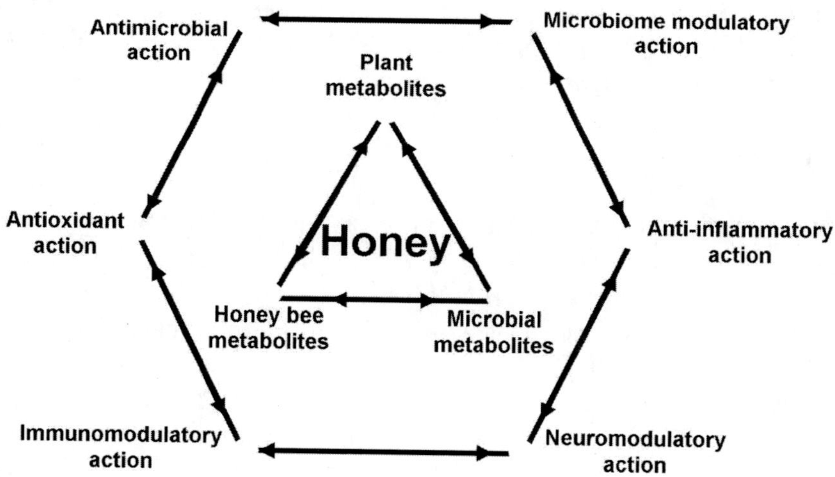

Figure 1. Honey as a natural postbiotic product.

All honeys made from various flower species have a postbiotic effect. Numerous studies on the composition and properties of honey have revealed that it is a ready-made natural multifunctional postbiotic (Table 1) (Pătruică and Mot, 2012; Horton et al., 2015; Olofsson et al., 2014; Olofsson et al., 2014; Olofsson and Vázquez, 2008; Vásquez et al., 2012).

Strong evidence for honey's postbiotic potential can be found in in vitro studies examining the effects of honey on the growth of probiotic bacteria and probiotic preparations (Rayes, 2012; Popa and Ustunol, 2011; Ustunol and Gandhi, 2001; Lucan et al., 2009; Schell et al., 2022; Rosendale et al., 2008; Shamala et al., 2000; Kajiwara et al., 2002; El-Arab et al., 2006; Li et al., 2020; Sanz et al., 2005; Jiang et al., 2020; de Melo et al., 2020). Honey supports and promotes the growth of probiotic *Bifidobacterium* and *Lactobacillus* species, including *B. longum*, *B. adolescentis*, *B. breve*, *B. bifidum*, *B. infantis*, *Lactobacillus acidophilus*, *Lactobacillus plantarum*, *Lactobacillus reuteri*, and *Lactobacillus rhamnosus* (Rosendale et al., 2008; Shamala et al., 2000; Kajiwara et al., 2002; El-Arab et al., 2006; Li et al., 2020; Haddadin et al., 2007; Schell et al., 2022). Honey's growth-promoting effect on bifidobacteria and lactobacilli is generally comparable to the effects of oligosaccharide postbiotics such as fructooligosaccharides, galactooligosaccharides, and inulin (Shin and Ustunol, 2005; Shamala et al., 2000; Kajiwara et al., 2002; Ustunol, 2001; Chick et al., 2001). Other research has discovered that honey not only promotes the growth of probiotic cultures, but it also increases the metabolism of bacterial strains from the human gut (Mohan et al., 2017; Schell et al., 2022). It is not surprising that different honeys have distinct postbiotic properties because oligosaccharide composition can influence postbiotic activity (Kolayli et al., 2012). Honey may contain oligosaccharides depending on the source (Sanz et al., 2004); for example, local New Zealand honey contained high levels of isomaltose and melesitose (Kolayli et al., 2012; Weston and Brocklebank, 1999; Schell et al., 2022), while raffinose was discovered in Italian honey (Oddo et al., 1995; Schell et al., 2022), influencing their postbiotic potential. Honeydew oligosaccharides have been demonstrated to increase populations of beneficial bifidobacteria and lactobacilli while lowering populations of potentially dangerous *bacteroides* and clostridia (Sanz et al., 2005; Schell et al., 2022). Honey-derived oligosaccharides had a postbiotic index comparable to commercial postbiotic fructooligosaccharides. Similarly, three Malaysian Tualang honeys that had been pre-treated to remove simple sugars promoted the growth of the probiotic *Bifidobacterium longum* (Jan and Mei, 2010; Schell et al., 2022).

The advent of multidrug antimicrobial resistance has aroused scientists' interest in complex natural substances having antibacterial effects, such as honey. Many factors contribute to honey's antibacterial effectiveness, including its high sugar content, low pH, and the presence of hydrogen peroxide produced by the bee enzyme glucose oxidase (da Silva et al., 2016; Anthimidou, Mossialos, 2013; Kafantaris et al., 2021). Non-peroxide components include the presence of phytochemicals such as methylglyoxal (Johnston et al., 2018; Kafantaris et al., 2021). Previous research has discovered that honey can influence a variety of biological processes in bacteria, including cell division, motility, biofilm formation, quorum sensing, protein synthesis, and oxidative stress response (Jenkins et al., 2011; Henriques et al., 2010; Lu et al., 2013; Lu et al., 2014; Roberts et al., 2015; Ahmed and Salih, 2019; Packer et al., 2012). Microarrays were used to look at the differences in gene expression of *Escherichia coli* cells after being treated with two Korean honeys (acacia and polyfloral). According to transcriptome studies, honey lowers genes involved in *E. coli* biofilm formation as well as virulence genes at low concentrations (Lee et al., 2011; Kafantaris et al., 2021). Furthermore, the antibacterial activity of Leptospermum medicinal honey against *E. coli* was investigated using microarray-based transcriptome analysis (Blair et al., 2009; Kafantaris et al., 2021). Leptospermum honey was found to have a multifactorial effect, with 78 (2%) genes upregulated and 46 (1%) genes downregulated more than twice when exposed to honey. The majority of genes that are up-regulated are involved in stress response, while the majority of genes that are down-regulated are involved in protein synthesis (Blair et al., 2009; Kafantaris et al., 2021). Another study on methicillin-resistant *Staphylococcus aureus* revealed that manuka honey had a substantial impact on the expression of virulence genes in MRSA. Manuka honey, in particular, significantly reduced transcription levels of virulence markers and regulators (e.g., fnb, lip, sec3, agr, sae, and sarV), reducing the ability of methicillin-resistant *Staphylococcus aureus* to initiate infection or biofilm formation (Jenkins et al., 2014; Kafantaris et al., 2021). Furthermore, a recent study used RNA sequencing in conjunction with cell biology techniques to analyze and explain the effects of manuka honey and its key components on the *P. aeruginosa* transcriptome (Bouzo et al., 2020; Kafantaris et al., 2021). As a result, *P. aeruginosa* cells were grown and treated with unprocessed manuka honey, artificial honey (sugar alone), pure methylglyoxal, and artificial honey augmented with methylglyoxal. Manuka honey boosts the expression of 138 genes while suppressing the expression of 97 genes involved in a variety of growth and adaption pathways, including the SOS response, quorum sensing, cell division, antibiotic resistance and susceptibility, cell wall, fatty acid, and phospholipid production. Surprisingly, no one component of honey was found to be solely responsible for its antibacterial effect (Bouzo et al., 2020; Kafantaris et al., 2021).

Numerous in vivo studies using animal models indicate that honey acts as a postbiotic, specifically by stimulating the population of probiotic bacteria, including *Bifidobacterium* spp. and *Lactobacillus* spp. (Shamala et al., 2000; El-Arab et al., 2006; Li et al., 2020; Wang et al., 2019; Schell et al., 2022), and also relieves symptoms of constipation and ulcerative *coli*tis (Li et al., 2020; Wang et al., 2019; Schell et al., 2022). Honey has also been demonstrated to boost the growth of recognized probiotics in shrimp, including *Microbavterium* spp., *Lactobacillus* spp., and *Neptumonas* spp.

(Hasyimi et al., 2020; Schell et al., 2022). Shrimp fed the honey postbiotic had higher levels of gut bacteria than shrimp fed the probiotic or synbiotic. Another study on the postbiotic effects of honey on *Vibrio parahaemolyticus*-infected Pacific white shrimp revealed that those fed honey during the infection phase had a lower pathogen burden and a greater survival rate than the control group (Fuandila et al., 2020). Honey's anti-inflammatory capabilities may contribute to its entire postbiotic potential because many gastrointestinal illnesses are associated with intestinal inflammation. Several studies on the anti-inflammatory characteristics of honey demonstrate that honey helps boost levels of anti-inflammatory cytokines while decreasing levels of pro-inflammatory cytokines (Blair et al., 2009; Ranneh et al., 2021; Vallianou et al., 2014). In rats with acetic acid-induced stomach ulcers, there was a significant increase in the concentrations of pro-inflammatory cytokines, tumor necrosis factor TNF-α, interleukin IL-1-β, and IL-6. After therapy with manuka honey, cytokine levels were substantially lower, ulcers healed faster, and acetic acid-induced oxidative damage was repaired (Almasaudi et al., 2017; Hadagali and Chua, 2014; Schell et al., 2022). Similarly, after treating rats with Egyptian honey for dextran sodium sulfate-induced ulcerative *coli*tis, blood levels of IL-1b and IL-6, as well as TNF-a, were significantly reduced in colon tissue samples (Nooh et al., 2016). Honey has been proposed to reduce inflammation by reducing reactive oxygen species, leukocyte infiltration, cyclooxygenase 1 and 2 (COX-1 and COX-2), and inducible nitric oxide synthase production (Vallianou et al., 2014; Hadagali and Chua, 2014). Polyphenols are the main components of honey that are responsible for its anti-inflammatory and antioxidant capabilities. Honey polyphenols have been shown to alter the intestinal microbiota of rats with ulcerative colitis, resulting in both a reduction in inflammation and the suppression of potentially hazardous organisms (Zhao et al., 2019). To date, just one human clinical trial has been done to explore the effects of daily honey consumption, specifically the safety of consuming manuka honey, which has stronger antibacterial activity than multifloral honey (Wallace et al., 2010). There were no significant changes in the number of the five major families of bacteria in the gut, although assessing postbiotic activity was not the primary focus of the study, and any effects may have been disguised by interactions with other meal components. The amount of honey used, as well as the honey and storage conditions (Schell et al., 2022).

Table 1. Postbiotic effects of various honeys

Honey type and source	Experimental approach	Postbiotic effect reported	References
Sundarban, Litchi, Cumin, and Eucalyptus (India)	ABTS radical decolorization, DPPH radical decolorization, FRAP, hydroxyl radical scavenging, and inhibition of lipid peroxidation	Antibacterial activities, inhibition against all the five bacteria (viz. *Escherichia coli*, *Klebsiella aerogens*, *Staphylococcus aureus*, *Salmonella typhi* and *Bacillus cereus*)	Goswami et al., 2017
Alfalfa and Eucalyptus (Australia)	Growth studies with growth media (WCA or NB), measuring the optical density	Increase in beneficial lactobacilli *Lactobacillus acidophilus*, *L. delbrueckii* subsp. *bulgaricus*, *L. plantarum*	Conway et al., 2010
Acacia and Chestnut (Croatia)	Agar disk diffusion assay, cultural enumeration (colony counts on agar plates)	Increase in beneficial *Bifidobacterium lactis* Bb-12 and *Bifidobacterium longum* Bb-46 and inhidition of *Listeria monocytogenes* FSL N1-017	Slacanac et al., 2012
Sage, Alfalfa and Sourwood (United States)	Agar disk diffusion assay, cultural enumeration (colony counts on agar plates)	Increase in beneficial *Lactobacillus delbrueckii* subsp. *bulgaricus*, L. *paracasei*, *Streptococcus thermophilus*, *Bifidobacterium adolescentis*, *B. infantis*, *B. longum*	Popa and Ustunol, 2011
Lime honey (Poland)	Shake-flask screening	Kynurenic acid in honey produced by yeasts *Yarrowia lipolytica*, *Candida magnolia*, or *Starmerella magnoliae* acted as G-protein-coupled receptor agonist, a NMDA receptor antagonist, a nicotinic antagonist, a neuroprotective agent for human	Beretta et al., 2007; Turski et al., 2009; Ziuzia et al., 2023
Honeydew (Spain)	Fecal bacteria fermentation	Increase in beneficial lactobacilli and bifidobacteria, reduction in enteric bacteria and *Bacteroides*.	Leeming et al., 2019; Schell et al., 2022
Buckwheat (China)	16S rDNA sequencing of V4 region	Increase in *Bifidobacterium* spp.	David et al., 2014; Schell et al., 2022
Juazeiro and Jurema-branca (Brazil)	Broth turbidity assay, with growth measured as turbidity	Increase in viable counts of *Bifidobacterium lactis* and *Lactobacillus acidophilus*	Tanes et al., 2021; Schell et al., 2022
Manuka (New Zealand)	Microplate growth bioassay, with growth measured as optical density (turbidity)	Increase in *Lactobacillus reuteri*, L. *rhamnosus* and *Bifidobacterium lactis*. Inhibition of pathogenic bacteria: *Escherichia coli*, *Salmonella typhi*, and *Staphylococcus aureus*	Gibson and Roberfroid, 1995; Schell et al., 2022

Table 1. (Continued)

Honey type and source	Experimental approach	Postbiotic effect reported	References
Clover (United States)	Microbroth dilution, with growth measured as optical density (turbidity)	Increase in *Bifidobacterium longum*, *B. adolescentis*, *B. breve*, *B. bifidum*, and *B. infantis*. Equally effective as commercial prebiotics: fructooligosaccharide, galactooligosaccharide, and inulin	Gibson and Manning, 2004; Schell et al., 2022
Clover (United States)	Microbroth dilution, with growth measured as optical density (turbidity)	Increase in two commercial *Bifidobacterium* spp. strains (in skim milk supplemented with honey)	Al-Sheraji et al., 2013; Schell et al., 2022
Sage, alfalfa and sourwood (United States)	Cultural enumeration (colony counts on agar plates)	Increase in *Streptococcus*, *Lactobacillus*, and *Bifidobacterium* strains	Lobo et al., 2010; Schell et al., 2022
Acacia and chestnut (Saudi Arabia)	Agar disk diffusion assay, cultural enumeration (colony counts on agar plates)	Increase of bifidobacteria and lactobacilli, specifically by reducing doubling time. Inhibition of pathogenic *Listeria monocytogenes*	Raschka and Daniel, 2005; Schell et al., 2022
Acacia and chestnut (Croatia)	Agar disk diffusion assay, cultural enumeration (colony counts on agar plates)	Increase in *Bifidobacterium lactis*	Nagpal and Kaur, 2011; Schell et al., 2022
Unidentified floral source (India)	Viable colony counts on agar plates using bifidobacteria isolated from infant fecal samples, and identified via phenotypic and molecular (PCR) methods	Increase in all *Bifidobacterium* isolates	Nooh and Nour-Eldien, 2016; Schell et al., 2022
Sourwood, alfalfa, and sage (Unspecified)	Microbroth dilution, with growth measured as optical density (turbidity)	Increase in five *Bifidobacterium* species of human intestinal origin (*B. longum*, *B. adolescentis*, *B. breve*, *B. bifidum*, and *B. infantis*). Inhibition of C. perfringens and E. aerofaciens.	Gill et al., 2006; Schell et al., 2022
Unidentified floral source (Jordan)	Colony counts (CFU/ml) calculated from optical density (turbidity) readings	Significant increase in *Bifidobacterium infantis* and *Lactobacillus acidophilus* of intestinal origin	Ottman et al., 2012; Schell et al., 2022

Honey type and source	Experimental approach	Postbiotic effect reported	References
Tualang and multifloral (Malaysia)	Honey samples pre-treated to remove simple sugars, remaining fraction used to supplement skim milk; bacterial enumeration (colony counts on agar plates)	Increase in *Bifidobacterium longum* by all honey fractions with simple sugars removed	Chick et al., 2001; Schell et al., 2022
Clover (Unspecified)	Growth of probiotic pure cultures in skim milk supplemented with various sweeteners measured via cultural enumeration (colony counts on agar)	Honey best supports growth of probiotic strains, with significant increase in *Bifidobacterium bifidum* and *Lactobacillus acidophilus* numbers	Mohan et al., 2017; Schell et al., 2022
Generic, unknown floral source (India)	Wistar strain male albino rats (n = 36); small and large intestine collection, suspension and viable cell count	Increase in *Lactobacillus acidophilus* and *Lactobacillus plantarum*	Grizard and Barthomeuf, 1999; Schell et al., 2022
Cotton (Egypt)	Swiss male albino mice (n = 42); cecum content collection, viable cell counts (bacterial enumeration on agar) of colonic bacteria	Increase in *Bifidobacterium* and *Lactobacillus*	Roberfroid et al., 2010; Schell et al., 2022
Jarrah (Australian floral source, purchased in China)	BALB/c mice (n = 30); 16S rRNA sequencing of V3–V4 region Fecal water content measured via weighing fecal samples before and after drying	Gut microbiota equilibrium re-established, specifically by increasing abundance of key bacterial groups in the gut, and suppressing harmful bacteria. Improvement in fecal water content, linked to alleviation of constipation	Chauhan and Chorawala, 2014; Schell et al., 2022
Prunella vulgaris, common name 'self-heal' (China)	Sprague Dawley male rats (n = 24) with induced *coli*tis; histological analysis of colon samples, intestinal mRNA analysis, gut microbial community analysis (from caeca) via 16S rRNA sequencing of the V3–V4 region	Decrease in Bacteroidetes, and increase in Firmicutes; and at genus level increases in the beneficial *Lactobacillus* spp., and decrease in Lachnospiraceae, which is associated with the pathological features of colitis. Overall reduction of symptoms associated with ulcerative colitis, mostly attributed to the abitlity of honey to modulate effects on gut microbiota	Haddadin et al., 2007; Schell et al., 2022

Table 1. (Continued)

Honey type and source	Experimental approach	Postbiotic effect reported	References
Unidentified floral source (Indonesia)	Pacific white shrimp fed honey (prebiotic), probiotic culture or synbiotic (combination of probiotic culture and honey); intestinal microbiota diversity analysis via DNA sequencing	Honey treatment most effective, showing increased intestinal microbiota diversity, and higher genus level abundance of beneficial (probiotic) bacteria. Honey-fed shrimp showed highest survival rate post infection with *Vibrio parahaemolyticus*	Weston and Brocklebank, 1999; Schell et al., 2022
Manuka (New Zealand) and multifloral (unspecified)	Pilot human clinical study where participants consumed daily dose (20 g) of honey; DNA from fecal sample sequenced for microbiota analysis	No significant changes (positive or negative) in gut microbiota populations, no antimicrobial effects of manuka honey on the beneficial populations of the gut	Wang et al., 2019; Schell et al., 2022

Overall, the honey bee proteome is currently understudied, owing to the low protein concentration (0.1-0.5%), which makes protein extraction difficult. The most common proteins in honey are MRJPs (Chua et al., 2015; Kafantaris et al., 2021), but there are other enzymes such as glucosidase (invertase), amylase (diastase), glucose oxidase, and others (Machado De-Melo et al., 2018). Proteins discovered in honey are frequently used as markers of authenticity, adulteration, and quality (Bilikova, 2015; Vaughn et al., 2008; Chua et al., 2013; Kafantaris et al., 2021). Almost all proteins found in honeys from chestnut, acacia, sunflower, eucalyptus, and orange were *Apis mellifera*-derived, including MRJP (MRJP 1-5), α-glucosidase, and defensin-1 (Di Girolamo, 2012; Kafantaris et al., 2021). SDS-PAGE and Western blotting revealed that honey's antibacterial activity is mediated by the antimicrobial peptide bee defensin-1 (Kwakman et al., 2010; Kafantaris et al., 2021). MRJP 1–5, α-glucosidase, glucose oxidase, profiling, and apizimin were detected in four different Italian honeys using 2D electrophoresis coupled with matrix-assisted laser desorption/ionization mass spectrometry (MALDI MS) (Rossano et al., 2012; Kafantaris et al., 2021). SDS-PAGE, native PAGE, and MS methods were used to identify MRJP 1–9, alpha-glucosidase, α-amylase, glucose oxidase, and transferrin 1 in honey (Borutinskaite et al., 2018; Zhang et al., 2019; Kafantaris et al., 2021). Honey from *Mimosa scabrella* Bentham can be detected by 2D electrophoresis, proteomics, and main component analysis (Azevedo et al., 2017; Kafantaris et al., 2021). Honeydew honey has 160 protein spots in its proteomic profile, whereas floral honey has 84 protein spots. Using the right proteins, this approach proved to be a useful tool for distinguishing between various forms of honey (45 matching points). Honey metabolomics has been used to identify origin, control quality, discover biomarkers, and authenticate honey. Nuclear magnetic resonance (NMR) spectroscopy has been used successfully to identify and categorize honey from a variety of floral sources and geographical origins (Beretta et al., 2008; LolLi et al., 2008; Donarski et al., 2008; Consonni and Cagliani, 2008; Kafantaris et al., 2021). In previous studies, NMR combined with chemometric analysis successfully differentiated four botanical honeys (chestnut, acacia, linden, and polyfloral) and six botanical honeys (acacia, linden, orange, eucalyptus, chestnut, and honeydew) (Schievano et al., 2010; Schievano et al., 2011; Kafantaris et al., 2021). Similarly, the use of chemometric techniques for 1H-NMR profiling has enabled the distinction of honeys produced in Greece, Brazil, South Africa, Zambia, and Slovakia (Karabagias, 2018; Boflo et al., 2012; Olawode et al., 2018; Kafantaris et al., 2021). In addition, NMR metabolomics technology was utilized to assess and categorize Vietnamese honey depending on its origin and quality. Several compounds were found that were unique to each honey sample examined (Luong et al., 2019; Kafantaris et al., 2021). NMR and ultra-high-performance liquid chromatography-quadrupole time-of-flight mass spectrometry (UHPLC-QTOF-MS) were used to classify raw stingless bee honey (Heterotrigona itama, Geniotrigona thoracica, and Tetrigona apicalis) (RazaLi et al., 2018; Kafantaris et al., 2021). D-fructofuranose (H. itama honey), α-d-glucose, d-xylose, and β-d-glucose (G. thoracica honey), and L-lactic acid, acetic acid, and L-alanine (T. apicalis honey) have all been identified as unique chemical indications of species origin (RazaLi et al., 2018; Kafantaris et al., 2021).

Microorganisms and plant metabolic products, such as phytohormones, have been identified in honey. Using sequential liquid-liquid extraction methods coupled with liquid chromatography-tandem mass spectrometry, 34 phytohormones were discovered in 14 types of honeys, of which 14 were cytokinins, 8 gibberellins, 5 brassinosteroids, indole-3-acetic acid, indole-3-butyric acid, abscisic acid, salicylic acid, jasmonic acid, jasmonoyl-leucine, and jasmonoyl-phenylalanine (Wang et al., 2017). Phytohormones can have an impact on plants, animals, and people. In the human body, gibberellic acid has anti-inflammatory qualities, but abscisic acid has depressive properties. Honey, which contains gibberellic and abscisic acids from plants and microbes, is an efficient postbiotic that can be utilized as a functional meal (Chanclud & Lacombe, 2017).

The Microbiome of Honey Bees

The honey bee (*A. mellifera*) is a useful model organism because its microbial community is highly adaptive to its host (Engel and Moran, 2013; Nowak et al., 2021). Although its microbiome is similar to that of mammals, its composition is substantially simpler. The fundamental similarities and differences between the honey bee and human gut microbiome have previously been discussed (Zheng et al., 2018; Nowak et al., 2021). Worker bees are commonly associated with hive maintenance and cleaning jobs, whereas newly emerged bees are usually associated with hive maintenance and cleaning chores. Adult bee interactions, comb contact, and bee bread consumption have all been investigated as potential routes of infection for freshly emerging bees (Li et al., 2017; Powell et al., 2014; Dong et al., 2020; Nowak et al., 2021). Representatives of the genera *Gilliamella*, *Frischella*, and *Snodgrassella* colonized the bee's intestines one day after hatching.

Lactobacillus, *Bifidobacterium*, and *Commensalibacter* colonized after three days, whereas *Gilliamella* numbers declined. Significant colonization of *L. kunkei* and *Bartonella* sp. occurred 12 days after emergence. *Bacteroides* sp., *Escherichia* sp., *Shigella* sp., and Porphyromonadaceae all declined between 19 and 25 days post emergence. The abundance of *Commensalibacter* sp. and *Bifidobacterium* sp. was reduced 25 days after emergence (Dong et al., 2020; Nowak et al., 2021). The honey bee microbiome is found in various parts of the gut, including the crop (which is located between the esophagus and the ventricle and is used to store and transport nectar to the hive; also known as the stomach or pouch); midgut; hindgut, which includes the ileum (a narrow tube with six longitudinal folds) and the lumen; and the distal rectum (Engel et al., 2012; Vásquez et al., 2012; Nowak et al., 2021). Only *Parasaccharibacter* sp. was detected in relative abundance in workers' hypopharyngeal glands (Corby-Harris et al., 2014; Nowak et al., 2021).

The intestines of adult workers are thought to be populated by specialized microorganisms from nine bacterial species clusters (Jones et al., 2017; Nowak et al., 2021). Each cluster is made up of interconnected bacterial strains. Host-adapted species that are extremely resistant to ambient oxygen predominate in honey bee microbial communities; hence, bacterial species transfer occurs through social contacts between hosts (Alberoni et al., 2016; Nowak et al., 2021).

Researchers showed that the intestine of honey bee workers is filled by nine clusters of bacterial species that account for 95–99.9% of the bacteria in almost all individuals using 16S rDNA community studies and total DNA metagenomics (Jones et al., 2017; Tola et al., 2020). *Snodgrasella alvi* (non-fermenting sugar bacteria that form a film directly on the intestinal wall; family Neisseriaceae) and *Gilliamella apicola* (bacteria capable of sugar fermentation that inhabit areas near the center of the intestinal lumen; family Orbaceae) are both members of the *Proteobacteria* phylum (Jones et al., 2017; Zheng et al., 2017; Tola et al., 2020; Nowak et al., 2021).

Lactobacillus Firm-4 and *Lactobacillus* Firm-5, both Gram-positive species belonging to the phylum Firmicutes, are widespread and numerous in the distal rectum (Tola et al., 2020; Jones et al., 2017; Nowak et al., 2021). Most adult workers have *Bifidobacterium asteroides* (although at substantially lower amounts) (Kwong and Moran, 2016; Jones et al., 2017; Bleau, 2020; Nowak et al., 2021). The most important microorganisms in bee intestines are clusters of bacterial species known as "nuclear bacteria" (Kešnerová, 2020; Nowak et al., 2021).

Other bacteria genera commonly found in honey bee digestive systems include *Apibacter*, *Asaia*, and *Acetobacter* (Raymann et al., 2018). In honey bee digestive tracts, certain rarer bacteria that can cause disease and death in honey bees, such as *Enterobacter*, *Klebsiella*, *Citrobacter*, and *Serratia*, have been found (Raymann et al., 2018). There are also less common or stable species of *Proteobacteria*: *Gammaproteobacteria Frischella* perrara (Orbaceae); *Alphaproteobacteria Parasaccharibacter apium*; *Bombella Favorum*; *Bombella mellum*; *Bombella apis* (family Acetobacteraceae, Alpha 2.2); and *Commensalibacter* sp. (Alpha 2.1) and *Bartonella apis* (Alpha 1) from the family Rhizobiaceae (Jones et al., 2017; Tola et al., 2020; Dong et al., 2020; Bleau, 2020; Kešnerová, 2016; Hilgarth et al., 2021; Nowak et al., 2021). *Apibacter* adventoris mensalis, a Bacteroidetes member, has also been detected in honey bee intestines (Kwong and Moran, 2016; Kwong et al., 2018; Nowak et al., 2021).

The honey bees contain 10 known taxa: four *Lactobacillus* sp. representatives, two *Gilliamella* species, one *Bifidobacterium* species, and one *Snodgrassella* species, which are believed to be part of the core gut microbiome of honey bees. *Frischella* sp. and *Bartonella* sp. taxa may vary depending on habitat (Subotic et al., 2019; Nowak et al., 2021). They are minor members of the digestive system of honey bees (Kešnerová, 2020; Nowak et al., 2021). The dominant phyla in honey bee gut are *Proteobacteria* (63.2%), Firmicutes (17.6%), with 15.9% *Lactobacillus* sp., *Actinobacteria* (4.1%), with 3.34% *Bifidobacterium* sp., and Bacteroidetes (1.7%), with 0.23% *Bacteroides* sp. (Wang et al., 2021; Wang et al., 2021; Nowak et al., 2021). A core member, *Lactobacillus* firm-4, was detected in 98.4% of the bees examined (Kešnerová et al., 2020; Nowak et al., 2021).

Lactobacilli exhibit excellent antioxidant and anti-inflammatory properties, as evidenced by the findings of *L. plantarum* H28 and *L. plantarum* H24 strains from honey bee digestive tracts (Kenfack et al., 2018; Niode et al., 2020). By boosting the expression of detoxification enzymes in the gut, the honeybee gut microbiota aids in the breakdown and detoxification of xenobiotics and pesticides (thiacloprid, imidacloprid, and fluvalinate) (Wu et al., 2020). Lactobacilli of the species *Lactobacillus kunkeei* and *Lactobacillus plantarum* (strains H28, H24, KX519413, KX519414, LP8, LP25, LP86, LP95, and LP100) with higher antioxidant capacity were recovered from honey bee intestines (Kenfack et al., 2018; Chandran and Keerthi, 2018; Hmood et al., 2019; Niode et al., 2020; Iorizzo et al., 2021). The lactic acid bacteria *Enterococcus faecalis* (HBE1, HBE3, HBE4), *Lactobacillus* brevis (HBE2), and *Lactobacillus casei* (HBE5) isolated from honeybee workers may represent new potential pharmacobiotics for the production of functional dietary foods that promote human health (Elzeini et al., 2021). As a result, the honeybee gut microbiome can be considered a source of bacteria potentially suitable for use as probiotic cultures, as most of them have enhanced antimicrobial, antioxidant, and anti-inflammatory effects and can survive in human and animal gastrointestinal tracts after exposure to stressful environmental conditions (Elzeini et al., 2021; Nowak A et al., 2021).

The gut microbiome of *Apis mellifera* was researched in Sub-Saharan African regions of Kenya, where beekeeping employs indigenous and traditional management practices that require very little human involvement in comparison to those used in Europe (Tola et al., 2020; Nowak et al., 2021). They confirmed that the major members of the honey bee gut microbiome belong to the genera *Gilliamella*, *Snodgrassella*, *Lactobacillus* (Firm-4 and Firm-5), *Bifidobacterium*, *Frischella*, *Commensalibacter*, *Bombella*, *Apibacter*, and *Bartonella*, and that *Frischella* sp. was the third most dominant genus (16.9%), while *Lactobacillus* (Firm-4 and Firm-5) showed lower abundance than demonstrated in other studies (Tola et al., 2020; Nowak et al., 2021). Fungal taxa found in honey bee digestive systems include *Saccharomyces*, *Zygosaccharomyces*, and *Candida* (Yun et al., 2018).

The Microbiome of Honey

Honey contains fewer microorganisms than other fermented foods. The majority of the microbiome in honey comes from pollen, flowers, soil, air, dust, and honey bee digestive tracts (Snowdon and Cliver, 1996; Snowdon and Cliver, 1996; Kafantaris et al., 2021). The honey microbiome consists of bacteria, yeasts, and molds that can change depending on their environment (Wen et al., 2017; Kafantaris et al., 2021). Several secondary microbiological contaminants can be added into honey during human processing (Snowdon and Cliver, 1996; Olaitan et al., 2007). Bacteria and fungus, plant-associated microorganisms present in plants and soil, can be transmitted to hives during pollination. Honey bee gut have been identified as a significant source of microbial transmission into honey. *Lactobacillus* and *Bifidobacterium* are key components of the honey bee gut microbiota and have been found to be universally preserved (Anderson et al., 2013; Raymann et al., 2018). These taxa have been found in honey and bee nectar (Olofsson and Vázquez, 2008). Although the gut microbiome may contribute to the microbial community in honey, many gut bacteria are only found in the gut and do not flourish in other environments. Only *L. kunkeei* and Acetobacteraceae (*Asaia* spp.) were found in extreme conditions such as honey and royal jelly (Martinson et al., 2012; Anderson et al., 2013; Vojvodic et al., 2013; Xiong et al., 2023).

The majority of bacterial species identified in honey were osmotolerant, xerotolerant, and acidotolerant, owing to honey's comparatively high sugar content, low water activity, and low pH (Brudzynski, 2021; Xiong et al., 2023). Most bacteria in honey are metabolically dormant because they are unlikely to flourish in honey. Some physicochemical features of honey, such as titratable acidity, water activity, and color, have been experimentally linked to the composition of the honey microbiome (Wen et al., 2017; Balzan et al., 2020; Kňazovická et al., 2019; Xiong et al., 2023). The honey microbiome may represent numerous bioindicators, including the agricultural and urban landscape, the microbial environment to which honey bees are exposed, and chemical contaminants along foraging routes (Rissato et al., 2007; Lambert et al., 2012). The honey microbiome can represent the hive's immune status, which is related to the immune system (Xiong et al., 2023). NGS metagenome sequencing can give a taxonomic classification of the honey microbiome as well as an indicator of overall hive health and honey provenance (Bovo et al., 2020; Xiong et al., 2023).

Previously, certain honeys had up to 108 colony-forming units per gram of viable lactic acid bacteria (Vásquez et al., 2012). During honey production, bees transfer bacteria from their gut microbiome into nectar, and therefore into honey. Many Enterobacteriaceae and Firmicutes have been discovered in flowers, including *Lactobacillus*, *Bacillus*, and *Weissella* spp., many of which are found in honey products and honey bee guts. *Lactobacillus* spp., *Bacillus* spp., *Streptococcus* spp., *Clostridium* spp., and Gram-negative bacteria are among the microorganisms transported from the gut to honey (Naseer et al., 2015; Olofsson et al., 2016; Kafantaris et al., 2021). Honey has also been reported to include *Achromobacter* spp., *Citrobacter* spp., *Enterobacter* spp., *Flavobacterium* spp., Proteus spp., and *Pseudomonas* spp. (Ahn et al., 2012; Kafantaris et al., 2021).

According to a study on the microbiome of stingless bee honey (Rosli et al., 2020; Xiong et al., 2023), *Lactobacillus malefermentans* is the most frequent species in honey. Lactobacilli may be lacking in some honeys because they disappear when the humidity falls below 18% during honey ripening (Ruiz-Argueso and Rodríguez-Navarro, 1975; Wen et al., 2017; Xiong et al., 2023). Other studies have discovered that the presence of *L. kunkeei* is intermittent and dependent on variables such as the source of the bloom and the time of year (Vásquez et al., 2012; Wen et al., 2017; Xiong et al., 2023). Unresolved Enterobacteriaceae were discovered in honey, most likely from the pollination environment because they are regularly recovered from forage bee crops (Corby-Harris et al., 2014; Xiong et al., 2023).

Most honeys have a similar bacterial composition, with *Bacillus* spp. and *Lactococcus* spp. being the most common phylotypes. Bacterial communities in honey were relatively conserved, although fungal communities were more diverse (Xiong et al., 2023). The bacterial microbiome did not change appreciably during the honey-ripening process. *Metschnikowia*, *Cladosporium*, and Alternaria were the most prevalent phylotypes in Vitex flowers, while *Metschnikowia*, *Phoma*, and *Candida* were the most common fungi in Vitex honey, suggesting significant divergence of fungal communities between flowers and honey (Wen et al., 2017; Kafantaris et al., 2021). Some plant-produced microorganisms, such as actinobacteria, are beneficial to bees (Kurek-Górecka et al., 2020). Although certain *Actinobacteria* spp. are plant pathogens, many of them protect honey bees and other insects by generating secondary chemicals that prevent fungal growth and spoilage (Mohr and Tebbe, 2006; Barke et al., 2010; Anderson et al., 2013). Certain secondary metabolites produced by lactic acid bacteria strains have been proven to combat spoilage microbes and pathogens while also improving hive health. *Lactobacillus kunkeei*, for example, protects bee colonies from illnesses like *Paenibacillus larvae* and *Nosema ceranae* (Arredondo et al., 2018; Xiong et al., 2023).

A recent study employed the Illumina MiSeq NGS platform to analyze the bacterial diversity of 30 honeys from Slovakia, Latvia, Switzerland, India, Japan, and Tanzania (Kňazovická et al., 2019; Kafantaris et al., 2021). There are 52 bacteria genera in all, which have been categorized into two groups. *Lactobacillus kunkei* and *L. apinorum* (obligate fructophiles) were the most prevalent bacteria in the first group, followed by *Bombella apis* and *Fructobacillus* spp. *Melissococcus plutonius*, a bee pathogen, and other pathogens such as *Enterococcus faecalis* were detected in the second group, most likely as a result of contamination of samples during collection, processing, and storage (Kňazovická et al., 2019; Kafantaris et al., 2021).

Lactobacilli *L. kunkei* is a common species found in flowers, fruits, and soil, as well as hive environs and fermented bee products (Anderson et al., 2013). *L. kunkei*i was discovered in honey bee bread using both culture-dependent and culture-independent techniques (Anderson et al., 2013). *L. kunkei*i is one of the fructophiles found in some honeys but not all (Xiong et al., 2023). Flowers, bee guts, and bee bread have all been found to contain *L. kunkei*ii (Anderson et al., 2013). The striking similarity of Firmicutes observed in flower nectar and honey obtained from beehives shows that horizontal transmission of these bacteria occurs during pollination (Vásquez et al., 2012).

Lactococcus lactis is another often detected bacterial species in honey, and it is found in all sequenced honeys (Xiong et al., 2023). Lactic acid bacteria are present in certain bee species due to horizontal transfer between hives and the environment. *Lactococcus* is a lactic acid bacterium that can ferment honey carbohydrates (fructose and glucose) and produce lactic acid. Lactic acid bacteria have previously been isolated from honey bee hives and bee products (Sinacori et al., 2014; Kňazovická et al., 2020; Xiong et al., 2023).

Serratia symbiotica accounts for 4.8% of the bacteria in polyfloral honeys from Italy (Bovo et al., 2020). *Serratia* is a large Hymenoptera genus (Dillon and Dillon, 2004; Xiong et al., 2023). *Serratia* in honey has a fascinating history as a secondary endosymbiont with aphids. *Serratia* may have originated from aphid honeydew, which was then fed to bees, resulting in honey production (Bovo et al., 2020; Xiong et al., 2023). Some *Serratia* species have been discovered as opportunistic honey bee diseases that may have a significant impact on hive health (Raymann et al., 2018; Xiong et al., 2023).

Honey frequently contains yeasts and molds (Kacániová et al., 2009; Ki, 2018; Kafantaris et al., 2021). *Bettsia*, *Yarrowia*, *Skoua*, *Zygosaccharomyces*, and *Metschnikowia* were the most prevalent fungal taxa detected in diverse types of honey. Similarly, the fungal profile of chasteberry honey is diverse, with the most prevalent genera being *Waitea*, *Phoma*, *Metschnikowia*, and *Cryptococcus*. *Metschnikowia* was discovered to be stable in mature chasteberry honey and dominant in chasteberry flowers. *Metschnikowia* and other yeasts in honey may have originated from nectar, which can be passed from flowers and fruits to honey bee products (Hong et al., 2001; Lievens et al., 2015; Xiong et al., 2023). *Waitea* and *Cryptococcus* may be absent from some honeys due to floral origin, as these two genera were discovered to be abundant in Vitex blossoms (Wen et al., 2017; Xiong et al., 2023). By culture methods, yeasts such as *Zygosaccharomyces* and *Debaryomyces* have been discovered as the most prevalent taxa in honey (Sinacori et al., 2014; Xiong et al., 2023). In a culture-independent ITS2 metabarcoding investigation, *Zygosaccharomyces* was the only species discovered in almost all honeys (Balzan et al., 2020; Xiong et al., 2023).

Cladosporium is a filamentous fungus that is abundant in the environment, and some of its species are potential plant diseases (Bensch et al., 2012). It is one of the most common plant-associated fungi discovered in honey. *Cladosporium* has been proposed to coexist with bees, be transmitted from plants or bees, and survive in bee products (Martinson et al., 2012). *Botrytis*, *Penicillium*, and *Mucor* are filamentous fungi found in plant pollen that are conveyed to honey bees and are frequently found in beebread (Disayathanoowat et al., 2020). Candida, *Cryptococcus*, *Kloeckera*, *Metschnikowia*, and *Rhodotorula* are some common yeast genera recovered from pollen and beebread (Gilliam et al., 1974).

Filamentous fungi such as *Aspergillus* are considered environmental contaminants in honey (Kacániová et al., 2009). According to a metagenomic study, *Aspergillus flavus* is the second most abundant fungus in polyfloral Italian honey (Bovo et al., 2020; Xiong et al., 2023). *Aspergillus flavus* is a honey bee pathogen that can cause stone fruit disease. It has been found in high proportions in some monofloral honeys, wildflower honeys, and manuka honeys. *Ascosphaera apis* is also the cause of calcareous disease (Vojvodic et al., 2013; Xiong et al., 2023). It has been discovered that the genus *Ascosphaera* sp. predominates in various wildflower honeys. However, the presence of hazardous fungi does not automatically mean that the hives are contaminated. During a two-year metagenomic study, none of the chosen colonies containing pathogenic fungal DNA had any of these symptoms (Bovo et al., 2020). For these infections to arise, certain environmental variables must be present, and the most dangerous fungus can only survive in honey as latent spores (Xiong et al., 2023).

Conclusion

Honey contains low-molecular-weight prebiotic oligosaccharides and polysaccharides. Honey oligosaccharides, like well-known commercial prebiotics, are not digested in the upper gastrointestinal tract but are fermented by beneficial bacteria in the human and animal large intestine, promoting their development and vitality. The prebiotic characteristics of honey are highlighted as depending on the plant from which it is derived. Fresh honey contains probiotics, which are healthy microorganisms that limit the growth and development of pathogenic and opportunistic microflora. It can also be a source of physiologically active chemicals with antimicrobial effects. Lactobacilli and bifidobacteria can persist in honey for up to 2–3 months after harvesting. The botanical origin of the honey, as well as the habitat and subspecies of honey bees, may impact the composition of the microflora of stock and fresh honey. Probiotic bacteria contribute in the development of honey bee resistance to unfavorable environmental variables by directly reducing pathogen growth and activating immune system components.

It is plausible to infer that honey is a postbiotic - fermented nectar that has been partially digested by bee enzymes and their symbiotic lactic acid bacteria and yeasts. Honey is characterized as a postbiotic functional product due to the presence of prebiotic compounds and probiotic microorganisms and their metabolites. Lactic acid bacteria and yeasts are symbionts of honey bees create metabolites that contribute to the production of organoleptic qualities of honey (taste, scent, consistency) as well as the range of its therapeutic capabilities using honey polysaccharides and oligosaccharides as substrates. A variety of factors influence the qualitative and quantitative composition of prebiotic sugars in honey and lactic acid bacteria, and thus bacterial metabolites, which explains why different types of honey have different medicinal properties. All microorganisms in the beneficial microbiota of bees have a direct antibacterial action as well as an indirect immunostimulatory effect, indicating that probiotic bacteria play an important role in bee illness.

Honey is a source of components for new postbiotic supplements for humans due to its high level of postbiotic activity toward healthy human intestinal flora and the antagonistic effect of fresh honey bacteria on human infections. The discovery of bacterial strains with high levels of antibacterial activity against antibiotic-resistant pathogens in honey and the intestinal microbiome raises the prospect of developing novel alternative techniques for combating therapeutically resistant pathogenic organisms. Because probiotic bacteria have antagonistic action against a wide range of pathogenic microorganisms, they can be used in medical and veterinary care to prevent and cure bee diseases.

Acknowledgment

This research received funding from the IDB RAS Government basic research program in 2023 No 0088-2021-0019 and 0088-2021-0008.

References

Adebolu, T. "Effect of natural honey on local isolates of diarrhea-causing bacteria in southwestern nigeria." *African Journal of Biotechnology* 4 (2005): 1172-74.

Ahn, J. H., I. P. Hong, J. I. Bok, B. Y. Kim, J. Song and H. Y. Weon. "Pyrosequencing analysis of the bacterial communities in the guts of honey bees apis cerana and apis mellifera in korea." *J Microbiol* 50 (2012): 735-45. 10.1007/s12275-012-2188-0. http://www.ncbi.nlm.nih.gov/pubmed/23124740.

Alberoni, D., F. Gaggia, L. Baffoni and D. Di Gioia. "Beneficial microorganisms for honey bees: Problems and progresses." *Applied Microbiology and Biotechnology* 100 (2016): 9469-82. 10.1007/s00253-016-7870-4. http://www.ncbi.nlm.nih.gov/pubmed/27717968.

Almasaudi, S. B., A. T. Abbas, R. R. Al-Hindi, N. A. El-Shitany, U. A. Abdel-Dayem, S. S. Ali, R. M. Saleh, S. K. Al Jaouni, M. A. Kamal and S. M. Harakeh. "Manuka honey exerts antioxidant and anti-inflammatory activities that promote healing of acetic acid-induced gastric ulcer in rats." *Evidence-Based Complementary and Alternative Medicine* 2017 (2017): 5413917. 10.1155/2017/5413917. http://www.ncbi.nlm.nih.gov/pubmed/28250794.

Alnaqdy, A., A. Al-Jabri, Z. Al Mahrooqi, B. Nzeako and H. Nsanze. "Inhibition effect of honey on the adherence of salmonella to intestinal epithelial cells in vitro." *International Journal of Food Microbiology* 103 (2005): 347-51. 10.1016/j.ijfoodmicro.2004.11.042. http://www.ncbi.nlm.nih.gov/pubmed/16099316.

Al-Sheraji, S. H., A. Ismail, M. Y. Manap, S. Mustafa, R. M. Yusof and F. A. Hassan. "Prebiotics as functional foods: A review." *Journal of Functional Foods* 5 (2013): 1542-53. 10.1016/j.jff.2013.08.009.

Al-Swayeh, O. A. and A. T. Ali. "Effect of ablation of capsaicin-sensitive neurons on gastric protection by honey and sucralfate." *Hepatogastroenterology* 45 (1998): 297-302. http://www.ncbi.nlm.nih.gov/pubmed/9496530.

Alvarez-Perez, S., C. M. Herrera and C. de Vega. "Zooming-in on floral nectar: A first exploration of nectar-associated bacteria in wild plant communities." *FEMS Microbiology Ecology* 80 (2012): 591-602. 10.1111/j.1574-6941.2012.01329.x. http://www.ncbi.nlm.nih.gov/pubmed/22324904.

Alvarez-Suarez, J. M., S. Tulipani, S. Romandini, E. Bertoli and M. Battino. "Contribution of honey in nutrition and human health: A review." *Mediterranean Journal of Nutrition and Metabolism* 3 (2009): 15-23. 10.1007/s12349-009-0051-6.

Al-Waili, N. S., M. Akmal, F. S. Al-Waili, K. Y. Saloom and A. Ali. "The antimicrobial potential of honey from united arab emirates on some microbial isolates." *Medical Science Monitor* 11 (2005): BR433-8. http://www.ncbi.nlm.nih.gov/pubmed/16319779.

Anderson, K. E., T. H. Sheehan, B. M. Mott, P. Maes, L. Snyder, M. R. Schwan, A. Walton, B. M. Jones and V. Corby-Harris. "Microbial ecology of the hive and pollination landscape: Bacterial associates from floral nectar, the alimentary tract and stored food of honey bees (apis mellifera)." *Plos One* 8 (2013): e83125. 10.1371/journal.pone.0083125. http://www.ncbi.nlm.nih.gov/pubmed/24358254.

Anthimidou, E. and D. Mossialos. "Antibacterial activity of greek and cypriot honeys against staphylococcus aureus and pseudomonas aeruginosa in comparison to manuka honey." *Journal of Medicinal Food* 16 (2013): 42-7. 10.1089/jmf.2012.0042. http://www.ncbi.nlm.nih.gov/pubmed/23134461.

Arredondo, D., L. Castelli, M. P. Porrini, P. M. Garrido, M. J. Eguaras, P. Zunino and K. Antunez. "Lactobacillus kunkeei strains decreased the infection by honey bee pathogens paenibacillus larvae and nosema ceranae." *Benef Microbes* 9 (2018): 279-90. 10.3920/BM2017.0075. http://www.ncbi.nlm.nih.gov/pubmed/29264966.

Azevedo, M. S., P. A. Valentim-Neto, S. K. T. Seraglio, C. F. P. da Luz, A. C. M. Arisi and A. C. O. Costa. "Proteome comparison for discrimination between honeydew and floral honeys from botanical species mimosa scabrella bentham by principal component analysis." *J Sci Food Agric* 97 (2017): 4515-19. 10.1002/jsfa.8317. http://www.ncbi.nlm.nih.gov/pubmed/28337740.

Badawy, O. F., S. S. Shafii, E. E. Tharwat and A. M. Kamal. "Antibacterial activity of bee honey and its therapeutic usefulness against escherichia coli o157:H7 and salmonella typhimurium infection." *Revue Scientifique et Technique* 23 (2004): 1011-22. 10.20506/rst.23.3.1543. http://www.ncbi.nlm.nih.gov/pubmed/15861897.

Badolato, M., G. Carullo, E. Cione, F. Aiello and M. C. Caroleo. "From the hive: Honey, a novel weapon against cancer." *European Journal of Medicinal Chemistry* 142 (2017): 290-99. 10.1016/j.ejmech.2017.07.064. http://www.ncbi.nlm.nih.gov/pubmed/28797675.

Balzan, M. V., R. Sadula and L. Scalvenzi. "Assessing ecosystem services supplied by agroecosystems in mediterranean europe: A literature review." *Land* 9 (2020): 245. 10.3390/land9080245.

Barke, J., R. F. Seipke, S. Gruschow, D. Heavens, N. Drou, M. J. Bibb, R. J. Goss, D. W. Yu and M. I. Hutchings. "A mixed community of actinomycetes produce multiple antibiotics for the fungus farming ant acromyrmex octospinosus." *BMC Biol* 8 (2010): 109. 10.1186/1741-7007-8-109. http://www.ncbi.nlm.nih.gov/pubmed/20796277.

Bensch, K., U. Braun, J. Z. Groenewald and P. W. Crous. "The genus cladosporium." *Stud Mycol* 72 (2012): 1-401. 10.3114/sim0003. http://www.ncbi.nlm.nih.gov/pubmed/22815589.

Beretta, G., E. Caneva and R. M. Facino. "Kynurenic acid in honey from arboreal plants: Ms and nmr evidence." *Planta Medica* 73 (2007): 1592-5. 10.1055/s-2007-993740. http://www.ncbi.nlm.nih.gov/pubmed/17999354.

Beretta, G., E. Caneva and R. M. Facino. "Kynurenic acid in honey from arboreal plants: Ms and nmr evidence." *Planta Medica* 73 (2007): 1592-5. 10.1055/s-2007-993740. http://www.ncbi.nlm.nih.gov/pubmed/17999354.

Beretta, G., E. Caneva, L. Regazzoni, N. G. Bakhtyari and R. Maffei Facino. "A solid-phase extraction procedure coupled to 1h nmr, with chemometric analysis, to seek reliable markers of the botanical origin of honey." *Analytica Chimica Acta* 620 (2008): 176-82. 10.1016/j.aca.2008.05.025. http://www.ncbi.nlm.nih.gov/pubmed/18558139.

Bilikova, K., T. Kristof Krakova, K. Yamaguchi and Y. Yamaguchi. "Major royal jelly proteins as markers of authenticity and quality of honey." *Arhiv Za Higijenu Rada i Toksikologiju* 66 (2015): 259-67. 10.1515/aiht-2015-66-2653. http://www.ncbi.nlm.nih.gov/pubmed/26751857.

Blair, S. E., N. N. Cokcetin, E. J. Harry and D. A. Carter. "The unusual antibacterial activity of medical-grade leptospermum honey: Antibacterial spectrum, resistance and transcriptome analysis." *European Journal of Clinical Microbiology & Infectious Diseases* 28 (2009): 1199-208. 10.1007/s10096-009-0763-z. http://www.ncbi.nlm.nih.gov/pubmed/19513768.

Bleau, N., S. Bouslama, P. Giovenazzo and N. Derome. "Dynamics of the honeybee (apis mellifera) gut microbiota throughout the overwintering period in canada." *Microorganisms* 8 (2020): 10.3390/microorganisms8081146. http://www.ncbi.nlm.nih.gov/pubmed/32751209.

Boffo, E. F., L. A. Tavares, A. C. T. Tobias, M. M. C. Ferreira and A. G. Ferreira. "Identification of components of brazilian honey by 1h nmr and classification of its botanical origin by chemometric methods." *Lwt* 49 (2012): 55-63. 10.1016/j.lwt.2012.04.024.

Bogdanov, S. "Nature and origin of the antibacterial substances in honey." *LWT - Food Science and Technology* 30 (1997): 748-53. 10.1006/fstl.1997.0259.

Bogdanov, S., T. Jurendic, R. Sieber and P. Gallmann. "Honey for nutrition and health: A review." *Journal of the American College of Nutrition* 27 (2008): 677-89. 10.1080/07315724.2008.10719745. http://www.ncbi.nlm.nih.gov/pubmed/19155427.

Bogdanov, S., K. Ruoff and L. Persano Oddo. "Physico-chemical methods for the characterisation of unifloral honeys: A review." *Apidologie* 35 (2004): S4-S17. 10.1051/apido:2004047.

Borutinskaite, V., G. Treigyte, V. Čeksteryte, B. Kurtinaitiene and R. Navakauskienė. "Proteomic identification and enzymatic activity of buckwheat (fagopyrum esculentum) honey based on different assays." *Journal of Food and Nutrition Research* 57 (2018):

Bouzo, D., N. N. Cokcetin, L. Li, G. Ballerin, A. L. Bottomley, J. Lazenby, C. B. Whitchurch, I. T. Paulsen, K. A. Hassan and E. J. Harry. "Characterizing the mechanism of action of an ancient antimicrobial, manuka honey, against pseudomonas aeruginosa using modern transcriptomics." *mSystems* 5 (2020): 10.1128/mSystems.00106-20. http://www.ncbi.nlm.nih.gov/pubmed/32606022.

Bovo, S., V. J. Utzeri, A. Ribani, R. Cabbri and L. Fontanesi. "Shotgun sequencing of honey DNA can describe honey bee derived environmental signatures and the honey bee hologenome complexity." *Sci Rep* 10 (2020): 9279. 10.1038/s41598-020-66127-1. http://www.ncbi.nlm.nih.gov/pubmed/32518251.

Brudzynski, K. "Honey as an ecological reservoir of antibacterial compounds produced by antagonistic microbial interactions in plant nectars, honey and honey bee." *Antibiotics (Basel)* 10 (2021): 10.3390/antibiotics10050551. http://www.ncbi.nlm.nih.gov/pubmed/34065141.

Carter, D. A., S. E. Blair, N. N. Cokcetin, D. Bouzo, P. Brooks, R. Schothauer and E. J. Harry. "Therapeutic manuka honey: No longer so alternative." *Front Microbiol* 7 (2016): 569. 10.3389/fmicb.2016.00569. http://www.ncbi.nlm.nih.gov/pubmed/27148246.

Chanclud, E. and B. Lacombe. "Plant hormones: Key players in gut microbiota and human diseases?" *Trends in Plant Science* 22 (2017): 754-58. 10.1016/j.tplants.2017.07.003. http://www.ncbi.nlm.nih.gov/pubmed/28843313.

Chandran, C. H. and T. R. Keerthi. "Probiotic potency of lactobacillus plantarum kx519413 and kx519414 isolated from honey bee gut." *FEMS Microbiology Letters* 365 (2018): 10.1093/femsle/fnx285. http://www.ncbi.nlm.nih.gov/pubmed/29319821.

Chauhan, S. V. and M. R. Chorawala. "Probiotics, prebiotics, and synbiotics." *International Journal of Pharmaceutical Sciences and Research* 3 (2014): 711-26.

Chick, H., H. S. Shin and Z. Ustunol. "Growth and acid production by lactic acid bacteria and bifidobacteria grown in skim milk containing honey." *Journal of Food Science* 66 (2001): 478-81. 10.1111/j.1365-2621.2001.tb16134.x.

Chua, L. S., J. Y. Lee and G. F. Chan. "Characterization of the proteins in honey." *Analytical Letters* 48 (2014): 697-709. 10.1080/00032719.2014.952374.

Chua, L. S., N. L. A. Rahaman, N. A. Adnan and T. T. Eddie Tan. "Antioxidant activity of three honey samples in relation with their biochemical components." *J Anal Methods Chem* 2013 (2013): 313798. 10.1155/2013/313798. https://doi.org/10.1155/2013/313798.

Conway, P. L., R. Stern and L. Tran. *The value-adding potential of prebiotic components of australian honey*. Barton, Australia: Rural Industries Research and Development Corporation, 2010, 30.

Cooper, R. A., L. Jenkins, A. F. Henriques, R. S. Duggan and N. F. Burton. "Absence of bacterial resistance to medical-grade manuka honey." *European Journal of Clinical Microbiology & Infectious Diseases* 29 (2010): 1237-41. 10.1007/s10096-010-0992-1. http://www.ncbi.nlm.nih.gov/pubmed/20549529.

Corby-Harris, V., P. Maes and K. E. Anderson. "The bacterial communities associated with honey bee (apis mellifera) foragers." *Plos One* 9 (2014): 10.1371/journal.pone.0095056.

Crane, E. *A book of honey*. Oxford, UK: Oxford University Press, 1980,

Crittenden, A. N. "The importance of honey consumption in human evolution." *Food and Foodways* 19 (2011): 257-73. 10.1080/07409710.2011.630618.

da Silva, P. M., C. Gauche, L. V. Gonzaga, A. C. Costa and R. Fett. "Honey: Chemical composition, stability and authenticity." *Food Chemistry* 196 (2016): 309-23. 10.1016/j.foodchem.2015.09.051. http://www.ncbi.nlm.nih.gov/pubmed/26593496.

David, L. A., C. F. Maurice, R. N. Carmody, D. B. Gootenberg, J. E. Button, B. E. Wolfe, A. V. Ling, A. S. Devlin, Y. Varma, M. A. Fischbach, *et al.* "Diet rapidly and reproducibly alters the human gut microbiome." *Nature* 505 (2014): 559-63. 10.1038/nature12820. http://www.ncbi.nlm.nih.gov/pubmed/24336217.

de Melo, F. H. C., F. Menezes, J. M. B. de Sousa, M. Dos Santos Lima, G. da Silva Campelo Borges, E. L. de Souza and M. Magnani. "Prebiotic activity of monofloral honeys produced by stingless bees in the semi-arid region of brazilian northeastern toward lactobacillus acidophilus la-05 and bifidobacterium lactis bb-12." *Food Research International* 128 (2020): 108809. 10.1016/j.foodres.2019.108809. http://www.ncbi.nlm.nih.gov/pubmed/31955768.

Di Girolamo, F., A. D'Amato and P. G. Righetti. "Assessment of the floral origin of honey via proteomic tools." *Journal of Proteomics* 75 (2012): 3688-93. 10.1016/j.jprot.2012.04.029. http://www.ncbi.nlm.nih.gov/pubmed/22571915.

Dillon, R. J. and V. M. Dillon. "The gut bacteria of insects: Nonpathogenic interactions." *Annu Rev Entomol* 49 (2004): 71-92. 10.1146/annurev.ento.49.061802.123416. http://www.ncbi.nlm.nih.gov/pubmed/14651457.

Disayathanoowat, T., H. Li, N. Supapimon, N. Suwannarach, S. Lumyong, P. Chantawannakul and J. Guo. "Different dynamics of bacterial and fungal communities in hive-stored bee bread and their possible roles: A case study from two commercial honey bees in china." *Microorganisms* 8 (2020): 10.3390/microorganisms8020264. http://www.ncbi.nlm.nih.gov/pubmed/32075309.

Donarski, J. A., S. A. Jones and A. J. Charlton. "Application of cryoprobe 1h nuclear magnetic resonance spectroscopy and multivariate analysis for the verification of corsican honey." *Journal of Agricultural and Food Chemistry* 56 (2008): 5451-6. 10.1021/jf072402x. http://www.ncbi.nlm.nih.gov/pubmed/18564849.

Dong, Z. X., H. Y. Li, Y. F. Chen, F. Wang, X. Y. Deng, L. B. Lin, Q. L. Zhang, J. L. Li and J. Guo. "Colonization of the gut microbiota of honey bee (apis mellifera) workers at different developmental stages." *Microbiol Res* 231 (2020): 126370. 10.1016/j.micres.2019.126370. http://www.ncbi.nlm.nih.gov/pubmed/31739261.

El-Soud, N. H. A. "Honey between traditional uses and recent medicine." *Macedonian Journal of Medical Sciences* 5(2) (2012): 10.3889/MJMS.1857-5773.2012.0213.

Elzeini, H. M., A. Ali, N. F. Nasr, M. Hassan, A. A. M. Hassan and Y. E. Elenany. "Probiotic capability of novel lactic acid bacteria isolated from worker honey bees gut microbiota." *FEMS Microbiology Letters* 368 (2021): 10.1093/femsle/fnab030. http://www.ncbi.nlm.nih.gov/pubmed/33705519.

Engel, P., V. G. Martinson and N. a. Moran. "Functional diversity within the simple gut microbiota of the honey bee." *Proceedings of the ldots* 109 (2012): 11002-07. 10.1073/pnas.1202970109.

Engel, P. and N. A. Moran. "Functional and evolutionary insights into the simple yet specific gut microbiota of the honey bee from metagenomic analysis." *Gut Microbes* 4 (2013): 60-65. 10.4161/gmic.22517.

Escuredo, O., I. Dobre, M. Fernandez-Gonzalez and M. C. Seijo. "Contribution of botanical origin and sugar composition of honeys on the crystallization phenomenon." *Food Chemistry* 149 (2014): 84-90. 10.1016/j.foodchem.2013.10.097. http://www.ncbi.nlm.nih.gov/pubmed/24295680.

Ezz El-Arab, A. M., S. M. Girgis, E. M. Hegazy and A. B. Abd El-Khalek. "Effect of dietary honey on intestinal microflora and toxicity of mycotoxins in mice." *BMC Complementary and Alternative Medicine* 6 (2006): 6. 10.1186/1472-6882-6-6. http://www.ncbi.nlm.nih.gov/pubmed/16533410.

Fuandila, N. N., W. Widanarni and M. Yuhana. "Growth performance and immune response of prebiotic honey fed pacific white shrimp litopenaeus vannamei to vibrio parahaemolyticus infection." *Journal of Applied Aquaculture* 32 (2019): 221-35. 10.1080/10454438.2019.1615593.

Gibson, G. R. and M. B. Roberfroid. "Dietary modulation of the human colonic microbiota: Introducing the concept of prebiotics." *J Nutr* 125 (1995): 1401-12. 10.1093/jn/125.6.1401. http://www.ncbi.nlm.nih.gov/pubmed/7782892.

Gill, S. R., M. Pop, R. T. Deboy, P. B. Eckburg, P. J. Turnbaugh, B. S. Samuel, J. I. Gordon, D. A. Relman, C. M. Fraser-Liggett and K. E. Nelson. "Metagenomic analysis of the human distal gut microbiome." *Science* 312 (2006): 1355-9. 10.1126/science.1124234. http://www.ncbi.nlm.nih.gov/pubmed/16741115.

Gilliam, M., D. B. Prest and H. L. Morton. "Fungi isolated from honey bees, apis mellifera, fed 2,4-d and antibiotics." *Journal of Invertebrate Pathology* 24 (1974): 213-7. 10.1016/0022-2011(74)90013-5. http://www.ncbi.nlm.nih.gov/pubmed/4413522.

Goswami, M., S. Bhattacharjee, S. Bhattacharyya and C. Rai. "Antioxidant and antimicrobial activities of four characteristic honey samples produced in west bengal (india)." *Journal of Chemical and Pharmaceutical Research* 9 (2017): 315-22. www.jocpr.com.

Grizard, D. and C. Barthomeuf. "Non-digestible oligosaccharides used as prebiotic agents: Mode of production and beneficial effects on animal and human health." *Reprod Nutr Dev* 39 (1999): 563-88. 10.1051/rnd:19990505. http://www.ncbi.nlm.nih.gov/pubmed/10619166.

Hadagali, M. D. and L. S. Chua. "The anti-inflammatory and wound healing properties of honey." *European Food Research and Technology* 239 (2014): 1003-14. 10.1007/s00217-014-2297-6.

Haddadin, M. S. Y., I. N. S. Jamal Abu and R. K. Robinson. "Effect of honey on the growth and metabolism of two bacterial species of intestinal origin." *Pakistan Journal of Nutrition* 6 (2007): 693-97. 10.3923/pjn.2007.693.697.

Haffejee, I. E. and A. Moosa. "Honey in the treatment of infantile gastroenteritis." *British Medical Journal (Clinical Research Ed.)* 290 (1985): 1866-7. 10.1136/bmj.290.6485.1866. http://www.ncbi.nlm.nih.gov/pubmed/3924286.

Hammond, E. N. and E. S. Donkor. "Antibacterial effect of manuka honey on clostridium difficile." *BMC Research Notes* 6 (2013): 188. 10.1186/1756-0500-6-188. http://www.ncbi.nlm.nih.gov/pubmed/23651562.

Hasyimi, W., W. Widanarni and M. Yuhana. "Growth performance and intestinal microbiota diversity in pacific white shrimp litopenaeus vannamei fed with a probiotic bacterium, honey prebiotic, and synbiotic." *Current Microbiology* 77 (2020): 2982-90. 10.1007/s00284-020-02117-w. http://www.ncbi.nlm.nih.gov/pubmed/32683466.

Henriques, A. F., R. E. Jenkins, N. F. Burton and R. A. Cooper. "The intracellular effects of manuka honey on staphylococcus aureus." *European Journal of Clinical Microbiology & Infectious Diseases* 29 (2010): 45-50. 10.1007/s10096-009-0817-2. http://www.ncbi.nlm.nih.gov/pubmed/19813035.

Hilgarth, M., J. Redwitz, M. A. Ehrmann, R. F. Vogel and F. Jakob. "Bombella favorum sp. Nov. And bombella mellum sp. Nov., two novel species isolated from the honeycombs of apis mellifera." *Int J Syst Evol Microbiol* 71 (2021): 10.1099/ijsem.0.004633. http://www.ncbi.nlm.nih.gov/pubmed/33439113.

Hmood, K. A., A. H. Habeeb and K. I. Al-Mhnna. "Antioxidant role of lactobacillus sp isolated from honey bee against histological effects of ochratoxin in vivo." *Al-Kufa University Journal for Biology* 11 (2019): 67-80.

Hong, S. G., J. Chun, H. W. Oh and K. S. Bae. "Metschnikowia koreensis sp. Nov., a novel yeast species isolated from flowers in korea." *Int J Syst Evol Microbiol* 51 (2001): 1927-31. 10.1099/00207713-51-5-1927. http://www.ncbi.nlm.nih.gov/pubmed/11594627.

Horton, M. A., R. Oliver and I. L. Newton. "No apparent correlation between honey bee forager gut microbiota and honey production." *PeerJ* 3 (2015): 1329. 10.7717/peerj.1329.

Iorizzo, M., Testa, B., Ganassi, S., Lombardi, S. J., Ianiro, M., Letizia, F., Succi, M., Tremonte, P., Vergalito, F., Cozzolino, A., Sorrentino, E., Petrarca, S., De Cristofaro, A., & Coppola, R. "Probiotic properties and potentiality of lactiplantibacillus plantarum strains for the biological control of chalkbrood disease." *J Fungi (Basel)* 7 (2021): 379. 10.3390/jof7050379. http://www.ncbi.nlm.nih.gov/pubmed/34066127.

Irish, J., S. Blair and D. A. Carter. "The antibacterial activity of honey derived from australian flora." *Plos One* 6 (2011): e18229. 10.1371/journal.pone.0018229. http://www.ncbi.nlm.nih.gov/pubmed/21464891.

Jan Mei, S., M. Mohd Nordin and A. Norrakiah. "Fructooligosaccharides in honey and effects of honey on growth of bifidobacterium longum bb 536." *International Food Research Journal* 17 (2010): 557-61.

Jenkins, R., N. Burton and R. Cooper. "Effect of manuka honey on the expression of universal stress protein a in meticillin-resistant staphylococcus aureus." *International Journal of Antimicrobial Agents* 37 (2011): 373-6. 10.1016/j.ijantimicag.2010. 11.036. http://www.ncbi.nlm.nih.gov/pubmed/21349691.

Jenkins, R., N. Burton and R. Cooper. "Proteomic and genomic analysis of methicillin-resistant staphylococcus aureus (mrsa) exposed to manuka honey in vitro demonstrated down-regulation of virulence markers." *Journal of Antimicrobial Chemotherapy* 69 (2014): 603-15. 10.1093/jac/dkt430. http://www.ncbi.nlm.nih.gov/ pubmed/24176984.

Jiang, L., M. H. Xie, G. J. Chen, J. T. Qiao, H. C. Zhang and X. X. Zeng. "Phenolics and carbohydrates in buckwheat honey regulate the human intestinal microbiota." *Evidence-Based Complementary and Alternative Medicine* 2020 (2020): Artn 6432942 10.1155/2020/6432942. <Go to ISI>://WOS:000522430800004.

Johnston, M., M. McBride, D. Dahiya, R. Owusu-Apenten and P. S. Nigam. "Antibacterial activity of manuka honey and its components: An overview." *AIMS microbiology* 4 (2018): 655-64. 10.3934/microbiol.2018.4.655. http://www.ncbi. nlm.nih.gov/pubmed/31294240.

Jones, J. C., C. Fruciano, F. Hildebrand, H. Al Toufalilia, N. J. Balfour, P. Bork, P. Engel, F. L. W. Ratnieks and W. O. H. Hughes. "Gut microbiota composition is associated with environmental landscape in honey bees." *Ecology and Evolution* 8 (2017): 441-51. 10.1002/ece3.3597.

Kacaniova, M., S. Pavlicova, P. Hascik, G. Kociubinski, V. Knazovicka, M. Sudzina, J. Sudzinova and M. Fikselova. "Microbial communities in bees, pollen and honey from slovakia." *Acta Microbiologica et Immunologica Hungarica* 56 (2009): 285-95. 10.1556/AMicr.56.2009.3.7. http://www.ncbi.nlm.nih.gov/pubmed/19789142.

Kafantaris, I., G. D. Amoutzias and D. Mossialos. "Foodomics in bee product research: A systematic literature review." *European Food Research and Technology* 247 (2020): 309-31. 10.1007/s00217-020-03634-5.

Karabagias, I. K. "A targeted metabolomic procedure for the identification of isophorone related compounds in honey." *Journal of Plant Biochemistry & Physiology* 06 (2018): 10.4172/2329-9029.1000210.

Kenfack, H. M. C., Z. F. Ngoufack, M. P. Kaktcham, R. Y. Wang, T. Zhu and L. Yin. "Safety and antioxidant properties of five probiotic lactobacillus plantarum strains isolated from the digestive tract of honey bees." *American Journal of Microbiological Research* 6 (2018): 1-8. 10.12691/ajmr-6-1-1.

Kešnerová, L., O. Emery, M. Troilo, J. Liberti, B. Erkosar and P. Engel. "Gut microbiota structure differs between honeybees in winter and summer." *ISME J* 14 (2020): 801-14. 10.1038/s41396-019-0568-8. http://www.ncbi.nlm.nih.gov/pubmed/31836840.

Kešnerová, L., R. Moritz and P. Engel. "Bartonella apis sp. Nov., a honey bee gut symbiont of the class alphaproteobacteria." *International Journal of Systematic and Evolutionary Microbiology* 66 (2016): 414-21. 10.1099/ijsem.0.000736.

Kňazovická, V. "Diversity of bacteria in slovak and foreign honey, with assessment of its physico-chemical quality and counts of cultivable microorganisms." *Journal of Microbiology, Biotechnology and Food Sciences* 9 (2019): 414-21. 10.15414/jmbfs.2019.9.special.414-421.

Kolayli, S., L. Boukraâ, H. Sahin and F. Abdellah. *Chapter 1. Sugars in honey*. London: UK: The Royal Society of Chemistry, 2012,

Kurek-Gorecka, A., M. Gorecki, A. Rzepecka-Stojko, R. Balwierz and J. Stojko. "Bee products in dermatology and skin care." *Molecules* 25 (2020): 10.3390/molecules 25030556. http://www.ncbi.nlm.nih.gov/pubmed/32012913.

Kuropatnicki, A. K., M. Kłósek and M. Kucharzewski. "Honey as medicine: Historical perspectives." *Journal of Apicultural Research* 57 (2018): 113-18. 10.1080/002 18839.2017.1411182.

Kwakman, P. H., A. A. te Velde, L. de Boer, D. Speijer, C. M. Vandenbroucke-Grauls and S. A. Zaat. "How honey kills bacteria." *FASEB journal : official publication of the Federation of American Societies for Experimental Biology* 24 (2010): 2576-82. 10.1096/fj.09-150789. http://www.ncbi.nlm.nih.gov/pubmed/20228250.

Kwong, W. K. and N. A. Moran. *Gut microbial communities of social bees*. 14. 2016.

Kwong, W. K., M. I. Steele and N. A. Moran. "Genome sequences of apibacter spp., gut symbionts of asian honey bees." *Genome Biology and Evolution* 10 (2018): 1174-79. 10.1093/gbe/evy076. http://www.ncbi.nlm.nih.gov/pubmed/29635372.

Lambert, O., M. Piroux, S. Puyo, C. Thorin, M. Larhantec, F. Delbac and H. Pouliquen. "Bees, honey and pollen as sentinels for lead environmental contamination." *Environ Pollut* 170 (2012): 254-9. 10.1016/j.envpol.2012.07.012. http://www.ncbi.nlm.nih.gov/pubmed/22842054.

Lee, J. H., J. H. Park, J. A. Kim, G. P. Neupane, M. H. Cho, C. S. Lee and J. Lee. "Low concentrations of honey reduce biofilm formation, quorum sensing, and virulence in escherichia coli o157:H7." *Biofouling* 27 (2011): 1095-104. 10.1080/08927014.2011.633704. http://www.ncbi.nlm.nih.gov/pubmed/22047137.

Li, J. H., J. D. Evans, W. F. Li, Y. Z. Zhao, G. DeGrandi-Hoffman, S. K. Huang, Z. G. Li, M. Hamilton and Y. P. Chen. "New evidence showing that the destruction of gut bacteria by antibiotic treatment could increase the honey bee's vulnerability to nosema infection." *Plos One* 12 (2017): e0187505. 10.1371/journal.pone.0187505. http://www.ncbi.nlm.nih.gov/pubmed/29125851.

Li, Y., S. Long, Q. Liu, H. Ma, J. Li, W. Xiaoqing, J. Yuan, M. Li and B. Hou. "Gut microbiota is involved in the alleviation of loperamide-induced constipation by honey supplementation in mice." *Food Sci Nutr* 8 (2020): 4388-98. 10.1002/fsn3.1736. http://www.ncbi.nlm.nih.gov/pubmed/32884719.

Lievens, B., J. E. Hallsworth, M. I. Pozo, Z. B. Belgacem, A. Stevenson, K. A. Willems and H. Jacquemyn. "Microbiology of sugar-rich environments: Diversity, ecology and system constraints." *Environ Microbiol* 17 (2015): 278-98. 10.1111/1462-2920.12570. http://www.ncbi.nlm.nih.gov/pubmed/25041632.

Lin, S. M., P. C. Molan and R. T. Cursons. "The in vitro susceptibility of campylobacter spp. To the antibacterial effect of manuka honey." *European Journal of Clinical Microbiology & Infectious Diseases* 28 (2009): 339-44. 10.1007/s10096-008-0630-3. http://www.ncbi.nlm.nih.gov/pubmed/18818958.

Lin, S. M., P. C. Molan and R. T. Cursons. "The controlled in vitro susceptibility of gastrointestinal pathogens to the antibacterial effect of manuka honey." *European Journal of Clinical Microbiology & Infectious Diseases* 30 (2011): 569-74. 10.1007/s10096-010-1121-x. http://www.ncbi.nlm.nih.gov/pubmed/21165664.

Lobo, V., A. Patil, A. Phatak and N. Chandra. "Free radicals, antioxidants and functional foods: Impact on human health." *Pharmacognosy Reviews* 4 (2010): 118-26. 10.4103/0973-7847.70902. http://www.ncbi.nlm.nih.gov/pubmed/22228951.

Lolli, M., D. Bertelli, M. Plessi, A. G. Sabatini and C. Restani. "Classification of italian honeys by 2d hr-nmr." *Journal of Agricultural and Food Chemistry* 56 (2008): 1298-304. 10.1021/jf072763c. http://www.ncbi.nlm.nih.gov/pubmed/18205311.

Lu, J., Carter, D. A., Turnbull, L., Rosendale, D., Hedderley, D., Stephens, J., Gannabathula, S., Steinhorn, G., Schlothauer, R. C., Whitchurch, C. B., & Harry, E. J. "The effect of new zealand kanuka, manuka and clover honeys on bacterial growth dynamics and cellular morphology varies according to the species." *Plos One* 8 (2013): e55898. 10.1371/journal.pone.0055898. http://www.ncbi.nlm.nih.gov/pubmed/23418472.

Lu, J., L. Turnbull, C. M. Burke, M. Liu, D. A. Carter, R. C. Schlothauer, C. B. Whitchurch and E. J. Harry. "Manuka-type honeys can eradicate biofilms produced by staphylococcus aureus strains with different biofilm-forming abilities." *PeerJ* 2 (2014): e326. 10.7717/peerj.326. http://www.ncbi.nlm.nih.gov/pubmed/24711974.

Lučan, M., V. Slačanac, J. Hardi, M. Krešimir, J. Babic, V. Krstanović and J. Marko. "Inhibitory effect of honey-sweetened goat and cow milk fermented with bifidobacterium lactis bb-12 on the growth of listeria monocytogenes." *Mljekarstvo* 59 (2009): 96–106.

Luong, V., N. Tam, D. Xuan and N. Tai. "Nmr based metabolomic approach for evaluation of vietnamese honey." *Vietnam Journal of Chemistry* 57 (2019): 712-16. 10.1002/vjch.2019000101.

Machado De-Melo, A., L. De Almeida-Muradian, M. Sancho and A. Pascual Maté. "Composition and properties of apis mellifera honey: A review." *Journal of Apicultural Research* 57 (2017): 1-33. 10.1080/00218839.2017.1338444.

Maddocks, S. E. and R. E. Jenkins. "Honey: A sweet solution to the growing problem of antimicrobial resistance?" *Future Microbiology* 8 (2013): 1419-29. 10.2217/fmb.13.105. http://www.ncbi.nlm.nih.gov/pubmed/24199801.

Manning, T. S. and G. R. Gibson. "Microbial-gut interactions in health and disease. Prebiotics." *Best Practice & Research: Clinical Gastroenterology* 18 (2004): 287-98. 10.1016/j.bpg.2003.10.008. http://www.ncbi.nlm.nih.gov/pubmed/15123070.

Martinson, V. G., J. Moy and N. A. Moran. "Establishment of characteristic gut bacteria during development of the honeybee worker." *Appl Environ Microbiol* 78 (2012): 2830-40. 10.1128/AEM.07810-11. http://www.ncbi.nlm.nih.gov/pubmed/22307297.

Miguel, M. G., M. D. Antunes and M. L. Faleiro. "Honey as a complementary medicine." *Integrative Medicine Insights* 12 (2017): 1178633717702869. 10.1177/1178633717702869. http://www.ncbi.nlm.nih.gov/pubmed/28469409.

Mohan, A., S. Y. Quek, N. Gutierrez-Maddox, Y. Gao and Q. Shu. "Effect of honey in improving the gut microbial balance." *Food Quality and Safety* 1 (2017): 107-15. 10.1093/fqsafe/fyx015.

Mohr, K. I. and C. C. Tebbe. "Diversity and phylotype consistency of bacteria in the guts of three bee species (apoidea) at an oilseed rape field." *Environ Microbiol* 8 (2006): 258-72. 10.1111/j.1462-2920.2005.00893.x. http://www.ncbi.nlm.nih.gov/pubmed/16423014.

Molan, P. "Why honey is effective as a medicine." *Bee World* 82 (2015): 22-40. 10.1080/0005772x.2001.11099498.

Nagpal, R. and A. Kaur. "Synbiotic effect of various prebiotics on in vitro activities of probiotic lactobacilli." *Ecology of Food and Nutrition* 50 (2011): 63-8. 10.1080/03670244.2011.539161. http://www.ncbi.nlm.nih.gov/pubmed/21888588.

Naseer, S., S. Khan and K. Azim. "Identification of cultivable bacteria from natural honey of different botanical origin." *Pakistan Journal of Biochemistry and Molecular Biology* 48 (2015): 53-56.

Niode, N. J., C. L. Salaki, L. J. M. Rumokoy and T. E. Tallei. "Lactic acid bacteria from honey bees digestive tract and their potential as probiotics." *Proceedings of the International Conference and the 10th Congress of the Entomological Society of Indonesia (Iccesi 2019)* 8 (2020): 236-41. <Go to ISI>://WOS:000558724300041.

Nooh, H. Z. and N. M. Nour-Eldien. "The dual anti-inflammatory and antioxidant activities of natural honey promote cell proliferation and neural regeneration in a rat model of colitis." *Acta Histochem* 118 (2016): 588-95. 10.1016/j.acthis.2016.06.006. http://www.ncbi.nlm.nih.gov/pubmed/27378376.

Nowak, A., D. Szczuka, A. Gorczynska, I. Motyl and D. Kregiel. "Characterization of apis mellifera gastrointestinal microbiota and lactic acid bacteria for honeybee protection-a review." *Cells* 10 (2021): 10.3390/cells10030701. http://www.ncbi.nlm.nih.gov/pubmed/33809924.

Olaitan, P. B., O. E. Adeleke and I. O. Ola. "Honey: A reservoir for microorganisms and an inhibitory agent for microbes." *African Health Sciences* 7 (2007): 159-65. 10.5555/afhs.2007.7.3.159. http://www.ncbi.nlm.nih.gov/pubmed/18052870.

Olawode, E. O., R. Tandlich and G. Cambray. "(1)h-nmr profiling and chemometric analysis of selected honeys from south africa, zambia, and slovakia." *Molecules* 23 (2018): 10.3390/molecules23030578. http://www.ncbi.nlm.nih.gov/pubmed/29510542.

Olofsson, T. C., M. Alsterfjord, B. Nilson, E. Butler and A. Vasquez. "Lactobacillus apinorum sp. Nov., lactobacillus mellifer sp. Nov., lactobacillus mellis sp. Nov., lactobacillus melliventris sp. Nov., lactobacillus kimbladii sp. Nov., lactobacillus helsingborgensis sp. Nov. And lactobacillus kullabergensis sp. Nov., isolated from the honey stomach of the honeybee apis mellifera." *International Journal of Systematic and Evolutionary Microbiology* 64 (2014): 3109-19. 10.1099/ijs.0.059600-0. http://www.ncbi.nlm.nih.gov/pubmed/24944337.

Olofsson, T. C., E. Butler, P. Markowicz, C. Lindholm, L. Larsson and A. Vasquez. "Lactic acid bacterial symbionts in honeybees - an unknown key to honey's antimicrobial and therapeutic activities." *International Wound Journal* 13 (2016): 668-79. 10.1111/iwj.12345. http://www.ncbi.nlm.nih.gov/pubmed/25195876.

Olofsson, T. C. and A. Vasquez. "Detection and identification of a novel lactic acid bacterial flora within the honey stomach of the honeybee apis mellifera." *Current Microbiology* 57 (2008): 356-63. 10.1007/s00284-008-9202-0. http://www.ncbi.nlm.nih.gov/pubmed/18663527.

Ottman, N., H. Smidt, W. M. de Vos and C. Belzer. "The function of our microbiota: Who is out there and what do they do?" *Front Cell Infect Microbiol* 2 (2012): 104. 10.3389/fcimb.2012.00104. http://www.ncbi.nlm.nih.gov/pubmed/22919693.

Packer, J. M., J. Irish, B. R. Herbert, C. Hill, M. Padula, S. E. Blair, D. A. Carter and E. J. Harry. "Specific non-peroxide antibacterial effect of manuka honey on the staphylococcus aureus proteome." *International Journal of Antimicrobial Agents* 40 (2012): 43-50. 10.1016/j.ijantimicag.2012.03.012. http://www.ncbi.nlm.nih.gov/pubmed/22580031.

Patruica, S. and D. Mot. "The effect of using prebiotic and probiotic products on intestinal micro-flora of the honeybee (apis mellifera carpatica)." *Bull Entomol Res* 102 (2012): 619-23. 10.1017/S0007485312000144. http://www.ncbi.nlm.nih.gov/pubmed/22459313.

Persano Oddo, L., M. G. Piazza, A. G. Sabatini and M. Accorti. "Characterization of unifloral honeys." *Apidologie* 26 (1995): 453-65. 10.1051/apido:19950602.

Popa, D. and Z. Ustunol. "Influence of sucrose, high fructose corn syrup and honey from different floral sources on growth and acid production by lactic acid bacteria and bifidobacteria." *International Journal of Dairy Technology* 64 (2011): 247-53. 10.1111/j.1471-0307.2011.00666.x.

Powell, J. E., V. G. Martinson, K. Urban-Mead and N. A. Moran. "Routes of acquisition of the gut microbiota of the honey bee apis mellifera." *Appl Environ Microbiol* 80 (2014): 7378-87. 10.1128/AEM.01861-14. http://www.ncbi.nlm.nih.gov/pubmed/25239900.

Ranneh, Y., A. M. Akim, H. A. Hamid, H. Khazaai, A. Fadel, Z. A. Zakaria, M. Albujja and M. F. A. Bakar. "Honey and its nutritional and anti-inflammatory value." *BMC Complement Med Ther* 21 (2021): 30. 10.1186/s12906-020-03170-5. http://www.ncbi.nlm.nih.gov/pubmed/33441127.

Raschka, L. and H. Daniel. "Mechanisms underlying the effects of inulin-type fructans on calcium absorption in the large intestine of rats." *Bone* 37 (2005): 728-35. 10.1016/j.bone.2005.05.015. http://www.ncbi.nlm.nih.gov/pubmed/16126464.

Rayes, A. A. H. "Enhancement of probiotic bioactivity by some prebiotics to produce bio-fermented milk." *Life Science Journal* 9 (2012): 2246-53.

Raymann, K., L. M. Bobay and N. A. Moran. "Antibiotics reduce genetic diversity of core species in the honeybee gut microbiome." *Molecular Ecology* 27 (2018): 2057-66. 10.1111/mec.14434. http://www.ncbi.nlm.nih.gov/pubmed/29164717.

Razali, M., Zainal, Z., Maulidiani, M., Shaari, K., Zamri, Z., Mohd Idrus, M., Khatib, A., Abas, F., Ling, Y., Rui, L., & Ismail, I. "Classification of raw stingless bee honeys by bee species origins using the nmr- and lc-ms-based metabolomics approach." *Molecules* 23 (2018): 10.3390/molecules23092160. http://www.ncbi.nlm.nih.gov/pubmed/30154302.

Rissato, S., M. Galhiane, M. Dealmeida, M. Gerenutti and B. Apon. "Multiresidue determination of pesticides in honey samples by gas chromatography–mass spectrometry and application in environmental contamination." *Food Chemistry* 101 (2007): 1719-26. 10.1016/j.foodchem.2005.10.034.

Roberfroid, M., G. R. Gibson, L. Hoyles, A. L. McCartney, R. Rastall, I. Rowland, D. Wolvers, B. Watzl, H. Szajewska, B. Stahl, *et al.* "Prebiotic effects: Metabolic and health benefits." *Br J Nutr* 104 Suppl 2 (2010): S1-63. 10.1017/S0007114510003363. http://www.ncbi.nlm.nih.gov/pubmed/20920376.

Roberts, A. E., S. E. Maddocks and R. A. Cooper. "Manuka honey reduces the motility of pseudomonas aeruginosa by suppression of flagella-associated genes." *Journal of Antimicrobial Chemotherapy* 70 (2015): 716-25. 10.1093/jac/dku448. http://www.ncbi.nlm.nih.gov/pubmed/25404649.

Rodriguez-Flores, M. S., O. Escuredo, M. Miguez and M. C. Seijo. "Differentiation of oak honeydew and chestnut honeys from the same geographical origin using chemometric methods." *Food Chemistry* 297 (2019): 124979. 10.1016/j.foodchem.2019.124979. http://www.ncbi.nlm.nih.gov/pubmed/31253311.

Rosendale, D. I., I. S. Maddox, M. C. Miles, M. Rodier, M. Skinner and J. Sutherland. "High-throughput microbial bioassays to screen potential new zealand functional food ingredients intended to manage the growth of probiotic and pathogenic gut bacteria." *International Journal of Food Science & Technology* 43 (2008): 2257-67. 10.1111/j.1365-2621.2008.01863.x.

Rosli, F. N., M. H. F. Hazemi, M. A. Akbar, S. Basir, H. Kassim and H. Bunawan. "Stingless bee honey: Evaluating its antibacterial activity and bacterial diversity." *Insects* 11 (2020): 10.3390/insects11080500. http://www.ncbi.nlm.nih.gov/pubmed/32759701.

Rossano, R., M. Larocca, T. Polito, A. M. Perna, M. C. Padula, G. Martelli and P. Riccio. "What are the proteolytic enzymes of honey and what they do tell us? A fingerprint analysis by 2-d zymography of unifloral honeys." *Plos One* 7 (2012): e49164. 10.1371/journal.pone.0049164. http://www.ncbi.nlm.nih.gov/pubmed/23145107.

Ruiz-Argueso, T. and A. Rodriguez-Navarro. "Microbiology of ripening honey." *Applied Microbiology* 30 (1975): 893-6. 10.1128/am.30.6.893-896.1975. http://www.ncbi.nlm.nih.gov/pubmed/16350044.

Saba, Z., M. Suzana and M. Anum. "Honey: Food or medicine." *Med Health*. 2013 (2013): 3-18.

Sanz, M. L., M. González, C. de Lorenzo, J. Sanz and I. Martínez-Castro. "Carbohydrate composition and physico chemical properties of artisanal honeys from madrid(spain):

Occurrence ofechium sp honey." *Journal of the Science of Food and Agriculture* 84 (2004): 1577-84. 10.1002/jsfa.1823.

Sanz, M. L., N. Polemis, V. Morales, N. Corzo, A. Drakoularakou, G. R. Gibson and R. A. Rastall. "In vitro investigation into the potential prebiotic activity of honey oligosaccharides." *Journal of Agricultural and Food Chemistry* 53 (2005): 2914-21. 10.1021/jf0500684. http://www.ncbi.nlm.nih.gov/pubmed/15826039.

Schell, K. R., K. E. Fernandes, E. Shanahan, I. Wilson, S. E. Blair, D. A. Carter and N. N. Cokcetin. "The potential of honey as a prebiotic food to re-engineer the gut microbiome toward a healthy state." *Frontiers in Nutrition* 9 (2022): 957932. 10.3389/fnut.2022.957932. http://www.ncbi.nlm.nih.gov/pubmed/35967810.

Schievano, E., E. Peggion and S. Mammi. "1h nuclear magnetic resonance spectra of chloroform extracts of honey for chemometric determination of its botanical origin." *Journal of Agricultural and Food Chemistry* 58 (2010): 57-65. 10.1021/jf9022977. http://www.ncbi.nlm.nih.gov/pubmed/19938861.

Schievano, E., M. Stocchero, E. Morelato, C. Facchin and S. Mammi. "An nmr-based metabolomic approach to identify the botanical origin of honey." *Metabolomics* 8 (2011): 679-90. 10.1007/s11306-011-0362-8.

Schramm, D. D., M. Karim, H. R. Schrader, R. R. Holt, M. Cardetti and C. L. Keen. "Honey with high levels of antioxidants can provide protection to healthy human subjects." *Journal of Agricultural and Food Chemistry* 51 (2003): 1732-5. 10.1021/jf025928k. http://www.ncbi.nlm.nih.gov/pubmed/12617614.

Seraglio, S. K. T., B. Silva, G. Bergamo, P. Brugnerotto, L. V. Gonzaga, R. Fett and A. C. O. Costa. "An overview of physicochemical characteristics and health-promoting properties of honeydew honey." *Food Research International* 119 (2019): 44-66. 10.1016/j.foodres.2019.01.028. http://www.ncbi.nlm.nih.gov/pubmed/30884675.

Shamala, T. R., Y. Shri Jyothi and P. Saibaba. "Stimulatory effect of honey on multiplication of lactic acid bacteria under in vitro and in vivo conditions." *Letters in Applied Microbiology* 30 (2000): 453-5. 10.1046/j.1472-765x.2000.00746.x. http://www.ncbi.nlm.nih.gov/pubmed/10849275.

Shin, H. S. and Z. Ustunol. "Carbohydrate composition of honey from different floral sources and their influence on growth of selected intestinal bacteria: An in vitro comparison." *Food Research International* 38 (2005): 721-28. 10.1016/j.foodres. 2005.01.007.

Sinacori, M., N. Francesca, A. Alfonzo, M. Cruciata, C. Sannino, L. Settanni and G. Moschetti. "Cultivable microorganisms associated with honeys of different geographical and botanical origin." *Food Microbiology* 38 (2014): 284-94. 10.1016/j.fm.2013.07.013. http://www.ncbi.nlm.nih.gov/pubmed/24290653.

Slačanac, V., M. lučan, J. Hardi, V. KrstanoviĆ and D. Koceva KomleniĆ. "Fermentation of honey-sweetened soymilk with bifidobacterium lactis bb-12 and bifidobacterium longum bb-46: Fermentation activity of bifidobacteria and in vitro antagonistic effect against listeria monocytogenes fsl n1-017." *Czech Journal of Food Sciences* 30 (2012): 321-29. 10.17221/190/2011-cjfs.

SN., S. "Honey regimen in gastrointestinal disorders." *Bulletin of Islamic Medicine* 1 (1981): 358–62.

Snowdon, J. A. and D. O. Cliver. "Microorganisms in honey." *International Journal of Food Microbiology* 31 (1996): 1-26. 10.1016/0168-1605(96)00970-1. http://www.ncbi.nlm.nih.gov/pubmed/8880294.

Subotic, S., A. M. Boddicker, V. M. Nguyen, J. Rivers, C. E. Briles and A. C. Mosier. "Honey bee microbiome associated with different hive and sample types over a honey production season." *Plos One* 14 (2019): e0223834. 10.1371/journal.pone.0223834. http://www.ncbi.nlm.nih.gov/pubmed/31703071.

Tanes, C., K. Bittinger, Y. Gao, E. S. Friedman, L. Nessel, U. R. Paladhi, L. Chau, E. Panfen, M. A. Fischbach, J. Braun, *et al.* "Role of dietary fiber in the recovery of the human gut microbiome and its metabolome." *Cell Host Microbe* 29 (2021): 394-407 e5. 10.1016/j.chom.2020.12.012. http://www.ncbi.nlm.nih.gov/pubmed/33440171.

Tola, Y. H., J. W. Waweru, G. D. D. Hurst, B. Slippers and J. C. Paredes. "Characterization of the kenyan honey bee (apis mellifera) gut microbiota: A first look at tropical and sub-saharan african bee associated microbiomes." *Microorganisms* 8 (2020): 10.3390/microorganisms8111721. http://www.ncbi.nlm.nih.gov/pubmed/33153032.

Turski, M. P., M. Turska, W. Zgrajka, D. Kuc and W. A. Turski. "Presence of kynurenic acid in food and honeybee products." *Amino Acids* 36 (2009): 75-80. 10.1007/s00726-008-0031-z. http://www.ncbi.nlm.nih.gov/pubmed/18231708.

Ustunol, Z. and H. Gandhi. "Growth and viability of commercial bifidobacterium spp. In honey-sweetened skim milk." *Journal of Food Protection* 64 (2001): 1775-9. 10.4315/0362-028x-64.11.1775. http://www.ncbi.nlm.nih.gov/pubmed/11726158.

Vahdat Shariatpanahi, Z., F. Jamshidi, J. Nasrollahzadeh, Z. Amiri and H. Teymourian. "Effect of honey on diarrhea and fecal microbiotain in critically ill tube-fed patients: A single center randomized controlled study." *Anesthesia and Pain Medicine* 8 (2018): e62889. 10.5812/aapm.62889. http://www.ncbi.nlm.nih.gov/pubmed/29868456.

Vallianou, N. G. "Honey and its anti-inflammatory, anti-bacterial and anti-oxidant properties." *General Medicine: Open Access* 02 (2014): 10.4172/2327-5146.1000132.

Vásquez, A., E. Forsgren, I. Fries, R. J. Paxton, E. Flaberg, L. Szekely and T. C. Olofsson. "Symbionts as major modulators of insect health: Lactic acid bacteria and honeybees." *Plos One* 7 (2012): e33188. 10.1371/annotation/3ac2b867-c013-4504-9e06-bebf3fa039d1. https://doi.org/10.1371/annotation/3ac2b867-c013-4504-9e06-bebf3fa039d1.

Vásquez, A., T. C. Olofsson and D. Sammataro. "A scientific note on the lactic acid bacterial flora in honeybees in the USA – a comparison with bees from sweden." *Apidologie* 40 (2008): 26-28. 10.1051/apido:2008063.

Vojvodic, S., S. M. Rehan and K. E. Anderson. "Microbial gut diversity of africanized and european honey bee larval instars." *Plos One* 8 (2013): e72106. 10.1371/journal.pone.0072106. http://www.ncbi.nlm.nih.gov/pubmed/23991051.

Wallace, A., S. Eady, M. Miles, H. Martin, A. McLachlan, M. Rodier, J. Willis, R. Scott and J. Sutherland. "Demonstrating the safety of manuka honey umf (r) 20+in a human clinical trial with healthy individuals." *British Journal of Nutrition* 103 (2010): 1023-28. 10.1017/S0007114509992777. <Go to ISI>://WOS:000277168100011.

Wang, K., J. Li, L. Zhao, X. Mu, C. Wang, M. Wang, X. Xue, S. Qi and L. Wu. "Gut microbiota protects honey bees (apis mellifera l.) against polystyrene microplastics exposure risks." *Journal of Hazardous Materials* 402 (2021): 123828. 10.1016/j.jhazmat.2020.123828. http://www.ncbi.nlm.nih.gov/pubmed/33254809.

Wang, K., Z. R. Wan, A. Q. Ou, X. W. Liang, X. X. Guo, Z. Y. Zhang, L. M. Wu and X. F. Xue. "Monofloral honey from a medical plant, prunella vulgaris, protected against dextran sulfate sodium-induced ulcerative colitis via modulating gut microbial populations in rats." *Food & Function* 10 (2019): 3828-38. 10.1039/c9fo00460b. <Go to ISI>://WOS:000476683600059.

Wang, Q., W. J. Cai, L. Yu, J. Ding and Y. Q. Feng. "Comprehensive profiling of phytohormones in honey by sequential liquid-liquid extraction coupled with liquid chromatography-mass spectrometry." *Journal of Agricultural and Food Chemistry* 65 (2017): 575-85. 10.1021/acs.jafc.6b04234. http://www.ncbi.nlm.nih.gov/pubmed/28032995.

Wen, Y., L. Wang, Y. Jin, J. Zhang, L. Su, X. Zhang, J. Zhou and Y. Li. "The microbial community dynamics during the vitex honey ripening process in the honeycomb." *Front Microbiol* 8 (2017): 1649. 10.3389/fmicb.2017.01649. http://www.ncbi.nlm.nih.gov/pubmed/28912763.

Weston, R. J. and L. K. Brocklebank. "The oligosaccharide composition of some new zealand honeys." *Food Chemistry* 64 (1999): 33-37. 10.1016/s0308-8146(98)00099-5.

Willix, D. J., P. C. Molan and C. G. Harfoot. "A comparison of the sensitivity of wound-infecting species of bacteria to the antibacterial activity of manuka honey and other honey." *J Appl Bacteriol* 73 (1992): 388-94. 10.1111/j.1365-2672.1992.tb04993.x. http://www.ncbi.nlm.nih.gov/pubmed/1447054.

Wu, Y., Y. Zheng, Y. Chen, S. Wang, Y. Chen, F. Hu and H. Zheng. "Honey bee (apis mellifera) gut microbiota promotes host endogenous detoxification capability via regulation of p450 gene expression in the digestive tract." *Microbial Biotechnology* 13 (2020): 1201-12. 10.1111/1751-7915.13579. http://www.ncbi.nlm.nih.gov/pubmed/32338446.

Xiong, Z. R., J. H. Sogin and R. W. Worobo. "Microbiome analysis of raw honey reveals important factors influencing the bacterial and fungal communities." *Front Microbiol* 13 (2022): 1099522. 10.3389/fmicb.2022.1099522. http://www.ncbi.nlm.nih.gov/pubmed/36713191.

Zhang, Y. Z., Y. F. Chen, Y. Q. Wu, J. J. Si, C. P. Zhang, H. Q. Zheng and F. L. Hu. "Discrimination of the entomological origin of honey according to the secretions of the bee (apis cerana or apis mellifera)." *Food Research International* 116 (2019): 362-69. 10.1016/j.foodres.2018.08.049. http://www.ncbi.nlm.nih.gov/pubmed/30716957.

Zhao, H., N. Cheng, W. Zhou, S. Chen, Q. Wang, H. Gao, X. Xue, L. Wu and W. Cao. "Honey polyphenols ameliorate dss-induced ulcerative colitis via modulating gut microbiota in rats." *Molecular Nutrition & Food Research* 63 (2019): e1900638. 10.1002/mnfr.201900638. http://www.ncbi.nlm.nih.gov/pubmed/31533201.

Zheng, H., M. I. Steele, S. P. Leonard, E. V. S. Motta and N. A. Moran. "Honey bees as models for gut microbiota research." *Lab Anim (NY)* 47 (2018): 317-25. 10.1038/s41684-018-0173-x. http://www.ncbi.nlm.nih.gov/pubmed/30353179.

Zheng, Y. Z., G. Deng, Q. Liang, D. F. Chen, R. Guo and R. C. Lai. "Antioxidant activity of quercetin and its glucosides from propolis: A theoretical study." *Sci Rep* 7 (2017): 7543. 10.1038/s41598-017-08024-8. http://www.ncbi.nlm.nih.gov/pubmed/28790397.

Ziuzia, P., Z. Janiec, M. Wrobel-Kwiatkowska, Z. Lazar and M. Rakicka-Pustulka. "Honey's yeast-new source of valuable species for industrial applications." *International Journal of Molecular Sciences* 24 (2023): 10.3390/ijms24097889. http://www.ncbi.nlm.nih.gov/pubmed/37175595.

Biographical Sketch

Rustem A. Ilyasov

Affiliation: Koltzov Institute of Developmental Biology, Department of Biological Sciences, Russian Academy of Sciences (IDB RAS) (Moscow, Russia).

Education: MSc in Bashkir State University, PhD and DSc in Institute of Biochemistry and Genetics of Ufa Federal Research Center, Russian Academy of Sciences (IBG UFRC RAS) (Ufa, Russia).

Business Address: Vavilova str. 26, 119334 Moscow, Russia.

Research and Professional Experience: Molecular geneticist, populational geneticist, molecular evolutionist, molecular biologist, bioinformaticist, entomologist, apiologist, microbiologist.

Professional Appointments: Leading Researcher of Developmental Neurobiology Laboratory.

Honors: developed honey bee Apis mellifera and Apis cerana subspecies genetically identification method.

Publications from the Last 3 Years:

1. Ilyasov, R. A., Lee, M. l., Takahashi, J. i., Kwon, H. W., Nikolenko, A. G. A revision of subspecies structure of western honey bee Apis mellifera. *Saudi Journal of Biological Sciences* 2020, *27*, 3615-3621. doi: 10.1016/j.sjbs.2020.08.001.

2. Ilyasov, R. A., Lee, M. L., Yunusbaev, U. B., Nikolenko, A. G., Kwon, H. W. Estimation of C-derived introgression into A. m. mellifera colonies in the Russian Urals using microsatellite genotyping. *Genes and Genomics* 2020, *42*, 987–996. doi: 10.1007/s13258-020-00966-0.
3. Lim, S., Yunusbaev, U. B., Ilyasov, R. A., Lee, H. S., Kwon, H. W. Abdominal contact of fluvalinate induces olfactory deficit in Apis mellifera. *Pesticide Biochemistry and Physiology* 2020, *164*, 221-227. doi: 10.1016/j.pestbp.2020.02.005.
4. Danilenko, V. N., Devyatkin, A. V., Marsova, M. V., Shibilova, M. U., Ilyasov, R. A., Shmyrev, V. I. Common inflammatory mechanisms in COVID-19 and Parkinson's diseases: the role of microbiome, pharmabiotics and postbiotics in their prevention. *Journal of Inflammation Research* 2021, *14*, 6349–6381. doi: 10.2147/JIR.S333887.
5. Ilyasov, R. A., Han, G. Y., Lee, M. L., Kim, K. W., Park, J. H., Takahashi, J. I., Kwon, H. W., Nikolenko, A. G. Phylogenetic relationships among honey bee subspecies Apis mellifera caucasia and Apis mellifera carpathica based on the sequences of the mitochondrial genome. *Russian Journal of Genetics* 2021, *57*, 697-710. doi: 10.1134/S1022795421060041.
6. Ilyasov, R. A., Han, G. Y., Lee, M. L., Kim, K. W., Proshchalykin, M. Y., Lelej, A. C., Park, J. H., Takahashi, J. I., Kwon, H. W., Nikolenko, A. G. Genetic properties and evolution of Asian honey bee Apis cerana ussuriensis from Primorsky Krai, Russia. *Russian Journal of Genetics* 2021, *57*, 557-571. doi: 10.1134/S1022795421050033.
7. Ilyasov, R. A., Lim, S., Lee, M. L., Kwon, H. W., Nikolenko, A. G. Effect of miticides amitraz and fluvalinate on reproduction and productivity of honey bee Apis mellifera. *Uludag Bee Journal (Uludağ Arıcılık Dergisi)* 2021, *21*, 21-30. doi: 10.31467/uluaricilik.883775.
8. Ilyasov, R. A., Takahashi, J. I., Proshchalykin, M. Y., Lelej, A. S., Lee, M. L., Kwon, H. W., Nikolenko, A. G. First evidence of presence of Varroa underwoodi mites on native Apis cerana colonies in Primorsky Territory of Russia based on COX1 gene. *Journal of Apicultural Science* 2021, *65*, 177-186. doi: 10.2478/JAS-2021-0014.
9. Kim, D. I., Ilyasov, R., Yunusbaev, U., Lee, S. H., Kwon, H. W. Behavioral and molecular responses of Aedes aegypti to ultrasound. *Journal of Asia-Pacific Entomology* 2021, *24*, 429-435. doi: 10.1016/j.aspen.2020.12.016.
10. Momeni, J., Parejo, M., Nielsen, R. O., Langa, J., Montes, I., Papoutsis, L., Farajzadeh, L., Bendixen, C., Căuia, E., Charrière, J. D., Coffey, M. F., Costa, C., Dall'Olio, R., De La Rúa, P., Drazic, M. M., Filipi, J., Galea, T., Golubovski, M., Gregorc, A., … Estonba, A. Authoritative subspecies diagnosis tool for European honey bees based on ancestry informative SNPs. *BMC Genomics* 2021, *22*, 101. doi: 10.1186/s12864-021-07379-7.
11. Danilenko, V. N., Ilyasov, R. A., Yunes, R. A., Yanenko, A. S., Kozlovsky, Y. E., Sverchkova, N. V., Kolomiets, E. I. Microbiome of animals: search for biologically active ingredients for the creation of probiotics and pharmabiotics. *Uspekhi Sovremennoi Biologii* 2022, *142*, 333-348. doi: 10.31857/S0042132422040056.

12. Danilenko, V. N., Yunes, R. A., Ilyasov, R. A., Kovtun, A. S., Yanenko, A. S., Kozlovsky, Y. E., Sidorenko, A. V., Kolomiets, E. I. Study of the human and animal microbiome as genetic and pharmacological resources for the development of innovative biotechnologies in medicine, animal husbandry and agro-industrial complex. *Uspekhi Sovremennoi Biologii* 2022, *142*, 315-332. doi: 10.31857/S0042132422040044.
13. García, C. A. Y., Rodrigues, P. J., Tofilski, A., Elen, D., McCormak, G. P., Oleksa, A., Henriques, D., Ilyasov, R., Kartashev, A., Bargain, C., Fried, B., & Pinto, M. A. Using the Software Deepwings© to Classify Honey Bees Across Europe Through Wing Geometric Morphometrics. *Insects* 2022, *13*, 1132. doi: 10.3390/insects13121132.
14. Ilyasov, R., Danilenko, V., Galin, R., Kwon, H., Yanbaev, Y., Yumaguzhin, F. Molecular genetic methods in apicultural science. *Bulletin of the Bashkir State Agrarian University* 2022, *62*, 69-83. doi: 10.31563/1684-7628-2022-62-2-69-83.
15. Ilyasov, R., Danilenko, V., Galin, R., Kwon, H., Yanbaev, Y., Yumaguzhin, F. Potential pharmabiotics obtained from the honey bee gut microbiome. *Bulletin of the Bashkir State Agrarian University* 2022, *62*, 84-90. doi: 10.31563/1684-7628-2022-62-2-84-91.
16. Ilyasov, R. A., Rašic, S., Takahashi, J., Danilenko, V. N., Proshchalykin, M. Y., Lelej, A. S., Sattarov, V. N., Thai, P. H., Raffiudin, R., Kwon, H. W. Genetic relationships and signatures of adaptation to the climatic conditions in populations of Apis cerana based on the polymorphism of the gene Vitellogenin. *Insects* 2022, *13*, 1053. doi: 10.3390/insects13111053.
17. Ilyasov, R. A., Takahashi, J. I., Lee, M. L., Proshchalykin, M. Y., Lelej, A. S., Kwon, H. W., Danilenko, V. N., Nikolenko, A. G. Characteristics of Varroa underwoodi mites (Acari: Varroidae) in the population of Apis cerana ussuriensis (Hymenoptera: Apidae) in the Primorsky Krai of Russia. *Biology Bulletin Reviews (Zhurnal obshchei biologii)* 2022, *12*, 516-526. doi: 10.1134/S2079086422050048.
18. Ilyasov, R. A., Yunes, R. A., Yanbaev, Y.A., Yumaguzhin, F. G., Galin, R. R., Khisamov, R. R., Kwon, H. W., Ilyasova, A. Y., Zainullin, R. A., Danilenko, V. N. Microbiome of farm animals as a source of pharmacological and genetic resources for the development of innovative biotechnologies in the agro-industrial complex. *Bulletin of the Bashkir State Agrarian University* 2022, *63*, 39-49. doi: 10.31563/1684-7628-2022-63-3-39-49.
19. Kaskinova, M., Gaifullina, L., Ilyasov, R., Lelej, A., Kwon, H.W., Thai, P.H., Saltykova, E. Genetic structure of Apis cerana populations from South Korea, Vietnam and the Russian Far East based on microsatellite and mitochondrial DNA polymorphism. *Insects* 2022, *13*, 1174. doi: 10.3390/insects13121174.
20. Grishina, Y. V., Vatlin, A. A., Mavletova, D. A., Odorskaya, M. V., Senkovenko, A. M., Ilyasov, R. A., Danilenko, V. N. Metabolites Potentially Determine the High Antioxidant Properties of Limosilactobacillus fermentum U-21. *BioTech* 2023, *12*, 39. doi: 10.3390/biotech12020039.
21. Sagitov, S., Ilyasov, R., Sattarov, V., Abdrakhimova, Y., Danilenko, V., Gazizova, N., Sattarova, A., Boguslavsky, D. Phenetic variation in honey bee (Apis mellifera) population of the Toratau Geopark, the Republic of Bashkortostan. *Uludag Bee*

Journal (Uludağ Arıcılık Dergisi) 2023, *23*, 115-127. doi: 10.31467/uluaricilik.1271880.

22. Vatlin, A. A., Bekker, O. B., Shur, K. V., Ilyasov, R. A., Shatrov, P. A., Maslov, D. A., Danilenko, V. N. Kanamycin and Ofloxacin Activate the Intrinsic Resistance to Multiple Antibiotics in Mycobacterium smegmatis. *Biology* 2023, *12*, 506. doi: 10.3390/biology12040506.

Chapter 4

Postbiotics as Dynamic Biomolecules and Their Role in Promoting Host Health Status

Samaneh Moradi[1]
Sara Bazzaz[1]
Kimia Dehghan Sanej[1]
Alireza Mohammadi[2]
Negar Astanehe[1]
Anahita Ghorbani Tajani[3]
Amin Abbasi[1]
Saeedeh Shojaee-Aliabadi[1,*]
and Hedayat Hosseini[1,*]
[1]Department of Food Science and Technology,
National Nutrition and Food Technology Research Institute,
Faculty of Nutrition Science and Food Technology,
Shahid Beheshti University of Medical Sciences, Tehran, Iran
[2]Department of Food Science and Technology, Faculty of Agriculture,
Tarbiat Modares University, Tehran, Iran
[3]Department of Animal Science, University of Wyoming, Laramie, Wyoming, USA

[*] Corresponding Author's Email: hedayat@sbmu.ac.ir.
[*] Corresponding Author's Email: saeedeh.shojaee@gmail.com.

In: Exploring Microbiotics in Health and Disease
Editor: Edward L. Stillman
ISBN: 978-8-89113-410-2

Abstract

Currently, postbiotics have been defined by the International Scientific Association of Probiotics and Prebiotics (ISAPP) as preparations of inanimate microorganisms and/or their components that are beneficial to the host's health. In other words, postbiotics can contain a wide variety of components, including metabolites, functional proteins, microbial cell fractions, cell lysates, short-chain fatty acids (SCFAs), extracellular polysaccharides (EPS), teichoic acid, pili-type structures, and muropeptides derived from peptidoglycans. Postbiotics can be used as a novel strategy in a variety of pharmaceutical products for preventive therapy and to enhance current therapeutic approaches. Furthermore, it can extend the shelf life of food products, retard deterioration, and improve the functional properties of foods. It is important to note that the affordability of the manufacture and use of postbiotics in different delivery systems emphasizes the significance of these components from a clinical, technological, and financial perspective. Research to date indicates that these components have biological activities including antimicrobial, antioxidant, anti-proliferation, anti-inflammatory, and immunomodulatory, and they may play an important role in regulating immune system function, enhancing therapies, and reducing their possible side effects in some cases of gastrointestinal disorders and chronic diseases. As a result, the consumption of foods or dietary supplements containing postbiotic components has been characterized as one of the most important strategies to improve host health status. An overview of the concept of postbiotics and their clinical role in host health is presented in this chapter.

Keywords: biological activities, cell-free supernatant, gastrointestinal disorders, postbiotics

Introduction

The gastrointestinal tract (GIT) serves as the primary immune organ, constituting roughly 70% of the immune system in the human body [1]. The intestinal surface area is around 300 to 400 square centimeters and is colonized by many colonies of live bacteria. The aforementioned surface is inhabited by an estimated 10^{14} bacteria, representing a diverse range of more than 500 distinct species [2]. The findings of clinical investigations have revealed that several factors, including the maternal gut microbiota structure, mode of delivery, caregiving practices during infancy, administration of antibiotics, low-fiber dietary patterns, chronic medical conditions, and anxiety, play significant roles in modulating the gut microbiota equilibrium [3]. In the context of a well-functioning gastrointestinal tract, there exists a mutually beneficial relationship between naturally occurring bacteria and the cells of the host organism. This connection serves to activate and foster the immunological responses inside the gut, playing a significant role in the preservation of homeostasis in the organism. The terms 'dysbiosis' and 'eubiosis' are used in the context of elucidating the state of health and microbial constitution inside the gastrointestinal tract. Specifically, 'dysbiosis' pertains to pathological circumstances, while 'eubiosis' characterizes the presence of advantageous microorganisms or probiotics [4, 5]. Dysbiosis refers to a state characterized by the presence of pathogenic microorganisms and their toxic metabolites, which leads to a decline in the abundance of helpful microorganisms and a subsequent reduction in immune function. This compromised immune response renders the host vulnerable to a range of both infectious and non-infectious disorders [3]. One of the primary strategies used to achieve eubiosis is the restoration of gut microbiota equilibrium by the ingestion of probiotics, which may be obtained from food sources or dietary supplements [6]. Probiotics refer to non-pathogenic microorganisms that, when consumed in adequate quantities, have been observed to confer beneficial effects on the health of the host [7]. These microorganisms encompass various genera, including bacteria such as *Bifidobacterium*, *Lactobacillus*, and *Bacillus*, as well as yeast genera such as *Kluyveromyces*, *Saccharomyces*, *Torulaspora*, and *Pichia* [8, 9]. The mechanisms of action of probiotic cells, as determined by the International Scientific Association for Probiotics and Prebiotics (ISAPP) consensus panel, can be categorized as strain-dependent, species-dependent, and prevalent among frequently studied probiotic genera. Strain-dependent mechanisms are infrequent and limited to a few strains within a specific species. Species-dependent mechanisms are commonly observed across most strains of a probiotic species, such as *Lactobacillus paracasei* or *Bifidobacterium infantis*. Additionally, certain mechanisms of action are prevalent among frequently investigated probiotic genera [10, 11]. The therapeutic efficacy of probiotics has been substantiated in the treatment of a wide range of diseases, particularly those affecting the gastrointestinal tract, both within and outside of it. These conditions include lactose intolerance, Necrotizing Enterocolitis (NEC), colorectal cancer, acute infectious diarrhea, ulcerative colitis, hepatic encephalopathy, antibiotic-associated diarrhea, and Irritable Bowel Syndrome (IBS) [12-14].

Despite the presence of positive indicators, there is a lack of evidence from extensive long-term clinical studies with a substantial statistical sample to support the notion that the use of probiotic products improves the health status of individuals who were previously in good health [15]. The guidelines established by the Food and Agriculture Organization (FAO) and the World Health Organization (WHO) in 2002 [16], along with the findings from case report studies, have suggested that certain probiotic cells, such as *Lactobacillus buchneri*, *Lactobacillus helveticus*, *Lactobacillus hilgardii*, *Streptococcus thermophilus*, *Bifidobacterium*, and *Bacillus*, when administered through different delivery systems like pharmaceuticals or foods, may potentially be associated with adverse side effects. These side effects include the existence of virulence factors, the transmission of resistance genes, disruptions in metabolic processes, the generation of biogenic amines, and the development of opportunistic infections. These concerns are particularly relevant in pediatric populations and in individuals with underlying medical conditions (**Figure 1**) [15, 17].

In recent times, there has been a growing interest in addressing the challenges associated with the utilization of live probiotic cells, particularly in relation to their clinical, technological, and economic attributes. As a result, alternative elements such as non-digestible fibers (prebiotics) and microbial-derived biomolecules (postbiotics) have emerged as potential solutions [18]. These agents are employed with the aim of restoring the balance of the gut microbiome and promoting eubiosis, which in turn facilitates the establishment of homeostasis [19, 20]. There is a growing body of evidence indicating that the primary health-promoting impacts of intestinal microbiota may be linked to their non-living byproducts, known as postbiotics. These postbiotics possess the ability to imitate the advantageous effects of live parent cells by utilizing comparable or distinct metabolic pathways (**Figure 2**) [21]. The term "postbiotic," despite being a recent development, has gained rapid acceptance in the field of food science as well as in the domains of host health and nutrition. This has led to significant interest in their potential application as nutraceuticals, functional foods, and pharmaceuticals within the food, pharmaceutical, and biotechnological industries [10, 22, 23]. The objectives of this chapter were to provide an overview of the concept and safety issues regarding postbiotics and to assess their biological roles in promoting host health status.

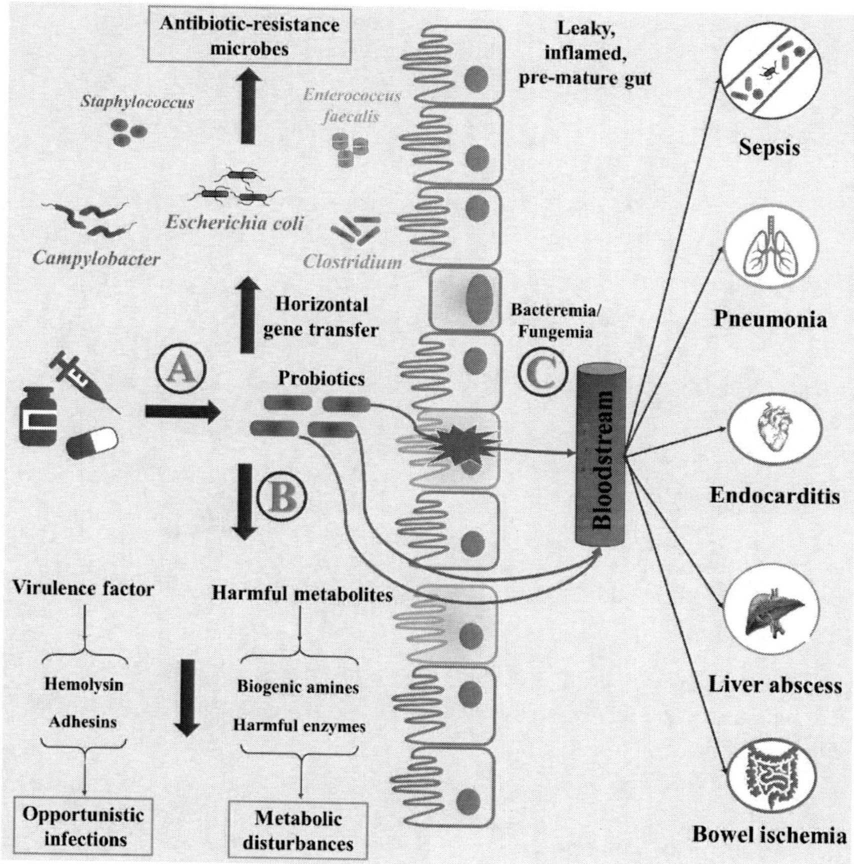

Figure 1. Schematic illustration of the potential risks associated with the (high) dietary intake of some probiotics in the at-risk individuals. (A) Spread (horizontal transfer) of antibiotic resistance genes in the gut microbial populations, which in turn leads to the development of antibiotic-resistant microbes; (B) Presence of virulence factors in probiotic microbial strains and their derived harmful metabolites may be associated with the opportunistic infections and metabolic disturbances; (C) Probiotic translocation from (leaky, inflamed and/or pre-mature) gut lumen to the bloodstream and subsequently into vital organs triggering generalized and localized infections.

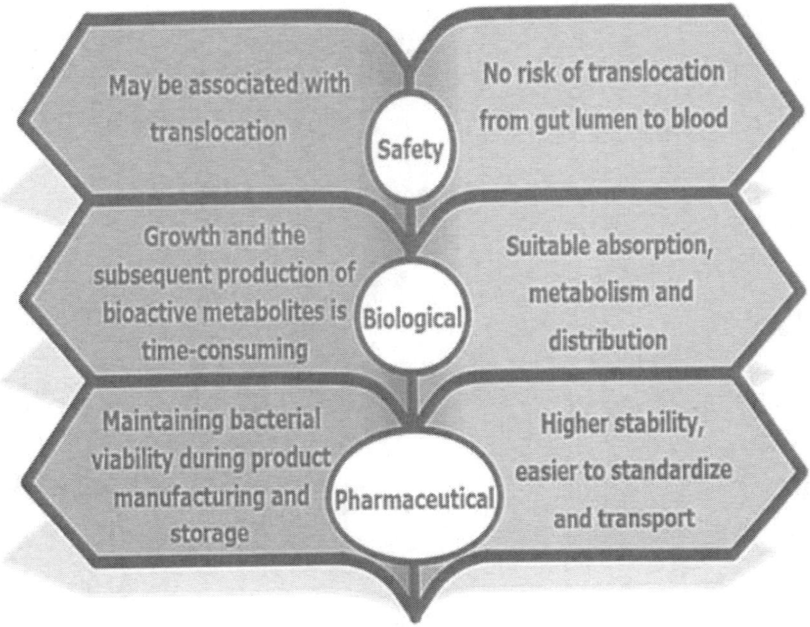

Figure 2. Advantages of postbiotics in terms of safety and biological properties as well as pharmaceutical relative to live probiotics (right column: postbiotics; left column: probiotics).

The Concepts of Postbiotics

In recent years, there has been a prevalent use of terminology such as 'biogenic', 'metabiotic', 'cell-free supernatant (CFS)', 'ghost probiotic', 'abiotic', 'pseudoprobiotic', and 'postbiotic' among researchers to characterize the non-living components of probiotic cells. Out of these options, the word 'postbiotic' is the most frequently used in scholarly literature [24-26]. The term 'postbiotic' is associated with inactive microbial cells, cellular components such as endo- and exo-polysaccharides, teichoic acids, peptidoglycan-derived muropeptides, and cell-surface proteins, as well as cell metabolites including enzymes, Short-Chain Fatty Acids (SCFAs), organic acids, and bacteriocins. These substances are produced by live probiotic cells during the process of fermentation, in response to gut circumstances, or released after cell lysis caused by physical and/or chemical inactivation. When administered in sufficient quantities, postbiotics provide various physiological health benefits to the host (**Figure 3**) [27, 28].

Functional Classification of Postbiotics

In light of the aforementioned potential side effects associated with the administration of probiotic products, it is imperative to explore alternative options that prioritize safety. One such alternative is the utilization of postbiotic components, which promote the growth of beneficial microorganisms residing in the gut and elicit similar physiological health advantages for the human host as live parent cells. Postbiotics may be categorized based on their primary constituents, including organic acids, lipids, carbohydrates, proteins, vitamins, and certain complex compounds, or by their physiological roles [25, 29].

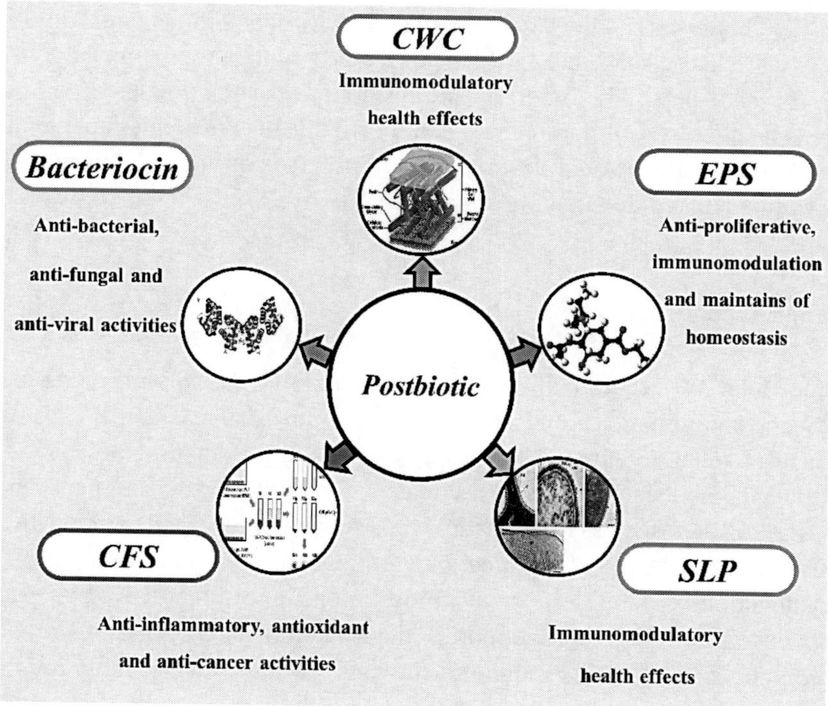

Figure 3. Main postbiotic constituents and their biological activities. Cell-Wall Constituents (CWC), Exopolysaccharides (EPS), Surface-Layer Proteins (SLP), Cell-Free Supernatants (CFS), and bacteriocins are the main postbiotic constituents that have key roles in maintaining the host's homeostasis through their biological activities.

Cell-Wall Constituents

Currently, there is a growing body of research indicating that the Cell-Wall Constituents (CWCs) found in probiotic cells have advantageous health properties and may be used in the development of a novel medicinal delivery method [30]. The primary constituents of the cell wall complex (CWC) that have been consistently discussed in several research are peptidoglycan and lipoteichoic acids, both of which possess immunomodulatory properties [31]. In an experimental paradigm including macrophage-like cells challenged with lipopolysaccharide (LPS), it was shown that peptidoglycans originating from different *Lactobacillus* species had a significant capacity to impede the discharge of inflammatory cytokines [32]. Furthermore, in the context of an animal model investigation, it was shown that the peptidoglycan originating from *L. rhamnosus* had the capability to stimulate innate immune reactions in mice that had weakened immune systems and were infected with *Streptococcus* spp. [33]. Based on the results of research conducted on pig intestinal epithelial cell lines, it has been shown that the postbiotics containing lipoteichoic acid generated *from L. plantarum* have considerable promise in stimulating anti-inflammatory responses [31].

Exopolysaccharides

Extracellular surface carbohydrate polymers, known as exopolysaccharides (EPSs), are commonly found on bacterial cell surfaces in either a capsular form or as released slime. These EPSs can contain a range of organic and inorganic components, including acetic acid, sulfate, acetylate, and phosphate [34, 35]. EPS offers a wide range of uses within the food and medical industries, including gel formation, utilization as thickening agents, emulsification capabilities, metal biosorption, and potential in cancer treatment [36, 37]. Furthermore, these compounds have favorable immunomodulatory and immune-protective properties, such as inhibiting the formation of bacterial biofilms and promoting the preservation of intestinal homeostasis [38]. The health-enhancing properties of EPS, as shown in both laboratory and animal research, are often attributed to EPS derivatives generated from different strains such as *Leuconostoc*, *Bacillus*, *Bifidobacterium*, and *Lactobacillus* strains [39, 40]. The findings of investigations conducted on immunological and epithelial cell cultures have shown that the EPS generated from *B. breve* and several *Lactobacillus* species exhibit significant immunomodulatory effects via their interaction with epithelial cells [41]. The exopolysaccharides produced by *B. longum* and *B. bifidum* have been found to promote the proliferation of *lactobacilli* and other advantageous anaerobic bacteria. Simultaneously, they inhibit the growth of harmful bacteria, including *Pseudomonas aeruginosa*, *Bacillus subtilis*, *Bacillus cereus*, *Staphylococcus aureus*, *Escherichia coli*, and *Salmonella* spp. [42, 43].

The work conducted by Zhang et al. (2017) [44] aimed to assess the adsorption capability of EPS generated by the marine bacteria *Alteromonas* sp. JL2810. It has been determined that the EPS has a notable capacity for adsorbing certain heavy metals (namely Cu^{2+}, Ni^{2+}, and Cr^{6+}), with its effectiveness being subject to the pH level of the surrounding media. Additionally, the findings obtained from the research using infrared spectrometry revealed that the functional groups of C=O, C-O-C, and O-H played a crucial role in the adsorption capacity of EPS towards the studied heavy metals. The researchers reached the conclusion that EPS, exhibiting a high capacity for adsorption, has the potential to serve as an innovative bio-resource for the elimination of heavy metals. In contrast, several EPSs include sugars that may be used within the food sector as novel additives to enhance the physicochemical and sensory characteristics of various goods [25, 45]. In general, exopolysaccharides have been found to have beneficial impacts on various biological processes, operating through diverse molecular pathways. For instance, EPSs possess the ability to regulate both innate and adaptive immune reactions, activate multiple types of immune cells such as T cells, B-lymphocytes, natural killer cells, and macrophages, induce apoptosis, and scavenge free radicals. These properties contribute to the immunomodulatory, antioxidant, and anticancer effects exerted by EPSs [46, 47].

Surface-Layer Proteins

The predominant composition of bacterial cell surfaces consists of a structured arrangement of proteins and glycoproteins known as Surface-Layer Proteins (SLPs). These SLPs form a porous layer that envelops and shields the cell surface [48]. The surface layer protein is often seen on the cellular membrane of probiotic microorganisms, namely within the *Lactobacillus* genus. The SLPA produced from *L. acidophilus* has significant health-promoting functions through interacting with immune cells and inducing immunomodulatory responses [49, 50]. The *L. helveticus*-derived SLP has a high capability for interacting with intestinal cells and reducing *E. coli* O157:H7 adherence, consequently enhancing mucosal homeostasis and preserving the effectiveness of the epithelial barrier [51] (**Figure 4**).

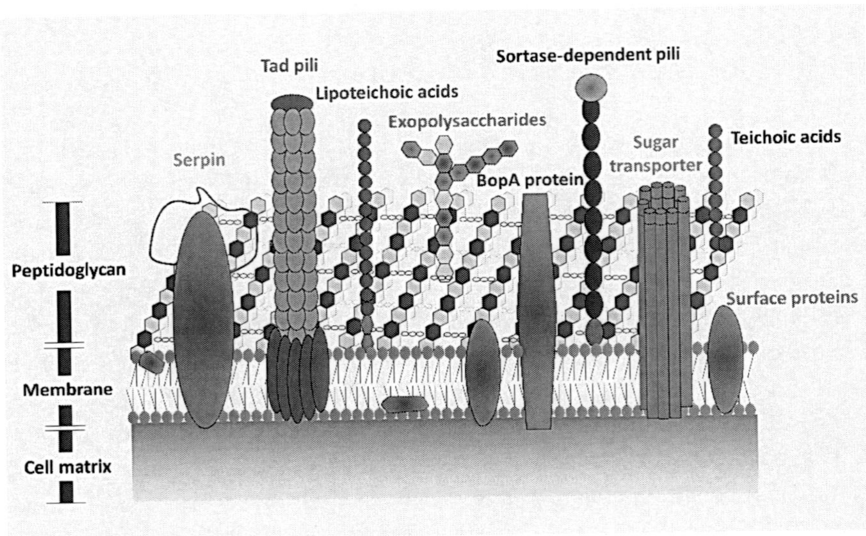

Figure 4. Schematic representation of probiotics' cell-wall constituents.

Cell-Free Supernatants (CFS)

The Cell Free-Supernatants (CFSs) produced from probiotic cells include a diverse array of substances, such as bacteriocins, diacetyl, hydrogen peroxide, organic acids (acetate, propionate, and butyrate), reuterin, and several other biomolecules [52, 53]. An increasing amount of data has shown the many health-promoting impacts of CFSs. Following the ingestion of food or supplements containing postbiotics, the aforementioned substances undergo an initial interaction with intestinal epithelial cells. Subsequently, in the second stage, they interact with immune cells. The nature of these interactions and their potential for stimulating anti-inflammatory and/or antioxidant properties depends on the origin of the postbiotics, which can consist of various probiotic cells [54]. In a laboratory-based investigation involving colon epithelial cells, the cell-free supernatant produced by *L. rhamnosus* GG showed significant efficacy in suppressing cytokine-induced cell death. Consequently, these probiotics have been suggested as a promising intervention for enhancing gastrointestinal homeostasis [55, 56]. In addition, it has been shown that CFS originating from probiotics has a significant capacity to impede the infiltration of infections. In accordance with this, Khodaii et al. (2017) demonstrated that CSF derived from *Lactobacilli* and *Bifidobacteria* has inhibitory effects on the invasion of Entero-Invasive *E. coli* (EIEC) strains when tested on T84 and Caco-2 colon cancer cell lines [57].

Bacteriocins

Bacteriocins, which are peptides with low molecular weight, have a significant function in the suppression of enteric pathogen proliferation [50, 58]. It is essential to acknowledge that, in addition to their antibacterial capabilities, several bacteriocins possess notable anti-fungal and anti-viral actions [59]. Numerous investigations conducted in both laboratory settings (*in vitro*) and living organisms (*in vivo*) have provided empirical evidence supporting the substantial antimicrobial efficacy of bacteriocins generated from Lactic Acid Bacteria. These bacteriocins have shown notable inhibitory effects on the proliferation and infection of several pathogenic bacterial strains, including but not limited to *Staphylococcus*, *Enterococcus*, *Bacillus*, *Clostridium*, and *Listeria* species [59, 60]. Bacteriocins possess several desirable properties that make them suitable components for functional food formulations. These properties include the ability to withstand high temperatures of up to 100°C, stability across a wide pH range of 3–10, resistance to the effects of salts, organic solvents, and enzymes, as well as the ability to maintain stability under refrigeration or freezing conditions [30, 59]. Nisin, generated from *Lactococcus* strains, is the only bacteriocin that has received approval for use by food companies. This lantibiotic is often employed as a preservative in many food items, including infant meals, canned soups, fisheries products, and dairy products [25]. The bacteriocins bifidocins and acidocin, which are derived from *Bifidobacteria*, exhibit a wide range of antimicrobial activity against gram-positive and gram-negative microbes by means of cell lysis mechanisms, especially in fermented food products [61, 62].

Postbiotics Effect on Human Health and Diseases

Numerous scientific studies have demonstrated the beneficial effects of probiotic-derived metabolites on human health. These substances have biological functions that have been extensively researched recently. The most important biological functions of postbiotics include immune modulation, antimicrobial activity, anticancer activity, and an alternative treatment for several human diseases. Postbiotics, as potential substitute elements, may be safer than their parent live cells, according to evidence. Additionally, because of their suitable economic, technological, and clinical characteristics, they could be used as helpful tools in the food and pharmaceutical industries to enhance health benefits [63].

Postbiotics and Immune System

Postbiotics have mostly been linked to immunomodulatory effects because they help to boost the adaptive and innate immune systems, keep the intestinal mucosal barrier strong, and stop pathogens with antimicrobial substances [64]. In this regard, several potential postbiotic processes for immune system modulation include: a) preventing the pathogens penetration into epithelial cells; b) stimulating expression in LTR; c) stimulating anti-inflammatory cytokine production and reducing pro-inflammatory cytokine production; d) suppressing the growth of pathogenic germs; e) preventing bacterial translocation; f) possessing a role in regulation of Th1- and Th2-mediated immune responses [65].

Pili and protein p40/p75, which are postbiotics made by Lactobacilli, are said to have immunomodulatory activity by protecting the intestinal barrier, promoting aggregation, bacteriocins, factor proteins, and S-layer proteins, and displaying antagonistic activity against pathogens [66]. It appears that changes in cell wall components such as peptidoglycan and lipoteichoic acid are linked to variations in the immunostimulant activity of various bacterial species and strains. It has been suggested that these bacteria modulate immune responses by increasing Th1-associated cytokines and decreasing Th2-related cytokines [67]. In another study, researchers investigated that peptidoglycans from three different Lactobacillus species (*Lactobacillus casei, Lactobacillus rhamnosus,* and *Lactobacillus acidophilus*) had a great ability to prevent the release of pro-inflammatory cytokines from macrophage-like cell types via the LPS-induced TLR-4 pathway [32]. However, in heat-inactivated probiotic strain combinations, including *Lactobacillus casei, Lactobacillus plantarum, Lactobacillus acidophilus, Lactobacillus rhamnosus, Streptococcus thermophilus, Bifidobacterium bifidum, and Saccharomyces boulardii,* intestinal cells were protected from *E. coli* infection by preventing an increase in paracellular permeability and the penetration of pathogens into the intestinal epithelium, maintaining membrane integrity, modulating the expression of cytokine genes, and ensuring the restoration of tight junction function [68]. Also, it was found that the probiotic bacteria "Streptococcus thermophilus CRL1190" and its exopolymeric substances make it harder for Helicobacter pylori to stick to human gastric adenocarcinoma epithelial cell lines (AGS cells) and reduce the inflammatory response. With these results, it has been hypothesized that *S. thermophilus* and its postbiotics protect the gastric mucosa and enhance the anti-inflammatory response by regulating cytokine IL-8 production [69]. In another study, the parabiotic Saccharomyces boulardii was given by mouth to mice with a model of intestinal obstruction. The results showed that heat-killed S. boulardii could protect the intestinal barrier by keeping the gut's permeability at a level that is normal for the body and by reducing the transfer of bacteria to E. coli ATCC 10536 and mucosal lesions [70]. In another study, researchers found that postbiotics in fermented infant formula with Lactobacillus paracasei CBA L74 could protect the host from intestinal pathogens by stopping the immune system's inflammatory cells and preventing colitis [71]. By oral administration to newborn mice infected with E. coli K1, some researchers reported the potential of postbiotics (a new protein called HM0539) made by Lactobacillus rhamnosus GG in the prevention and treatment of diseases associated with intestinal barrier dysfunction and demonstrated that HM0539 enhances the development of neonatal intestinal defense mechanisms and is sufficient to suppress the pathogenesis of E. coli K1. They also found that HM0539 had the ability to prevent LPS/D-galactosamine-induced bacterial translocation, dextran sodium sulfate (DSS)-induced colitis, and liver injury [72].

Additionally, it was discovered that postbiotics created by inactivating probiotics had immunomodulatory activity that was greater than that of probiotics. For instance, the activity of immunomodulation appears to be increased by the production of heat shock proteins (Hsp) during the heating process [73]. *Lactobacillus casei* (LcZ) (heat-inactivated and suspended in PBS at 106 CFU/ml) increases the expression of pro-inflammatory cytokines and transcription of TLR9, TLR4, TLR3, and TLR2, enhancing macrophage-mediated innate immune responses [74]. Results of studies conducted on inactive and live forms of *Bacillus subtilis* FPTB13 and *Bacillus amyloliquefaciens* FPTB16 showed that the inactive preparations enhanced the secretion of cellular immune parameters more than the live preparations [75]. Furthermore, a study in mice revealed that heat-inactivated combinations of LAB (two heat treatments were performed: 100°C for 30 minutes and 121°C for 15 minutes) increased the immunomodulatory activity of macrophage cells more than the same combination (*Enterococcus faecium*, *Lactobacillus plantarum*, *Lactobacillus acidophilus*, and *Lactobacillus fermentum*) containing live strains [76]. *Lactobacillus acidophilus* A2, *Lactobacillus salivarius* A6, and *Lactobacillus gasseri* A5 (heat-inactivated and suspended at 106 cells/ml in PBS) were also postbiotics with immunomodulatory activity *in vitro*. These non-living microbes change Th1-mediated immune responses by stimulating the growth of IL-10 and IL-12 p70, the production of IFN-ɣ by splenocytes, and the release of IL-12 p70 by dendritic cells. The mechanism by which LAB strains induce different responses in dendritic cells remains unclear, but immunomodulatory responses appear to be strain-dependent [77]. Both the probiotic and the metabiotic *Lactobacillus gasseri* TMC0356 showed immunomodulatory effects *in vitro*. The metabiotic *Lactobacillus gasseri* TMC0356 caused a greater increase in IL-12 production in macrophages compared to the probiotic, suggesting that heat treatment increased the strain's ability to activate IL-12 production in macrophages, such that the postbiotic form was greater than the original bacterial form to apply immunomodulatory effects [78].

Thus, postbiotics have immunomodulatory activities that ensure the health of the host. Therefore, they may be a safer alternative for immunocompromised individuals such as transplanted patients, the elderly and premature infants, and they may eliminate various probiotic disadvantages (**Figure 5**) [65].

Postbiotics and Maintenance of Intestinal Barrier

The epithelial barrier is the main line of defense of the intestinal tract, consisting of an adhesive layer of intestinal cells, a mucosal layer, and antimicrobial peptides, which can prevent epithelial damage caused by pathogenic bacteria and their toxins, as well as foreign antigens or other harmful substances [19]. Related research findings support the idea that the uptake of beneficial microbes (in a food/supplement matrix) may be a suitable strategy for gut barrier maintenance [79, 80]. In this regard, there is a significant correlation between probiotics and postbiotics and gut barrier function; the main mechanisms include the repair of mucosal damage caused by several pathological factors and the inhibition of cytokine-induced epithelial damage [81]. Probiotics' ability to maintain the intestinal barrier may be greatly influenced by their unique cell structures rather than their metabolic processes. In this regard, an animal model study showed that the *S. boulardii*-derived CWSs have a significant capacity to protect the intestinal barrier by maintaining gut permeability while reducing microbial translocation [82]. In addition, the presence of a large number of postbiotic components of *S. thermophilus*, *L. bulgaricus*, and *L. acidophilus* (1109 cells/ml) in functional yogurt can effectively inhibit intestinal barrier damage caused by various antigens by activating pro-inflammatory cytokines to induce nitric oxide (NO) synthesis [83].

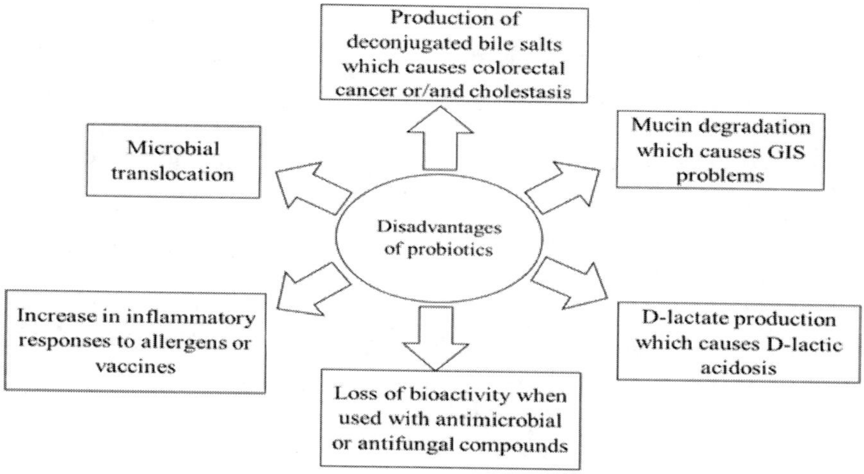

Figure 5. Some disadvantages of probiotics for immune system and microbiota.

Postbiotics and Treatment of Colitis

Colitis is a chronic inflammatory disease that affects normal intestinal function [84]. Some postbiotics derived from *Bifidobacterium* and *Lactobacillus* strains have a positive effect on host health by preventing the progression of colitis [85]. An *in vitro* study of cell samples from patients with colitis revealed postbiotics derived from B. breve and B. bifidum have a significant anti-inflammatory effect on peripheral blood mononuclear cells. In this context, administration of postbiotics stimulated the production of IL-10, an anti-inflammatory cytokine that plays a key role in the regulation of inflammatory responses, in peripheral blood mononuclear cells and prevented IL-8 (a cytokine associated with inflammation) in intestinal epithelial cells [73]. ColibiogenVR is a commercial postbiotic product derived from *Escherichia coli*, mainly containing amino acids, peptides, fatty acids, and polysaccharides. Modulation of colibiogen uptake improves colitis and overall health in a mouse model. Therefore, the use of postbiotic ingredients with health-promoting effects in commercial products is a new field in the treatment of colitis [25].

Postbiotics and Treatment of Necrotizing Enterocolitis

Necrotizing enterocolitis (NEC) is the most common and serious gut disease that usually occurs in the intestines of premature infants in the second to third week of their lives, with a 30% mortality rate [86]. NEC is characterized by invasion of pathogenic microorganisms, mucosal damage, inflammation, local infection, and full-thickness necrosis, ultimately leading to significant damage to the intestinal cell wall. Common symptoms of NEC may include bloating, decreased appetite and physical activity, vomiting of bile, and blood in the stool [31, 87]. In addition, the financial burden of NEC is very high, up to $1 billion per year in developed countries such as the United States [88]. Substantial evidence supports that NEC is a multifactorial disease, and several factors directly related to the development of severe inflammation and intestinal damage play a key role in the development and progression of NEC, especially in infants and children, although the exact pathophysiology is not completely clear [89]. Conventional NEC therapy is not effective enough to provide supportive care at the time of diagnosis, so researchers focused on the characteristics of new NEC prevention strategies. In this case, the administration of probiotics and their biological by-products (postbiotics) is considered an effective strategy to reduce the risk of NEC expansion in at-risk preterm infants [90]. Postbiotics can modulate gut microbiota composition, improve gut barrier integrity and immune system function, improve NEC treatment efficacy, and reduce its side effects in patients due to their antibacterial, antioxidant, anti-inflammatory, and immunomodulatory properties [9, 89, 91]. Despite significant progress, more research is needed to fully understand how to use postbiotics as an effective therapy to treat or prevent NEC in preterm infants [92].

Postbiotics and Treatment of Gastrointestinal Cancer

Cancer is one of the most common disorders of the gastrointestinal tract and is considered a multifactorial disease characterized by excessive (irregular and/or uncontrolled) cell growth [93]. Patients with cancer are usually treated with immunotherapy, radiation therapy, surgery, or chemotherapy based on 5-fluorouracil. In some cases, these common treatments can cause side effects like systemic toxicity, resistance to chemotherapy, and a return of the cancer [94]. In this case, a growing body of epidemiological evidence supports the positive effects of beneficial gut microbes and their postbiotics on breast, bladder, liver, colon, and gastric cancer [95]. The ability of postbiotic components to interact with host immune cells through a variety of G protein-coupled receptors (GPRs), which in turn activate multiple signaling pathways, enhance innate immune responses, and decrease inflammation (as a potent tumor development factor), is largely responsible for their antitumor activity [96]. Several studies have revealed the potential function of postbiotics in cancer prevention and treatment, mainly in gastrointestinal cancers [97]. A unique feature of epibiotic components is their ability to differentiate between normal and neoplastic cells, thereby promoting normal cell proliferation but inhibiting angiogenesis and stimulating the apoptotic response of cancer cells [98]. In this regard, butyrate acts as a histone deacetylase (HDAC) inhibitor, a new class of anticancer drugs with opposing effects on normal and cancerous colon cells. In normal colon cells, it acts as an oxidative energy source, but due to its accumulation in the nucleus, it can inhibit the growth of colon cancer cells and act as an HDAC inhibitor due to the Warburg effect and inefficient metabolism [99]. Furthermore, clinical results suggest that beneficial gut microbes and postbiotics derived from them may be valuable tools to promote the efficacy of cancer treatment [100, 101] through reducing abdominal pain, diarrhea severity, vomiting, atrophy, stomatitis, nerve damage, vascular damage, intestinal toxicity, and skin erythema compared to subjects who received placebo [102]. Therefore, postbiotics have received considerable attention from the scientific community due to their active role in regulating the cell cycle, stimulating differentiation, and regulating proapoptotic pathways, and are considered a new approach for adjuvant therapy in cancer individuals [103-105]. Furthermore, more preclinical and clinical studies are needed to develop suitable carriers and delivery methods, assess the biological fate of orally administered postbiotics, and investigate the precise mechanisms of cell death responses *in vivo* [106].

Postbiotics and Treatment of Diarrhea

A common gastrointestinal condition that typically results from viral and microbial infections is diarrhea. Conventional cancer treatments such as radiation therapy can also cause radiation-induced diarrhea in radiation oncology patients [107]. A large number of clinical studies have shown that probiotics and their derived postbiotics continue to play an important role in reducing the symptoms of diarrhea [108]. Several scientific reports have shown a positive correlation between the consumption of postbiotic supplements derived from *Lactobacillus plantarum* and a reduced incidence of diarrhea. Possible mechanisms for this phenomenon include changes in mucosal structure (increased digestibility and villi size) and an increase in the beneficial intestinal microbiota population [109]. Regular use of postbiotic capsules (derived from *Lactobacillus acidophilus* LB), containing approximately 5 billion non-viable cells, in patients with chronic diarrhea shortened the disease cycle and improved stool stability, bloating, abdominal discomfort, and the perception of incomplete evacuation [110]. In a clinical study of patients receiving treatment for diarrhea (oral rehydration solution), the addition of a postbiotic powder derived from *Lactobacillus acidophilus* LB to the oral rehydration solution significantly shortened the duration of illness to one day [111]. Therefore, postbiotics may serve as a promising treatment for diarrhea without serious side effects.

Postbiotics and Treatment of Pediatric Diseases

The mammalian gut contains one of the densest microbial communities known, with microbial cells outnumbering the eukaryotic cells that constitute their hosts [112]. This gut microbial community contributes to food digestion and the production of important components (such as secondary bile acids and different postbiotic components such as vitamins and short-chain fatty acids) and plays a key role in direct and host-mediated defense functions to resist the invasion of pathogenic microorganisms [91, 113]. Today, new sequencing technologies allow for a more detailed study of the intestinal microbiota and signs of intestinal dysbiosis, especially in pediatrics [19]. According to recent findings, the evolutionary state of the intestinal mucosa (mature or immature), the composition and balance of the gut microbiota, as well as the balance between dysbiosis conditions and gut eubiosis in infants, are major factors directly related to health promotion and the development of associated serious diseases such as sepsis, infantile colic, and necrotizing enterocolitis [114]. At birth, microbes colonize the entire body surface and are strongly involved in the development of the immune system. In newborns, the gut microbiota is first formed by nutrients and immune system (maternal immunoglobulin A (IgA)) components in milk and then changes during weaning when solid food is consumed, creating a new phase in the growth and development of the intestinal microbiota that is characterized by a large increase in bacterial numbers and the formation of a composition associated with the adult [115]. Alnabani et al. (2019) studied the function (reactivity) of the intestinal immune system in the first weeks of life and in adulthood in a mouse model. They determined that during the weaning phase, the gut microbiota stimulates a strong immune response, a well-planned "weaning response". Preventing this immune reaction (the weaning response) in turn leads to the formation of pathological imprints and increases the susceptibility to developing chronic diseases such as allergic inflammation, cancer, and colitis later in life [112].

From a "therapeutic microbiology" perspective, probiotic strategies could be an alternative therapy for intestinal diseases. In this context, among different *Lactobacillus* and *Bifidobacterium* genera, the species of B. breve, as the predominant species colonizing the gut of breast-fed infants and isolated from breast milk, is widely used in the prevention and/or treatment of pediatric diseases due to its biological functions (immunomodulatory and antimicrobial effects) and safety properties (non-transmitted drug resistance and cytotoxicity) [116]. On the other hand, one of the most important issues related to infants is the colonization of commensal intestinal bacteria, which can be influenced and modified by adding exogenous probiotic strains to the infant gut ecosystem, thus supporting safe alternative medicine such as prebiotic and postbiotic ingredients, for example, in neonates to treat infantile colic or enteral nutrition [114]. In this case, Martinelli et al. (2017), in an open randomized controlled trial, evaluated the efficacy of a standardized extract of *Melissa officinalis*, *Matricaria chamomilla*, inactivated *L. acidophilus* HA122, and simethicone as a control agent for infantile colic treatment. They determined that the administration of *Melissa officinalis* and *Matricaria chamomilla* extracts in combination with inactivated *L. acidophilus* HA122 significantly reduced the average daily crying duration compared with simethicone in children aged between two weeks and four months old [117]. In addition, Vandenplas et al. (2017), in a pilot study, evaluated the safety and efficacy of a medical device containing the intestinal mucosa protector xyloglucan and inactivated *B. breve* SGB01 and *L. reuteri* SGL01 (at a dose of 10^{10} CFU/g) and a lactase supplement as comparators in the treatment of 46 infants (3 to 16 weeks of age) with symptoms of infantile colic. The results showed a significant reduction in the average time of crying episodes, which in turn raised the possibility of the combined use of xyloglucan and postbiotic components to prevent and/or treat infant colic and any adverse side effects, although larger statistical samples are needed in future randomized controlled trials [118].

Postbiotics and Treatment of Lactose Intolerance

Based on the available evidence, postbiotics may play an effective role in reducing lactose intolerance symptoms. Lactose intolerance is a common gut disease worldwide. In Asia, the prevalence of this disease is estimated at 50% and even 100% in some Asian countries [118]. It can be diagnosed by symptoms such as swelling, bloating, nausea, abdominal pain, vomiting, diarrhea, and abdominal distention after consuming lactose and the hydrogen breath test (HBT) [119]. A study by Rampengan et al. (2010) investigated the effect of sachets containing postbiotic compounds (Dialac) on lactose-intolerant children. This study used the HBT test, and a range above 20 ppm was considered lactose intolerance. The results revealed a meaningful reduction in the HBT scale in patients and concluded that postbiotic sachets have acceptable potential to reduce symptoms and improve the status of lactose-intolerant children [120].

Postbiotics and Treatment of Celiac Diseases

An abnormal immune system response to gluten consumption results in celiac disease (CD), a systemic disease that primarily affects the small intestine [121]. It occurs in genetically predisposed individuals (non-HLA and HLA-DQ2/DQ8 positive genes) and is influenced by environmental triggers, including viral infections, certain glutens, and gut microbiota dysbiosis [122]. Gluten is inadequately digested in the human gut, with or without celiac disease. Unabsorbed gluten peptides pass through the mucosa of the small intestine. When gluten peptides enter the submucosa of the small intestine, human transglutaminase 2 (tTG) deamidates gluten peptides with its particular activity, thereby increasing the binding affinity to HLA DQ8 molecules and human leukocyte antigen (HLA) DQ2, followed by an inflammatory response in the patients [123]. The only treatment currently being used for this disease is a lifelong gluten-free diet. The role of gut microbiota in CD has recently been described. Numerous cross-sectional studies compared the microbiota of patients and controls and described different degrees of dysbiosis in celiac disease patients before and after a gluten-free diet. The microbiota has substantial functions in stimulating, training, and modulating the host immune system, so its modifications are often associated with immune feedback and inflammation [124]. Changes in the microbiota were found in CD cases. Interestingly, the microbiota in patients with celiac disease can change at different stages of the disease. Non-CD patients had different microbiota profiles between celiac disease on a gluten-containing diet (GCD-CD) and celiac disease on a gluten-free diet (GFD-CD). The occurrence of incremental changes in the microbial populations of *Lachnospriraceae*, *Victivallaceae*, *Escherichia coli*, *Enterobacteriaceae*, *Clostridiaceae*, *Coriobacteriaceae*, *Slackia*, ML615J-28, and unclassified species of *Clostridiales* and a reduction in *Eubacterium hallii*, *Lachnospriraceae*, *Faecalibacterium prausnitzii*, *Bifidobacterium*, *Anaerostipes hadrus*, *Clostridium lituseburense*, *Lactobacillus Veillonellaceae*, *Roseburia faecis*, and *Blautia wexlerae* in celiac disease patients in the acute stage of the disease stimulates gut dysbiosis conditions [125]. Protective microbiota such as *Bifidobacteria*, *Lactobacillus, Streptococcus and Firmicutes* were lower in CD patients compared to healthy controls. The ability of several postbiotic metabolites to inhibit gliadin activity has been studied in cultured gut epithelial cells. The most widely used cell line is Caco2, a gut epithelial cell line derived from human colorectal adenocarcinoma, although these transformed cells have the ability to transform into gut epithelial cells *in vitro*. Once separated, they provide tight junctions and absorption. The ability to inhibit the effects of gliadin and gliadin peptides on Caco2 cells was tested daily in *in vitro* experiments with Caco2 cells. Sano M. et al. (2014) have shown that the epigenetic LP CBA L74 is able to reduce the entry of gliadin peptides into Caco2 cells. They observed that LP CBA L74 could ferment numerous different types of grain. The effect of LP CBA L74 on the entry of P31-43 after fermentation was investigated using fermented oat, wheat, and rice. Penetration of P31-43-liss was reduced after treatment with fermented wheat (FI reduction of 24%), oats (FI reduction of 56%), and rice (FI reduction of 35%). These data suggest that the effect of LP CBA L74 on P31-43 liss entry persists after fermentation of different grains and that it may be due to compounds produced during the fermentation process rather than live bacteria [126]. Gallo M. and his colleagues looked into whether controlling the pH during rice fermentation with Lactobacillus paracasei CBA L74 could increase bacterial growth, make more lactic acid, and stop P31-43 from getting into Caco2 cells. During rice fermentation, pH control significantly increased lactic acid production. Even if P31-43-liss is taken out of the cells and the pH is controlled, fermented rice can still stop it from getting in. This creates a memory in the cells that can stop P31-43-liss from getting in within a few hours. These results may have nutritional value, suggesting that the effects of certain postbiotics may persist even after they exit the intestinal environment [127]. Recently, Freire R. and colleagues investigated the role of microbiota-derived biomolecules in modulating epithelial feedback to gluten using intestinal organoids obtained from duodenal biopsies in celiac and non-celiac patients. They utilized three bacterial by-products: lactate, butyrate, and PSA derived from Bacteroides fragilis. The authors investigated the expression of genes associated with altered gut barrier function in CD. Butyrate significantly increased the expression of *CLDN18*, *MUC5AC*, *MUC6*, and *TFF1* in celiac disease organoids. PSA only significantly increased the expression of *CLDN18*, while lactate did not alter the expression of genes related to the analyzed gut barrier function. Similar gene regulation was also observed in NC organoids. Furthermore, they investigated the effect of bacterial byproducts on cytokine release from gliadin-contaminated CD monolayers. All of the by-products help protect the body as a whole by reducing the release of pro-inflammatory cytokines caused by the digestion of gliadin by pepsin and trypsin (PTG). However, only butyrate and lactate significantly reduced IL15 and IFN cytokine secretion in celiac disease [128]. So, it looks like postbiotics are very good at stopping gliadin and gliadin peptides from working in gut epithelial cells in a lab. Postbiotics appear to be effective in several ways, aimed at preventing gluten-induced inflammation. The use of *in vitro* patient-derived organoids to model the pathogenesis of CD may become a new tool for further research in the treatment and prevention of celiac disease. Taken together, this evidence suggests that postbiotics can be used to prevent inflammation in at-risk patients with CD. However, only *in vivo* trials can validate this strategy [119].

Postbiotics and Treatment of Allergy

One of the clinical applications of postbiotics in food and nutrition is their effective role in the treatment of food allergies. Food allergy is a disorder of the immune system that significantly affects the quality of life of patients [129]. The prevalence of food allergy-related clinical symptoms, particularly in developed countries, has shown a significant upward trend over the past two decades, which is also economically necessary [91, 130]. According to the observations of several food studies, more than 170 foods are associated with food allergies, the most important of which are aquatic products such as fish and oyster shells and dairy products such as milk, eggs, wheat, nuts, soybeans, and seeds [131, 132]. Various studies have focused on the health-promoting role of gut microbiota and have reported direct and complex relationships between gut microbiota composition and immune function. In this context, where the gut environment is dominated by beneficial microbiota (especially probiotics), they contribute to food allergy symptoms in infected individuals by making contact with epithelial cells and the immune system [133]. According to evidence, various postbiotic metabolites, such as short-chain fatty acids, have a significant effect on reducing food allergy symptoms. These postbiotics stimulate host immune cell responses and decrease host susceptibility to harmless antigens [134]. Short-chain fatty acid postbiotics derived from *Bifidobacterium* and *Lactobacillus*, although they are an important source of energy for intestinal cells, bind to G protein-coupled receptors (on colonocytes, intestinal epithelium, and the immune system), stimulate epithelial-dendritic cells and macrophages to make interleukin 10, and promote the development of regulatory T-lymphocytes (Treg) in mesenteric lymph nodes, ultimately suppressing inflammatory responses and food allergies [135]. Given the active role of postbiotics in establishing a consistent relationship with the immune system and inducing an appropriate immune response to desensitize the host to the presence of certain antigenic agents and decrease inflammatory symptoms, they consider a new strategy to alleviate food allergies [119].

Postbiotics and Oral Health

The functional mechanism of probiotics is associated with the generation of compounds such as organic acids, bacteriocins, hydrogen peroxide, and fatty acids [23, 136]. These compounds are currently being produced in the laboratory and have health effects when consumed in sufficient quantities [25]. Moreover, they are considered promising alternative antibiotics due to their antibacterial activity [9, 137]. One of postbiotics' most important and impressive components is thought to be organic acids. Lactic acid, which is produced during fermentation, can effectively control pathogenicity [138]. Bacteriocins are peptides with antibacterial activity. These compounds are resistant to heat, acids, and alkalis and can prevent the growth of pathogens in the gastrointestinal tract. The mechanism of action of bacteriocins is in the bacterial plasma membrane [139]. In addition, fatty acids, which are one of the components of postbiotics, also have an antibacterial effect. Long-chain fatty acids such as eicosapentaenoic acid are effective against gram-positive bacteria. Fatty acids can kill bacteria in a number of ways, such as by making membranes more permeable, destroying bacterial cells, changing the structure and activity of enzymes, stopping electron transport chains from working, and changing the shape and function of sensitive parts like proteins [140]. H_2O_2 (hydrogen peroxide) is another antimicrobial agent whose antimicrobial action is because of its strong oxidizing effect on bacterial cells and the destruction of protein structures in their cytoplasm [141]. The beneficial role of some probiotics in improving oral health and preventing oral diseases has been investigated in some studies [142]. The antimicrobial properties of probiotics are thought to be related to the production of antibacterial compounds such as hydrogen peroxide and organic acids, as well as antifungal compounds such as fatty acids and bacteriocins [143]. In addition, *L. reuteri* has been reported to produce water-soluble antibacterial compounds, such as reuterin and reutecyclin, which have antagonistic effects [144]. These compounds are resistant to proteolytic and lipolytic enzymes and retain their function over a wide pH range [145]. The strain of *S. dentisani*, isolated from the oral cavity of caries-free individuals, can also generate bacteriocin and can be considered another useful probiotic [146]. Furthermore, in a three-month clinical trial, a probiotic strain of *Streptococcus salivarius* M18, which also produces bacteriocins, was shown to decrease cavity formation in children [147].

Some bacteria, such as *Streptococcus sanguinis* and *Streptococcus uberis*, were absent in subgingival plaque samples from patients with localized juvenile periodontitis and refractory periodontitis [148]. At the same time, they were also present in subgingival plaque samples from healthy individuals. These strains were shown to inhibit the growth of *A. actinomycetemcomitans* and other periodontal pathogens by producing hydrogen peroxide [149]. Bacteria (*Lactobacillus* spp., *Streptococcus mutans, and Streptococcus sobrinus*) have been suggested to cause a decrease in pH and demineralization of teeth. This is due to the organic acids produced in biofilms by the fermentation of these bacteria [150, 151]. On the other hand, as mentioned above, one of the mechanisms by which probiotics inhibit the growth of pathogenic bacteria is through the production of organic acids. One may therefore wonder whether the presence of these acids causes a further decrease in pH and an increase in dental caries. Various studies have shown that salivary pH was significantly higher in the probiotic-treated group than in the control group. The findings of this study are consistent with the results of several other studies reporting an increase in pH after consumption of yogurt and curd-containing probiotics [152]. It can be assumed that the increase in pH after the use of probiotics is due to the competition between probiotics and pathogenic bacteria, resulting in a decrease in their number. A decrease in the number of acidogenic pathogens leads to a decrease in acid production, which leads to an increase in salivary pH. Because cavities are affected by pH imbalances, these results may be important. Storage and safety issues have attracted attention as probiotic foods have become popular in recent years. Probiotic strains for the treatment of bacterial diseases must have certain properties. For example, probiotics should not cause disease or predispose individuals to other diseases by disrupting the ecosystem in which they live [153]. They should also be screened and tested for overall safety, such as for antibiotic resistance genes and genes associated with potential invasion [154]. Given these concerns about live bacteria consumption, we should consider a safe and suitable alternative that offers the same biological health advantages as probiotics [25]. Evidence from *in vitro* and *in vivo* studies shows that postbiotics are clinically safe and have therapeutic and beneficial effects when used in appropriate amounts and over a long period of time [155]. Postbiotics can be a safe and cost-effective alternative to probiotics in the pharmaceutical and food industries due to their safety profile, long shelf life (up to 5 years), non-toxic effect, standardization, and easier transportation [91, 104, 142].

Safety Aspects of Postbiotics

The intricate network of the human microbiota plays a significant role in determining human health and disease status. The abundant bacterial population found in the gut, estimated to be around 10^{14} CFU/g, has the potential to impact both metabolic functions and the immune system, acting as a defense mechanism against various pathogens [89, 156]. Given the increasing food and feed demands due to modern population growth, ensuring the quality and safety of food and feed products is crucial for societal well-being. Numerous studies have provided credible evidence showcasing the advantageous effects of bacteria, particularly those in the gut. However, it's important to note that probiotics might not be entirely safe for vulnerable groups such as infants, the elderly, or immunosuppressed individuals. In these cases, adverse effects, gastrointestinal symptoms, the transfer of antibiotic-resistant genes from probiotics to the normal microbiota, and systemic infections could occur [157, 158].

Presently, emerging evidence from recent studies suggests that the viability of probiotics isn't the sole determinant for conferring health benefits [25], offering a potential strategy to mitigate risks associated with probiotic consumption. Addressing safety concerns and establishing regulatory guidelines for postbiotics and related functional foods should be based on an assessment of potential risks and safety considerations. Despite the fact that most probiotic foods contain strains of *Lactobacillus* spp. and/or *Bifidobacterium* spp., which are rarely associated with clinical infections [159], probiotic products are generally perceived as safe, albeit with some risks for specific groups of people. Despite these potential risks linked to bacterial consumption in food, certain beneficial bacteria like LAB and *Bifidobacteria* can serve as effective tools against pathogens and spoilage microorganisms, as they can compete with harmful bacteria and produce beneficial compounds, thus enhancing food safety and shelf life [160]. In light of the positive and negative effects associated with different bacteria, the concept of postbiotics has emerged as a potential solution to counteract the negative aspects of probiotics. However, it's crucial to consider the specific probiotic strains and fermentation methods used in postbiotic production [89], as well as the safety aspects related to postbiotic consumption. While postbiotic consumption is a relatively new approach, there is currently no clinical or epidemiological evidence of associated risks. The absence of live microorganisms theoretically eliminates the risk of infection. Nonetheless, *in vitro* and *in vivo* studies have investigated the effects of postbiotics on various cells, blood parameters, metabolic biomarkers, and gut mucosa. *In vitro* studies are valuable tools for understanding interactions between host cells and bacteria, including both commensal and pathogenic types [161]. These studies not only shed light on potential mechanisms of action but also provide a foundation for subsequent animal and human research to explore postbiotic applications. However, the translation of *in vitro* findings to real-world scenarios can be limited, and species-specific effects must be considered, necessitating *in vivo* studies to confirm the effects observed *in vitro*. Several studies have examined the effects of postbiotics on cancer cell lines. For instance, research has demonstrated that heat-killed cells and postbiotics derived from different *Lactobacillus* strains can inhibit the growth of cancer cells [162]. Similarly, the cytotoxicity of cell extracts from *Lactobacillus* strains has been evaluated, revealing their potential to inhibit the proliferation of cancer cells [163]. In other studies, postbiotics produced by *Lactobacillus plantarum* strains induced antiproliferative and apoptotic effects on cancer cells in a dose- and time-dependent manner [95]. The potential molecular mechanisms behind these effects include the modulation of gene expressions associated with metastasis and apoptosis [164].

Animal models have been employed to investigate the effects of postbiotics as well. In a mice model, postbiotics from *Lactobacillus reuteri* were shown to mitigate liver damage induced by lipopolysaccharides [165]. Similarly, postbiotic supplementation from *Lactobacillus plantarum* RG14 in newly weaned lambs improved weight gain, nutrient intake, and microbial activity in the gut, along with enhanced production of mucosal antibodies and antimicrobial peptides [166]. In broiler chickens, postbiotic administration resulted in decreased inflammatory responses and improved growth performance [137]. Besides animal models, studies have explored postbiotic effects in humans as well. For instance, clinical reports have demonstrated the safety and potential benefits of postbiotic supplementation in infants and adults, including improvements in gastrointestinal functioning [161]. Furthermore, substances derived from postbiotic fermentation, such as short-chain fatty acids, peptides, and vitamins, have been recognized as potential alternatives for managing infectious diseases in aquaculture settings [167]. The gut epithelial barrier serves as the first line of defense against external threats, and maintaining its integrity is essential for overall health. Dysfunction in this barrier can lead to a "leaky gut," allowing harmful substances to enter the body. Strengthening the intestinal barrier can promote well-being, making postbiotics promising candidates for this purpose [168]. It's worth noting that the positive effects of fermented foods on the gastrointestinal tract don't solely come from live microorganisms but can also be attributed to the products of fermentation [169]. The mechanisms underlying the effects of postbiotics on gut barrier integrity have been investigated in various studies. The proteins p40 and p75 from postbiotics derived from *Lactobacillus rhamnosus* GG, for example, play a role in preventing damage, inhibiting apoptosis, and stimulating the proliferation of intestinal epithelial cells [27]. These proteins have been recognized as pivotal players in the function of probiotics and their metabolites [170].

Conclusion

In conclusion, postbiotics hold the potential to contribute to overall well-being through various mechanisms, although their precise mode of action remains to be fully elucidated. The studies mentioned above reinforce the safety and potential benefits of postbiotic consumption at appropriate dosages and concentrations.

References

[1] Denev, P., Kratchanova, M., Ciz, M., Lojek, A., Vasicek, O., Nedelcheva, P., Blazheva, D., Toshkova, R., Gardeva, E., Yossifova, L., Hyrsl, P., and Vojtek, L. (2014). Biological activities of selected polyphenol-rich fruits related to immunity and gastrointestinal health. *Food Chemistry.*, 157, 37-44.

[2] Hsiao, W. W. L., Metz, C., Singh, D. P., and Roth, J. (2008). The microbes of the intestine: an introduction to their metabolic and signaling capabilities. *Endocrinol Metab Clin North Am.*, 37(4), 857-71.

[3] Moludi, J., Alizadeh, M., Lotfi Yagin, N., Pasdar, Y., Nachvak, S. M., Abdollahzad, H., and Tabaei, A. S. (2018). New insights on atherosclerosis: A cross-talk between endocannabinoid systems with gut microbiota. *J Cardiovasc Thorac Res.*, 10(3), 129-37.

[4] Khan, N., Mendonca, L., Dhariwal, A., Fontes, G., Menzies, D., Xia, J., Divangahi, M., and King, I. L. (2019). Intestinal dysbiosis compromises alveolar macrophage immunity to Mycobacterium tuberculosis. *Mucosal immunology.*, 12(3), 772.

[5] Hosseini, H., Abbasi, A., Sabahi, S., Akrami, S., and Yousefi-Avarvand, A. (2023). Assessing the Potential Biological Activities of Postbiotics Derived from Saccharomyces cerevisiae: An *In Vitro* Study. *Probiotics and Antimicrobial Proteins.*, 1-17.

[6] Abbasi, A., Aghebati-Maleki, A., Yousefi, M., and Aghebati-Maleki, L. (2021). Probiotic intervention as a potential therapeutic for managing gestational disorders and improving pregnancy outcomes. *Journal of Reproductive Immunology.*, 143, 103244.

[7] Haghshenas, B., Haghshenas, M., Nami, Y., Khosroushahi, A. Y., Abdullah, N., Barzegari, A., Rosli, R., and Hejazi, M. S. (2016). Probiotic assessment of Lactobacillus plantarum 15HN and Enterococcus mundtii 50H isolated from traditional dairies microbiota. *Advanced pharmaceutical bulletin.*, 6(1), 37.

[8] Saber, A., Alipour, B., Faghfoori, Z., and Yari Khosroushahi, A. (2017). Cellular and molecular effects of yeast probiotics on cancer. *Critical reviews in microbiology.*, 43(1), 96-115.

[9] Rad, A., Abbasi, A., Javadi, A., Pourjafar, H., Javadi, M., and Khaleghi, M. (2020). Comparing the microbial quality of traditional and industrial yoghurts. *Biointerface Research in Applied Chemistry.*, 10(4), 6020-5.

[10] Cuevas-González, P., Liceaga, A., and Aguilar-Toalá, J., (2020). Postbiotics and Paraprobiotics: From concepts to applications. *Food Research International.*, 109502.

[11] Abbasi, A., Bazzaz, S., Da Cruz, A. G., Khorshidian, N., Saadat, Y. R., Sabahi, S., Ozma, M. A., Lahouty, M., Aslani, R., and Mortazavian, A. M. (2023). A Critical

Review on Akkermansia muciniphila: Functional Mechanisms, Technological Challenges, and Safety Issues. *Probiotics and Antimicrobial Proteins.*, 1-23.

[12] Mohamadshahi, M., Veissi, M., Haidari, F., Shahbazian, H., Kaydani, G. A., and Mohammadi, F. (2014). Effects of probiotic yogurt consumption on inflammatory biomarkers in patients with type 2 diabetes. *BioImpacts: BI.*, 4(2), 83.

[13] Maia, L. P., Levi, Y. L. d. A. S., do Prado, R. L., Santinoni, C. d. S., and Marsicano, J. A. (2019). Effects of probiotic therapy on serum inflammatory markers: A systematic review and meta-analysis. *Journal of Functional Foods.*, 54, 466-78.

[14] Karimi, N., Jabbari, V., Nazemi, A., Ganbarov, K., Karimi, N., Tanomand, A., et al. (2020). Thymol, cardamom and Lactobacillus plantarum nanoparticles as a functional candy with high protection against Streptococcus mutans and tooth decay. *Microbial Pathogenesis.*, 104481.

[15] Cohen, P. A. (2018). Probiotic safety—no guarantees. *JAMA internal medicine.*, 178(12), 1577-8.

[16] Joint, F. (2002). *WHO working group report on drafting guidelines for the evaluation of probiotics in food.* London, Ontario, Canada., 30.

[17] Ordóñez, J. L., Troncoso, A. M., García-Parrilla, M. D. C., and Callejón, R. M. (2016). Recent trends in the determination of biogenic amines in fermented beverages–A review. *Analytica chimica acta.*, 939, 10-25.

[18] Abbasi, A., Sanej, K. D., Moradi, S., Bazzaz, S., Esmaeili, A., Ghafourian, K., et al. (2023). Bioactive Compounds and Biological Activities of Allium sativum L. *Bioactive Compounds in the Storage Organs of Plants*: Springer, p. 1-40.

[19] Piqué, N., Berlanga, M., and Miñana-Galbis, D. (2019). Health benefits of heat-killed (Tyndallized) probiotics: an overview. *International journal of molecular sciences.*, 20(10), 2534.

[20] Rad, A. H., Maleki, L. A., Kafil, H. S., Zavoshti, H. F., and Abbasi, A. (2020). Postbiotics as novel health-promoting ingredients in functional foods. *Health Promotion Perspectives.*, 10(1), 3.

[21] Guéniche, A., Bastien, P., Ovigne, J. M., Kermici, M., Courchay, G., Chevalier, V., Breton, L., and Castiel-Higounenc, I. (2010). *Bifidobacterium longum* lysate, a new ingredient for reactive skin. *Experimental dermatology.*, 19(8), e1-e8.

[22] Rad, A., Abbasi, A., Kafil, H., and Ganbarov, K. (2020). Potential Pharmaceutical and Food Applications of Postbiotics: A review. *Current pharmaceutical biotechnology.*

[23] Homayouni Rad, A., Samadi Kafil, H., Fathi Zavoshti, H., Shahbazi, N., and Abbasi, A. (2020). Therapeutically Effects of Functional Postbiotic Foods. *Clinical Excellence.*, 10(2), 33-52.

[24] de Almada, C. N., Almada, C. N., Martinez, R. C., and Sant'Ana, A. S. (2016). Paraprobiotics: evidences on their ability to modify biological responses, inactivation methods and perspectives on their application in foods. *Trends in food science & technology.*, 58, 96-114.

[25] Aguilar-Toalá, J., Garcia-Varela, R., Garcia, H., Mata-Haro, V., González-Córdova, A., Vallejo-Cordoba, B., and Hernández-Mendoza, A. (2018). Postbiotics: An evolving term within the functional foods field. *Trends in Food Science & Technology.*, 75, 105-14.

[26] Homayouni, Rad, A., Aghebati, Maleki, L., Samadi, Kafil, H., and Abbasi, A. (2020). Postbiotics: A novel strategy in food allergy treatment. *Critical Reviews in Food Science and Nutrition.*, 1-8.

[27] Cicenia, A., Scirocco, A., Carabotti, M., Pallotta, L., Marignani, M., and Severi, C. (2014). Postbiotic activities of lactobacilli-derived factors. *Journal of clinical gastroenterology.*, 48, S18-S22.

[28] Rai, A. K., Pandey, A., and Sahoo, D. (2018). Biotechnological potential of yeasts in functional food industry. Trends in food science & technology.

[29] Homayouni-rad, A., Fathi-zavoshti, H., Douroud, N., Shahbazi, N., and Abbasi, A. (2020). Evaluating the Role of Postbiotics as a New Generation of Probiotics in Health and Diseases. *Journal of Ardabil University of Medical Sciences.*, 19(4), 381-99.

[30] Sarkar, A., and Mandal, S. (2016). Bifidobacteria—Insight into clinical outcomes and mechanisms of its probiotic action. *Microbiological research.*, 192, 159-71.

[31] Kim, K. W., Kang, S. S., Woo, S. J., Park, O. J., Ahn, K. B., Song, K. D., Lee, H. K., Yun, C. H., and Han, S. H. (2017). Lipoteichoic acid of probiotic Lactobacillus plantarum attenuates poly I: C-induced IL-8 production in porcine intestinal epithelial cells. *Frontiers in microbiology.*, 8, 1827.

[32] Wu, Z., Pan, D., Guo, Y., Sun, Y., and Zeng, X. (2015). Peptidoglycan diversity and anti-inflammatory capacity in Lactobacillus strains. *Carbohydrate Polymers.*, 128, 130-7.

[33] Kolling, Y., Salva, S., Villena, J., and Alvarez, S. (2018). Are the immunomodulatory properties of Lactobacillus rhamnosus CRL1505 peptidoglycan common for all Lactobacilli during respiratory infection in malnourished mice? *PloS one.*, 13(3), e0194034.

[34] Poli, A., Anzelmo, G., and Nicolaus, B. (2010). Bacterial exopolysaccharides from extreme marine habitats: production, characterization and biological activities. *Marine drugs.*, 8(6), 1779-802.

[35] Abbasi, A., Bazzaz, S., Ibrahim, S. A., Hekmatdoost, A., Hosseini, H., Sabahi, S., Sheykhsaran, E., Saadat, Y. R., Ozma, M. A., and Lahouty, M. (2023). A Critical Review on the Gluten-Induced Enteropathy/Celiac Disease: Gluten-Targeted Dietary and Non-Dietary Therapeutic Approaches. *Food Reviews International.*, 1-41.

[36] Manivasagan, P., and Kim, S. K. (2014). Extracellular polysaccharides produced by marine bacteria. *Advances in food and nutrition research.*, 72, Elsevier, p. 79-94.

[37] Freitas, F., Alves, V. D., and Reis, M. A. (2011). Advances in bacterial exopolysaccharides: from production to biotechnological applications. *Trends in biotechnology.*, 29(8), 388-98.

[38] Whitfield, G. B., Marmont, L. S., and Howell, P. L. (2015). Enzymatic modifications of exopolysaccharides enhance bacterial persistence. *Frontiers in microbiology.*, 6, 471.

[39] Castro-Bravo, N., Wells, J. M., Margolles, A., and Ruas-Madiedo, P. (2018). Interactions of surface exopolysaccharides from Bifidobacterium and Lactobacillus within the intestinal environment. *Frontiers in microbiology.*, 9.

[40] Saadat, Y. R., Khosroushahi, A. Y., and Gargari, B. P. (2019). A comprehensive review of anticancer, immunomodulatory and health beneficial effects of the lactic acid bacteria exopolysaccharides. *Carbohydrate polymers*., 217, 79-89.

[41] Patten, D. A., Leivers, S., Chadha, M. J., Maqsood, M., Humphreys, P. N., Laws, A. P., and Collett, A. (2014). The structure and immunomodulatory activity on intestinal epithelial cells of the EPSs isolated from Lactobacillus helveticus sp. Rosyjski and Lactobacillus acidophilus sp. 5e2. *Carbohydrate research*., 384, 119-27.

[42] Liu, Z., Zhang, Z., Qiu, L., Zhang, F., Xu, X., Wei, H., and Tao, X. (2017). Characterization and bioactivities of the exopolysaccharide from a probiotic strain of Lactobacillus plantarum WLPL04. *Journal of dairy science*., 100(9), 6895-905.

[43] Wu, M. H., Pan, T. M., Wu, Y. J., Chang, S. J., Chang, M. S., and Hu, C. Y. (2010). Exopolysaccharide activities from probiotic Bifidobacterium: Immunomodulatory effects (on J774A. 1 macrophages) and antimicrobial properties. *International journal of food microbiology*., 144(1), 104-10.

[44] Zhang, Z., Cai, R., Zhang, W., Fu, Y., and Jiao, N. (2017). A novel exopolysaccharide with metal adsorption capacity produced by a marine bacterium Alteromonas sp. JL2810. *Marine drugs*., 15(6), 175.

[45] Moghaddas, Kia, E., Ghasempour, Z., Ghanbari, S., Pirmohammadi, R., and Ehsani, A. (2018). Development of probiotic yogurt by incorporation of milk protein concentrate (MPC) and microencapsulated Lactobacillus paracasei in gellan-caseinate mixture. *British Food Journal*., 120(7), 1516-28.

[46] Rahbar, Saadat, Y., Pourghassem, Gargari, B., Shahabi, A., Nami, Y., and Yari Khosroushahi, A. (2020). Prophylactic role of Lactobacillus Paracasei exopolysaccharides on colon cancer cells through apoptosis not ferroptosis. *Pharmaceutical Sciences*.

[47] Rad, A. H., Maleki, L. A., Kafil, H. S., Zavoshti, H. F., and Abbasi, A. (2020). Postbiotics as Promising Tools for Cancer Adjuvant Therapy. Tabriz University of Medical Sciences.

[48] Hynönen, U., and Palva, A. (2013). Lactobacillus surface layer proteins: structure, function and applications. *Applied microbiology and biotechnology*., 97(12), 5225-43.

[49] Konstantinov, S. R., Smidt, H., de Vos, W. M., Bruijns, S. C., Singh, S. K., Valence, F., et al. (2008). S layer protein A of *Lactobacillus acidophilus* NCFM regulates immature dendritic cell and T cell functions. *Proceedings of the National Academy of Sciences*., 105(49), 19474-9.

[50] Gareau, M. G., Sherman, P. M., and Walker, W. A. (2010). Probiotics and the gut microbiota in intestinal health and disease. *Nature reviews Gastroenterology & hepatology*., 7(9), 503.

[51] Johnson-Henry, K. C., Hagen, K. E., Gordonpour, M., Tompkins, T. A., and Sherman, P. M. (2007). Surface-layer protein extracts from *Lactobacillus helveticus* inhibit enterohaemorrhagic *Escherichia coli* O157: H7 adhesion to epithelial cells. *Cellular microbiology*., 9(2), 356-67.

[52] Bianchi, F., Dall'Asta, M., Del Rio, D., Mangia, A., Musci, M., and Scazzina, F. (2011). Development of a headspace solid-phase microextraction gas

chromatography–mass spectrometric method for the determination of short-chain fatty acids from intestinal fermentation. *Food Chemistry.*, 129(1), 200-5.

[53] Lukic, J., Chen, V., Strahinic, I., Begovic, J., Lev-Tov, H., Davis, S. C., Tomic-Canic, M., and Pastar, I. (2017). Probiotics or pro-healers: the role of beneficial bacteria in tissue repair. *Wound Repair and Regeneration.*, 25(6), 912-22.

[54] De Marco, S., Sichetti, M., Muradyan, D., Piccioni, M., Traina, G., Pagiotti, R., and Pietrella, D. (2018). Probiotic cell-free supernatants exhibited anti-inflammatory and antioxidant activity on human gut epithelial cells and macrophages stimulated with LPS. *Evidence-Based Complementary and Alternative Medicine.*, 2018.

[55] Bermudez-Brito, M., Plaza-Díaz, J., Munoz-Quezada, S., Gomez-Llorente, C., and Gil, A. (2012). Probiotic mechanisms of action. *Annals of Nutrition and Metabolism.*, 61(2), 160-74.

[56] Yan, F., Cao, H., Cover, T. L., Whitehead, R., Washington, M. K., and Polk, D. B. (2007). Soluble proteins produced by probiotic bacteria regulate intestinal epithelial cell survival and growth. *Gastroenterology.*, 132(2), 562-75.

[57] Khodaii, Z., Ghaderian, S. M. H., and Natanzi, M. M. (2017). Probiotic bacteria and their supernatants protect enterocyte cell lines from enteroinvasive Escherichia coli (EIEC) invasion. *International journal of molecular and cellular medicine.*, 6(3), 183.

[58] do Carmo, M. S., itapary, dos Santos, C., Araújo, M. C., Girón, J. A., Fernandes, E. S., and Monteiro-Neto, V. (2018). Probiotics, mechanisms of action, and clinical perspectives for diarrhea management in children. *Food & function.*, 9(10), 5074-95.

[59] Juturu, V., and Wu, J. C. (2018). Microbial production of bacteriocins: Latest research development and applications. *Biotechnology advances.*

[60] Corr, S. C., Li, Y., Riedel, C. U., O'Toole, P. W., Hill, C., and Gahan, C. G. (2007). Bacteriocin production as a mechanism for the antiinfective activity of Lactobacillus salivarius UCC118. *Proceedings of the National Academy of Sciences.*, 104(18), 7617-21.

[61] Bali, V., Panesar, P. S., and Bera, M. B. (2016). Trends in utilization of agro-industrial byproducts for production of bacteriocins and their biopreservative applications. *Critical reviews in biotechnology.*, 36(2), 204-14.

[62] Liu, G., Ren, L., Song, Z., Wang, C., and Sun, B. (2015). Purification and characteristics of bifidocin A, a novel bacteriocin produced by Bifidobacterium animals BB04 from centenarians' intestine. *Food control.*, 50, 889-95.

[63] Aghebati-Maleki, L., Hasannezhad, P., Abbasi, A., and Khani, N. (2021). Antibacterial, antiviral, antioxidant, and anticancer activities of postbiotics: a review of mechanisms and therapeutic perspectives. *Biointerface Res Appl Chem.*, 12, 2629-45.

[64] De Marco, S., Sichetti, M., Muradyan, D., Piccioni, M., Traina, G., Pagiotti, R., et al. (2018). Probiotic Cell-Free Supernatants Exhibited Anti-Inflammatory and Antioxidant Activity on Human Gut Epithelial Cells and Macrophages Stimulated with LPS. *Evidence-Based Complementary and Alternative Medicine.*, 2018, 1756308.

[65] Yeşilyurt, N., Yılmaz, B., Ağagündüz, D., and Capasso, R. (2021). Involvement of probiotics and postbiotics in the immune system modulation. *Biologics.*, 1(2), 89-110.

[66] Teame, T., Wang, A., Xie, M., Zhang, Z., Yang, Y., Ding, Q., Gao, C., Olsen, R. E., Ran, C., and Zhou, Z. (2020). Paraprobiotics and Postbiotics of Probiotic Lactobacilli, Their Positive Effects on the Host and Action Mechanisms: A Review. *Frontiers in Nutrition.*, 7.

[67] Ou, C. C., Lin, S. L., Tsai, J. J., and Lin, M. Y. (2011). Heat-Killed Lactic Acid Bacteria Enhance Immunomodulatory Potential by Skewing the Immune Response toward Th1 Polarization. *Journal of Food Science.*, 76(5), M260-M7.

[68] Servi, B. d., and Ranzini, F. (2017). Protective efficacy of antidiarrheal agents in a permeability model of Escherichia coli-infected CacoGoblet® cells. *Future Microbiology.*, 12(16), 1449-55.

[69] Marcial, G., Villena, J., Faller, G., Hensel, A., and de Valdéz, G. F. (2017). Exopolysaccharide-producing Streptococcus thermophilus CRL1190 reduces the inflammatory response caused by Helicobacter pylori. *Beneficial microbes.*, 8(3), 451-61.

[70] Generoso, S. V., Viana, M. L., Santos, R. G., Arantes, R. M. E., Martins, F. S., Nicoli, J. R., Machado, J. A. N., Correia, M. I. T. D., and Cardoso, V. N. (2011). Protection against increased intestinal permeability and bacterial translocation induced by intestinal obstruction in mice treated with viable and heat-killed Saccharomyces boulardii. *European Journal of Nutrition.*, 50(4), 261-9.

[71] Zagato, E., Mileti, E., Massimiliano, L., Fasano, F., Budelli, A., Penna, G., and Rescigno, M. (2014). *Lactobacillus paracasei* CBA L74 metabolic products and fermented milk for infant formula have anti-inflammatory activity on dendritic cells *in vitro* and protective effects against colitis and an enteric pathogen *in vivo*. *PloS one.*, 9(2), e87615.

[72] Gao, J., Li, Y., Wan, Y., Hu, T., Liu, L., Yang, S., et al. (2019). A novel postbiotic from Lactobacillus rhamnosus GG with a beneficial effect on intestinal barrier function. *Frontiers in microbiology.*, 10, 477.

[73] de Almada, C. N., Almada, C. N., Martinez, R. C. R., and Sant'Ana, A. S. (2016). Paraprobiotics: Evidences on their ability to modify biological responses, inactivation methods and perspectives on their application in foods. *Trends in Food Science & Technology.*, 58, 96-114.

[74] Wang, Y., Xie, J., Wang, N., Li, Y., Sun, X., Zhang, Y., and Zhang, H. (2013). *Lactobacillus casei* Zhang modulate cytokine and Toll-like receptor expression and beneficially regulate poly I: C-induced immune responses in RAW264.7 macrophages. *Microbiology and Immunology.*, 57(1), 54-62.

[75] Kamilya, D., Baruah, A., Sangma, T., Chowdhury, S., and Pal, P. (2015). Inactivated Probiotic Bacteria Stimulate Cellular Immune Responses of Catla, Catla catla (Hamilton) *In Vitro*. *Probiotics and Antimicrobial Proteins.*, 7(2), 101-6.

[76] Chen, C. Y., Tsen, H. Y., Lin, C. L., Lin, C. K., Chuang, L. T., Chen, C. S., and Chiang, Y. C. (2013). Enhancement of the immune response against *Salmonella* infection of mice by heat-killed multispecies combinations of lactic acid bacteria. *Journal of Medical Microbiology.*, 62(11), 1657-64.

[77] Chuang, L., Wu, K. G., Pai, C., Hsieh, P. S., Tsai, J. J., Yen, J. H., and Lin, M. Y. (2007). Heat-Killed Cells of Lactobacilli Skew the Immune Response Toward T Helper 1 Polarization in Mouse Splenocytes and Dendritic Cell-Treated T Cells. *Journal of Agricultural and Food Chemistry*., 55(26), 11080-6.

[78] Miyazawa, K., He, F., Kawase, M., Kubota, A., Yoda, K., and Hiramatsu, M. (2011). Enhancement of immunoregulatory effects of Lactobacillus gasseri TMC0356 by heat treatment and culture medium. *Letters in Applied Microbiology*., 53(2), 210-6.

[79] Martín, R., Chamignon, C., Mhedbi-Hajri, N., Chain, F., Derrien, M., Escribano-Vázquez, U., et al. (2019). The potential probiotic *Lactobacillus rhamnosus* CNCM I-3690 strain protects the intestinal barrier by stimulating both mucus production and cytoprotective response. *Scientific reports*., 9(1), 5398.

[80] Abbasi, A., Sanej, K. D., Mohammadi, A., Moradi, S., Nayeri, B. D., Bazzaz, S., and Hosseini, H. *The Role of Postbiotics in Food Safety Promotion*.

[81] Hou, Q., Ye, L., Liu, H., Huang, L., Yang, Q., Turner, J. R., and Yu, Q. (2018). *Lactobacillus* accelerates ISCs regeneration to protect the integrity of intestinal mucosa through activation of STAT3 signaling pathway induced by LPLs secretion of IL-22. *Cell Death & Differentiation*., 25(9), 1657-70.

[82] Generoso, S. V., Viana, M. L., Santos, R. G., Arantes, R. M., Martins, F. S., Nicoli, J. R., Machado, J. A. N., Correia, M. I. T. D., and Cardoso, V. N. (2011). Protection against increased intestinal permeability and bacterial translocation induced by intestinal obstruction in mice treated with viable and heat-killed Saccharomyces boulardii. *European journal of nutrition*., 50, 261-9.

[83] Zeng, J., Jiang, J., Zhu, W., and Chu, Y. (2016). Heat-killed yogurt-containing lactic acid bacteria prevent cytokine-induced barrier disruption in human intestinal Caco-2 cells. *Annals of microbiology*., 66(1), 171-8.

[84] Xiao, X., Kim, J., Sun, Q., Kim, D., Park, C. S., Lu, T. S., and Park, Y. (2015). Preventive effects of cranberry products on experimental colitis induced by dextran sulphate sodium in mice. *Food chemistry*., 167, 438-46.

[85] Wasilewska, E., Zlotkowska, D., and Wroblewska, B. (2019). Yogurt starter cultures of Streptococcus thermophilus and Lactobacillus bulgaricus ameliorate symptoms and modulate the immune response in a mouse model of dextran sulfate sodium-induced colitis. *Journal of Dairy Science*., 102(1), 37-53.

[86] Puri, P. (2018). *Pediatric Surgery: General Principles and Newborn Surgery*. Springer.

[87] Homayouni-rad, A., Aghebati-Maleki, L., Samadi-Kafil, H., Abbasi, A., and Khani, N., (2021). Postbiotics as a safe alternative to live probiotic bacteria in the food and pharmaceutical industries. *HBI_Journals*., 26, 132-57.

[88] Hodzic, Z., Bolock, A. M., and Good, M. (2017). The role of mucosal immunity in the pathogenesis of necrotizing enterocolitis. *Frontiers in pediatrics*., 5, 40.

[89] Mosca, F., Gianni, M. L., and Rescigno, M. (2019). Can postbiotics represent a new strategy for NEC? Probiotics and Child Gastrointestinal Health: Advances in Microbiology, *Infectious Diseases and Public Health*, Volume 10., 37-45.

[90] Patel, R. M., and Underwood, M. A. editors. (2018). Probiotics and necrotizing enterocolitis. *Seminars in pediatric surgery*, Elsevier.

[91] Homayouni Rad, A., Aghebati, Maleki, L., Samadi, Kafil, H., and Abbasi, A. (2021). Postbiotics: A novel strategy in food allergy treatment. *Critical reviews in food science and nutrition*., 61(3), 492-9.

[92] Abbasi, A., Rad, A. H., Ghasempour, Z., Sabahi, S., Kafil, H. S., Hasannezhad, P., Saadat, Y. R., andShahbazi, N. (2022). The biological activities of postbiotics in gastrointestinal disorders. *Critical Reviews in Food Science and Nutrition*., 62(22), 5983-6004.

[93] Abbasi, A., Rad, A. H., Maleki, L. A., Kafil, H. S., and Baghbanzadeh, A. (2023). Antigenotoxicity and Cytotoxic Potentials of Cell-Free Supernatants Derived from Saccharomyces cerevisiae var. boulardii on HT-29 Human Colon Cancer Cell Lines. *Probiotics and Antimicrobial Proteins*., 1-13.

[94] Yu, B., Wang, Z., Almutairi, L., Huang, S., and Kim, M. H. (2020). Harnessing iron-oxide nanoparticles towards the improved bactericidal activity of macrophage against Staphylococcus aureus. *Nanomedicine: Nanotechnology, Biology and Medicine*., 24, 102158.

[95] Chuah, L. O., Foo, H. L., Loh, T. C., Mohammed Alitheen, N. B., Yeap, S. K., Abdul, Mutalib, N. E., Rahim, R. A., and Yusoff, K. (2019). Postbiotic metabolites produced by Lactobacillus plantarum strains exert selective cytotoxicity effects on cancer cells. *BMC complementary and alternative medicine*., 19, 1-12.

[96] Venegas, D. P., Marjorie, K., Landskron, G., González, M. J., Quera, R., Dijkstra, G., Harmsen, H. J. M., Faber, K. N., and Hermoso, M. A. (2019). Corrigendum: Short chain fatty acids (SCFAs)-mediated gut epithelial and immune regulation and its relevance for inflammatory bowel diseases. *Frontiers in Immunology*., 10.

[97] Schwartz, D. J., Rebeck, O. N., and Dantas, G. (2019). Complex interactions between the microbiome and cancer immune therapy. *Critical reviews in clinical laboratory sciences*., 56(8), 567-85.

[98] Davis, C. D., and Milner, J. A. (2009). Gastrointestinal microflora, food components and colon cancer prevention. *The Journal of nutritional biochemistry*., 20(10), 743-52.

[99] Donohoe, D. R., Collins, L. B., Wali, A., Bigler, R., Sun, W., and Bultman, S. J. (2012). The Warburg effect dictates the mechanism of butyrate-mediated histone acetylation and cell proliferation. *Molecular cell.*, 48(4), 612-26.

[100] Ou, J., Carbonero, F., Zoetendal, E. G., DeLany, J. P., Wang, M., Newton, K., Gaskins, H. R., and O'Keefe, S. J. D. (2013). Diet, microbiota, and microbial metabolites in colon cancer risk in rural Africans and African Americans. *The American journal of clinical nutrition*., 98(1), 111-20.

[101] Wang, K., Li, W., Rui, X., Chen, X., Jiang, M., and Dong, M. (2014). Characterization of a novel exopolysaccharide with antitumor activity from Lactobacillus plantarum 70810. *International journal of biological macromolecules*., 63, 133-9.

[102] Österlund, P., Ruotsalainen, T., Korpela, R., Saxelin, M., Ollus, A., Valta, P., Kouri, M., Elomaa, I., and Joensuu, H. (2007). *Lactobacillus* supplementation for diarrhoea related to chemotherapy of colorectal cancer: a randomised study. *British journal of cancer*., 97(8), 1028-34.

[103] Kurata, N., Tokashiki, N., Fukushima, K., Misao, T., Hasuoka, N., Kitagawa, K., Mashimo, M., Regan, J. W., Murayama, T., and Fujino, H. (2019). Short chain fatty acid butyrate uptake reduces expressions of prostanoid EP4 receptors and their mediation of cyclooxygenase-2 induction in HCA-7 human colon cancer cells. *European Journal of Pharmacology*., 853, 308-15.

[104] Rad, A. H., Aghebati-Maleki, L., Kafil, H. S., and Abbasi, A. (2021). Molecular mechanisms of postbiotics in colorectal cancer prevention and treatment. *Critical reviews in food science and nutrition*., 61(11), 1787-803.

[105] Abbasi, A., Aghebati-Maleki, L., and Homayouni-Rad, A. (2022). The promising biological role of postbiotics derived from probiotic Lactobacillus species in reproductive health. *Critical Reviews in Food Science and Nutrition*., 62(32), 8829-41.

[106] Abbasi, A., Hajipour, N., Hasannezhad, P., Baghbanzadeh, A., and Aghebati-Maleki, L. (2022). Potential *in vivo* delivery routes of postbiotics. *Critical Reviews in Food Science and Nutrition*., 62(12), 3345-69.

[107] Linn, Y. H., Thu, K. K., and Win, N. H. H. (2019). Effect of probiotics for the prevention of acute radiation-induced diarrhoea among cervical cancer patients: a randomized double-blind placebo-controlled study. *Probiotics and antimicrobial proteins*., 11, 638-47.

[108] Lai, H. H., Chiu, C. H., Kong, M. S., Chang, C. J., and Chen, C. C. (2019). Probiotic Lactobacillus casei: Effective for Managing Childhood Diarrhea by Altering Gut Microbiota and Attenuating Fecal Inflammatory Markers. *Nutrients*., 11(5), 1150.

[109] Loh, T. C., Choe, D. W., Foo, H. L., Sazili, A. Q., and Bejo, M. H. (2014). Effects of feeding different postbiotic metabolite combinations produced by Lactobacillus plantarum strains on egg quality and production performance, faecal parameters and plasma cholesterol in laying hens. *BMC veterinary research*., 10, 1-9.

[110] Xiao, S. D., De Zhang, Z., Lu, H., Jiang, S. H., Liu, H. Y., Wang, G. S., Xu, G. M., Zhang, Z. B., Lin, G. J., and Wang, G. L. (2003). Multicenter, randomized, controlled trial of heat-killed *Lactobacillus acidophilus* LB in patients with chronic diarrhea. *Advances in therapy*., 20, 253-60.

[111] Liévin-Le, Moal, V., Sarrazin-Davila, L. E., and Servin, A. L., (2007). An experimental study and a randomized, double-blind, placebo-controlled clinical trial to evaluate the antisecretory activity of Lactobacillus acidophilus strain LB against nonrotavirus diarrhea. *Pediatrics*., 120(4), e795-e803.

[112] Al Nabhani, Z., Dulauroy, S., Marques, R., Cousu, C., Al Bounny, S., Déjardin, F., Sparwasser, T., Bérard, M., Cerf-Bensussan, N., and Eberl, G. (2019). A weaning reaction to microbiota is required for resistance to immunopathologies in the adult. *Immunity*., 50(5), 1276-88. e5.

[113] Sonnenburg, J. L., and Bäckhed, F. (2016). Diet–microbiota interactions as moderators of human metabolism. *Nature*., 535(7610), 56-64.

[114] Daelemans, S., Peeters, L., Hauser, B., and Vandenplas, Y. (2018). Recent advances in understanding and managing infantile colic. F1000Research., 7.

[115] Subramanian, S., Huq, S., Yatsunenko, T., Haque, R., Mahfuz, M., Alam, M. A., et al. (2014). Persistent gut microbiota immaturity in malnourished Bangladeshi children. *Nature*., 510(7505), 417-21.

[116] Bozzi Cionci, N., Baffoni, L., Gaggìa, F., and Di Gioia, D. (2018). Therapeutic microbiology: the role of Bifidobacterium breve as food supplement for the prevention/treatment of paediatric diseases. *Nutrients.*, 10(11), 1723.

[117] Martinelli, M., Ummarino, D., Giugliano, F. P., Sciorio, E., Tortora, C., Bruzzese, D., et al. (2017). Efficacy of a standardized extract of Matricariae chamomilla L., *Melissa officinalis* L. and tyndallized *Lactobacillus acidophilus* (HA 122) in infantile colic: An open randomized controlled trial. *Neurogastroenterology & Motility.*, 29(12), e13145.

[118] Vandenplas, Y., Bacarea, A., Marusteri, M., Bacarea, V., Constantin, M., and Manolache, M. (2017). Efficacy and safety of APT198K for the treatment of infantile colic: a pilot study. *Journal of Comparative Effectiveness Research.*, 6(2), 137-44.

[119] Sabahi, S., Homayouni Rad, A., Aghebati-Maleki, L., Sangtarash, N., Ozma, M. A., Karimi, A., Hosseini, H., and Abbasi, A. (2022). Postbiotics as the new frontier in food and pharmaceutical research. *Critical Reviews in Food Science and Nutrition.*, 1-28.

[120] Rampengan, N. H., Manoppo, J., and Warouw, S. M. (2010). Comparison of efficacies between live and killed probiotics in children with lactose malabsorption. *Southeast Asian J Trop Med Public Health.*, 41(2), 474-81.

[121] Rubio-Tapia, A., and Murray, J. A. (2019). Updated guidelines by the European Society for the Study of Coeliac Disease. SAGE Publications Sage UK: London, England, p. 581-2.

[122] Caio, G., Volta, U., Sapone, A., Leffler, D. A., De Giorgio, R., Catassi, C., and Fasano, A. (2019). Celiac disease: a comprehensive current review. *BMC medicine.*, 17, 1-20.

[123] Molberg, Ø., Mcadam, SN., Körner, R., Quarsten, H., Kristiansen, C., Madsen, L., et al. (1998). Tissue transglutaminase selectively modifies gliadin peptides that are recognized by gut-derived T cells in celiac disease. *Nature medicine.*, 4(6), 713-7.

[124] Belkaid, Y., and Hand, T. W. (2014). Role of the microbiota in immunity and inflammation. *Cell.*, 157(1), 121-41.

[125] Nadal, I., Donant, E., Ribes-Koninckx, C., Calabuig, M., and Sanz, Y. (2007). Imbalance in the composition of the duodenal microbiota of children with coeliac disease. *Journal of medical microbiology.*, 56(12), 1669-74.

[126] Sarno, M., Lania, G., Cuomo, M., Nigro, F., Passannanti, F., Budelli, A., et al. (2014). *Lactobacillus paracasei* CBA L74 interferes with gliadin peptides entrance in Caco-2 cells. *International Journal of food sciences and nutrition.*, 65(8), 953-9.

[127] Gallo, M., Nigro, F., Passannanti, F., Nanayakkara, M., Lania, G., Parisi, F., Salameh, D., Budelli, A., Barone, M. V., and Nigro, R. (2019). Effect of pH control during rice fermentation in preventing a gliadin P31-43 entrance in epithelial cells. *International Journal of Food Sciences and Nutrition.*, 70(8), 950-8.

[128] Freire, R., Ingano, L., Serena, G., Cetinbas, M., Anselmo, A., Sapone, A., Sadreyev, R. I., Fasano, A., and Senger, S. (2019). Human gut derived-organoids provide model to study gluten response and effects of microbiota-derived molecules in celiac disease. *Scientific reports.*, 9(1), 7029.

[129] Paparo, L., Nocerino, R., Di Scala, C., Della Gatta, G., Di Costanzo, M., Buono, A., Bruno, C., and Canani, R. B. (2019). Targeting food allergy with probiotics. *Probiotics and Child Gastrointestinal Health: Advances in Microbiology, Infectious Diseases and Public Health*, Volume 10., 57-68.

[130] López-Fandiño, R. (2020). Role of dietary lipids in food allergy. *Critical reviews in food science and nutrition*., 60(11), 1797-814.

[131] Gupta, R. S., Springston, E. E., Warrier, M. R., Smith, B., Kumar, R., Pongracic, J., and Holl, J. L. (2011). The prevalence, severity, and distribution of childhood food allergy in the United States. *Pediatrics*., 128(1), e9-e17.

[132] Sabahi, S., Abbasi, A., and Mortazavi, S. A. (2022). Characterization of cinnamon essential oil and its application in Malva sylvestris seed mucilage edible coating to the enhancement of the microbiological, physicochemical and sensory properties of lamb meat during storage. *Journal of Applied Microbiology*., 133(2), 488-502.

[133] Prince, B. T., Mandel, M. J., Nadeau, K., and Singh, A. M. (2015). Gut microbiome and the development of food allergy and allergic disease. *Pediatric Clinics*., 62(6), 1479-92.

[134] Nowak-Węgrzyn, A., and Chatchatee, P. (2017). Mechanisms of tolerance induction. *Annals of Nutrition and Metabolism*., 70(Suppl. 2), 7-24.

[135] Luu, M., Monning, H., and Visekruna, A. (2020). Exploring the molecular mechanisms underlying the protective effects of microbial SCFAs on intestinal tolerance and food allergy. *Frontiers in immunology*., 11, 1225.

[136] Żółkiewicz, J., Marzec, A., Ruszczyński, M., and Feleszko, W. (2020). Postbiotics—a step beyond pre-and probiotics. *Nutrients*., 12(8), 2189.

[137] Johnson, C. N., Kogut, M. H., Genovese, K., He, H., Kazemi, S., and Arsenault, R. J. (2019). Administration of a postbiotic causes immunomodulatory responses in broiler gut and reduces disease pathogenesis following challenge. *Microorganisms*., 7(8), 268.

[138] Baird, B., Lucia, L., Acuff, G., Harris, K., and Savell, J. (2006). Beef hide antimicrobial interventions as a means of reducing bacterial contamination. *Meat science*., 73(2), 245-8.

[139] Šušković, J., Kos, B., Beganović, J., Leboš, Pavunc, A., Habjanič, K., and Matošić, S. (2010). Antimicrobial activity–the most important property of probiotic and starter lactic acid bacteria. *Food Technology and Biotechnology*., 48(3), 296-307.

[140] Yoon, B. K., Jackman, J. A., Valle-González, E. R., and Cho, N. J. (2018). Antibacterial free fatty acids and monoglycerides: biological activities, experimental testing, and therapeutic applications. *International journal of molecular sciences*., 19(4), 1114.

[141] Osborn, H., and Akoh, C. (2002). Structured lipids-novel fats with medical, nutraceutical, and food applications. *Comprehensive reviews in food science and food safety*., 1(3), 110-20.

[142] Homayouni Rad, A., Pourjafar, H., and Mirzakhani, E. (2023). A comprehensive review of the application of probiotics and postbiotics in oral health. *Frontiers in Cellular and Infection Microbiology*., 13, 1120995.

[143] Twetman, L., Larsen, U., Fiehn, N. E., Stecksén-Blicks, C., and Twetman, S. (2009). Coaggregation between probiotic bacteria and caries-associated strains: an *in vitro* study. *Acta Odontologica Scandinavica.*, 67(5), 284-8.

[144] Ganzle, M. G., Höltzel, A., Walter, J., Jung, G. n., and Hammes, W. P. (2000). Characterization of reutericyclin produced by Lactobacillus reuteri LTH2584. *Applied and environmental microbiology.*, 66(10), 4325-33.

[145] Rodriguez, E., Arques, J., Rodriguez, R., Nunez, M., and Medina, M. (2003). Reuterin production by lactobacilli isolated from pig faeces and evaluation of probiotic traits. *Letters in applied microbiology.*, 37(3), 259-63.

[146] López-López, A., Camelo-Castillo, A., Ferrer, M. D., Simon-Soro, Á., and Mira, A. (2017). Health-associated niche inhabitants as oral probiotics: the case of Streptococcus dentisani. *Frontiers in microbiology.*, 8, 379.

[147] Di Pierro, F., Zanvit, A., Nobili, P., Risso, P., and Fornaini, C. (2015). Cariogram outcome after 90 days of oral treatment with Streptococcus salivarius M18 in children at high risk for dental caries: results of a randomized, controlled study. *Clinical, cosmetic and investigational dentistry.*, 107-13.

[148] Trüper, H. G., and De'Clari, L. (1997). Taxonomic note: necessary correction of specific epithets formed as substantives (nouns)"in apposition". *International Journal of Systematic Bacteriology.*, 47(3), 908-9.

[149] Niels, N. L. (2006). Reclassification of Actinobacillus actinomycetemcomitans, Haemophilus aphrophilus, Haemophilus paraphrophilus and Haemophilus segnis as Aggregatibacter actinomycetemcomitans gen. nov., comb. nov., Aggregatibacter aphraphilus comb. nov. and Aggregatibacter segnis comb. nov., and emended description of Aggregatibacter aphrophilus to include V factor-dependent and V factor-independent isolates. *Int J Syst Evol Microbiol.*, 56, 2135-46.

[150] Simon, L. (2007). The role of Streptococcus mutans and oral ecology in the formation of dental caries.

[151] Conrads, G., de Soet, J. J., Song, L., Henne, K., Sztajer, H., Wagner-Döbler, I., and Zeng, A. P. (2014). Comparing the cariogenic species *Streptococcus sobrinus* and *S. mutans* on whole genome level. *Journal of oral microbiology.*, 6(1), 26189.

[152] Srivastava, S., Saha, S., Kumari, M., and Mohd, S. (2016). Effect of probiotic curd on salivary pH and Streptococcus mutans: a double blind parallel randomized controlled trial. *Journal of clinical and diagnostic research: JCDR.*, 10(2), ZC13.

[153] Hillman, J., Brooks, T., Michalek, S., Harmon, C., Snoep, J., and van Der Weijden, C. (2000). Construction and characterization of an effector strain of Streptococcus mutans for replacement therapy of dental caries. *Infection and immunity.*, 68(2), 543-9.

[154] Meurman, J. H., and Stamatova, I., (2007). Probiotics: contributions to oral health. *Oral diseases.*, 13(5), 443-51.

[155] Dinić, M., Lukić, J., Djokić, J., Milenković, M., Strahinić, I., Golić, N., and Begović, J. (2017). *Lactobacillus fermentum* postbiotic-induced autophagy as potential approach for treatment of acetaminophen hepatotoxicity. *Frontiers in microbiology.*, 8, 594.

[156] Abbasi, A., Saadat, T. R., and Saadat, Y. R. (2022). Microbial exopolysaccharides–β-glucans–as promising postbiotic candidates in vaccine adjuvants. *International Journal of Biological Macromolecules.*

[157] Sotoudegan, F., Daniali, M., Hassani, S., Nikfar, S., and Abdollahi, M. (2019). Reappraisal of probiotics' safety in human. *Food and Chemical Toxicology.*, 129, 22-9.

[158] Abbasi, A., Sabahi, S., Bazzaz, S., Tajani, A. G., Lahouty, M., Aslani, R., and Hosseini, H. (2023). An edible coating utilizing Malva sylvestris seed polysaccharide mucilage and postbiotic from Saccharomyces cerevisiae var. boulardii for the preservation of lamb meat. *International Journal of Biological Macromolecules.*, 246, 125660.

[159] Wright, Av. (2005). Regulating the safety of probiotics-the European approach. *Current pharmaceutical design.*, 11(1), 17-23.

[160] Gaggìa, F., Mattarelli, P., and Biavati, B. (2010). Probiotics and prebiotics in animal feeding for safe food production. *International journal of food microbiology.*, 141, S15-S28.

[161] Wegh, C. A., Geerlings, S. Y., Knol, J., Roeselers, G., and Belzer, C. (2019). Postbiotics and their potential applications in early life nutrition and beyond. *International journal of molecular sciences.*, 20(19), 4673.

[162] Sadeghi-Aliabadi, H., Mohammadi, F., Fazeli, H., and Mirlohi, M. (2014). Effects of Lactobacillus plantarum A7 with probiotic potential on colon cancer and normal cells proliferation in comparison with a commercial strain. *Iranian Journal of Basic Medical Sciences.*, 17(10), 815.

[163] Awaisheh, S., Obeidat, M., Al-Tamimi, H., Assaf, A., El-Qudah, J., and Rahahleh, R. (2016). *In vitro* cytotoxic activity of probiotic bacterial cell extracts against Caco-2 and HRT-18 colorectal cancer cells. *Milk Science International-Milchwissenschaft.*, 69(7), 33-7.

[164] Maghsood, F., Johari, B., Rohani, M., Madanchi, H., Saltanatpour, Z., and Kadivar, M. (2020). Anti-proliferative and anti-metastatic potential of high molecular weight secretory molecules from probiotic Lactobacillus reuteri cell-free supernatant against human colon cancer stem-like cells (HT29-ShE). *International Journal of Peptide Research and Therapeutics.*, 26, 2619-31.

[165] Cui, Y., Qi, S., Zhang, W., Mao, J., Tang, R., Wang, C., Liu, J., Luo, X. M., and Wang, H. (2019). *Lactobacillus reuteri* ZJ617 culture supernatant attenuates acute liver injury induced in mice by lipopolysaccharide. *The Journal of Nutrition.*, 149(11), 2046-55.

[166] Izuddin, W. I., Loh, T. C., Samsudin, A. A., Foo, H. L., Humam, A. M., and Shazali, N. (2019). Effects of postbiotic supplementation on growth performance, ruminal fermentation and microbial profile, blood metabolite and GHR, IGF-1 and MCT-1 gene expression in post-weaning lambs. *BMC veterinary research.*, 15(1), 1-10.

[167] Ang, C. Y., Sano, M., Dan, S., Leelakriangsak, M., and Lal, T. M. (2020). Postbiotics applications as infectious disease control agent in aquaculture. *Biocontrol science.*, 25(1), 1-7.

[168] Anderson, R. C. (2019). Are postbiotics the long sought-after solution for a leaky gut? *The Journal of nutrition.*, 149(11), 1873-4.

[169] Maguire, M., and Maguire, G. (2019). Gut dysbiosis, leaky gut, and intestinal epithelial proliferation in neurological disorders: towards the development of a new therapeutic using amino acids, prebiotics, probiotics, and postbiotics. *Reviews in the Neurosciences.*, 30(2), 179-201.

[170] Bermudez-Brito, M., Plaza-Díaz, J., Muñoz-Quezada, S., Gómez-Llorente, C., and Gil, A. (2012). Probiotic mechanisms of action. *Annals of Nutrition and Metabolism.*, 61(2), 160-74.

Chapter 5

Postbiotics as a Novel Dietary-Based Approach in Celiac Disease

Amin Abbasi, PhD
Maedeh Jabarzadeh Marand, MSc
Sara Razaghi, MSc
Sahand Sohrabi[*], MSc
and Hedayat Hosseini[†], PhD
Department of Food Science and Technology,
National Nutrition and Food Technology Research Institute,
Faculty of Nutrition Science and Food Technology,
Shahid Beheshti University of Medical Sciences, Tehran, Iran

Abstract

Celiac disease (CD), also known as chronic intestinal enteropathy, is an autoimmune disease that affects the small intestine. It is triggered by the consumption of gluten protein, particularly its gliadin component, in susceptible individuals. The most common treatment for celiac patients is a gluten-free diet. However, studies have shown that this diet may not always effectively improve the symptoms of celiac disease. Additionally, the economic and psychological burden of adhering to a strict gluten-free diet can negatively impact a person's quality of life. Therefore, there is a need to change the current treatment process. Research has suggested that the use of pre-, pro-, and post-biotics can help reduce inflammation caused by small intestine immunity and improve the health of celiac

---

[*] Corresponding Author's Email: hedayat@sbmu.ac.ir.
[†] Corresponding Author's Email: sahandsohrabi@sbmu.ac.ir.

In: Exploring Microbiotics in Health and Disease
Editor: Edward L. Stillman
ISBN: 978-8-89113-410-2

patients. Postbiotics are compounds that result from the secretions of living bacteria or are released from the bacterial cell after lysis. They include various metabolites such as bioactive peptides, bacteriocins, extracellular polysaccharides, enzymes, organic acids, and fatty acids. Studies have shown that postbiotics can improve the health and quality of life of individuals. Most of these studies have been conducted on the Caco-2 cell line, which suggests that postbiotics can disrupt the inflammatory response process triggered by gliadin. This disruption can prevent or reduce the entry of gliadin peptides into Caco-2 cells, thereby preventing the harmful effects of this protein on celiac patients. Consequently, postbiotic compounds with safety profile and unique function in degradation of gluten peptides and promotion of the intestinal cell integrity can be considered novel and accessible approach in celiac diet-based therapy.

Keywords: celiac disease, postbiotic, bioactive peptides, bacteriocins, diet-based therapy

Introduction

Celiac disease (CD) is an autoimmune disorder that manifests as a chronic enteropathy and affects the small intestine, particularly the duodenum [1, 2]. The abnormal response of the immune system to a peptide antigen derived from gluten protein leads to the development of symptoms of this systemic disease [1]. As wheat is one of the most commonly consumed grains worldwide, most reports and studies on celiac disease focus on its gluten protein. However, it is important to consider other prolamins, such as hordein from barley and secalin from rye, in the pathogenesis of celiac disease [3]. This disease is widely distributed in all regions of the world and is considered an epidemic that affects all parts of the world. Approximately 1.1 to 1.7 percent of the global population suffer from the consequences of this disease, with women being more affected than men [2]. Genetic sensitivity, exposure to external stimuli such as gluten allergen protein, viral infections, and dysbiosis of the digestive system are among the factors that make individuals susceptible to celiac disease [1]. When discussing genetic sensitivity in individuals, it can be noted that although approximately 30 to 40 percent of the population are HLA-DQ2/DQ8 positive, as previously mentioned, only 1 to 1.5 percent of them develop the celiac disease phenotype. This statistic suggests that environmental factors or the presence of other genes may play a role in individuals' susceptibility to celiac disease [1]. In individuals with a genetic predisposition to celiac disease, these peptides derived from incomplete digestion of gluten proteins can pass through the intestinal epithelial cells and reach the lamina propria where they can trigger an inflammatory pathway, ultimately resulting in the development of the disease [3]. Celiac disease is typically a chronic inflammation that occurs in the small intestine, resulting in an increase in the number of lymphocytes located in the epithelial area (IEL), which initiates the inflammatory pathway associated with this disease. Therefore, major symptoms of this disease include chronic diarrhea and intestinal cramps [1, 2]. If these symptoms are accompanied by atrophy and destruction of intestinal microvilli, malabsorption of nutrients can occur, leading to nutritional deficiencies and related disorders. Common consequences of this disease include anemia and osteoporosis, which may be caused by nutritional deficiencies resulting from the malabsorption of food [2].

When children are suspected of having this disease but do not exhibit clear symptoms, it is necessary to perform a biopsy of the small intestine tissue to ensure an accurate diagnosis. One diagnostic criterion for this disease involves the shortening of intestinal villi resulting from atrophy in a specific area of the small intestine and an increase in the proliferation of crypt cells [1]. If left untreated, celiac disease can result in premature death and the development of various types of intestinal lymphomas. Furthermore, chronic inflammatory bowel disease or celiac disease is associated with other chronic illnesses, including type 1 diabetes and mental disorders such as schizophrenia [2]. Interestingly, poor digestion of gluten protein in the human intestine and digestive system occurs regardless of whether the individual has celiac disease or not [1]. One aspect that receives significant attention in the study of celiac disease is the influence of an individual's environment on the development of underlying factors of this disease. However, our current knowledge is insufficient to fully understand the physio-pathological connections of this disease [4].

Throughout evolution, the human body has adapted to coexist with microbes that have colonized various regions of the human body. Microbes that naturally inhabit the human body are referred to as microbiota. In addition to bacteria, microbiota also include viruses, protozoa, fungi, and single-celled organisms. Microorganisms cover different parts of the human body from the early stages of birth, including the oral and ear cavities, various parts of the digestive system, respiratory and urinary-reproductive tracts. The human digestive system not only provides nutrients to the body but also serves as a source of nutrients for microorganisms [2]. Probiotics are beneficial bacteria that naturally inhabit the human digestive system, especially the intestinal region. The role of probiotics in the occurrence of various metabolic diseases has been studied and investigated. Probiotics in the digestive system metabolize dietary fibers that are not digested by digestive enzymes. Short-chain fatty acids such as butyrate, propionate, and acetate are produced from the fermentation of fiber polysaccharides [1]. Native microorganisms present in the digestive system not only strive to maintain their own survival in the highly competitive environment of the gut but also prevent colonization and invasion by newly ingested bacteria. These microorganisms exert their protective effects through a mechanism of competitive exclusion [2]. For years, researchers have studied the importance of the microbiome in the human digestive system and its various functions, including maintaining intestinal homeostasis and regulating inflammatory responses caused by dietary factors [5]. Every healthy individual has a unique gut microbiota. The Firmicutes and Bacteroidetes bacteria are the two main bacteria that make up about 90% of the total gut microbiome population. Numerous studies have reported a close relationship between the metabolism of gluten and peptides derived from incomplete digestion of gliadin protein with the gut microbiota [2]. Numerous studies have shown that dysbiosis is one of the major causes of celiac disease. In fact, this imbalance that occurs in the human gastrointestinal microbiota is the basis for many chronic diseases, including celiac disease [5, 6]. In 2016, Caminero and colleagues discovered that bacteria present in the digestive system and gut microbiota have the ability to reduce the immune response of gluten on T cells through its hydrolysis [7]. Other researchers have also reported the microbial flora of other areas of the digestive system, including the mouth, in the hydrolysis of gluten. In another study, it has been shown that oral administration of *Lactococcus lactis* can increase tolerance to antigenic peptides derived from incomplete digestion of gliadin protein in an animal model [8, 9]. After numerous studies, researchers concluded that dysbiosis of the colon and duodenum is associated with celiac disease [2]. Postbiotics are bacterial metabolites that are either secreted by bacteria outside the cell or released into the environment after bacterial cell lysis [2]. Postbiotics include both non-viable probiotics and metabolites that are secreted or released as a result of bacterial lysis by these microorganisms [1]. Metabolites such as short-chain fatty acids, microbial peptides, and organic acids are among the products classified as postbiotics. Enzymes, extracellular polysaccharides, and bacteriocins also fall into this category [1, 2]. It has been shown that postbiotics have the potential to exert their health-promoting effects on the host body if consumed in sufficient quantities [1-3].

Postbiotics have the advantage of being more stable and safe compared to probiotics. Additionally, since these compounds do not contain live bacteria, they do not pose a risk of infection or induce acute or chronic inflammatory responses in the human body. Postbiotics can suppress the inflammatory pathway caused by peptides derived from incomplete digestion of gliadin protein through various mechanisms, thereby improving the quality of life for celiac patients and reducing the symptoms associated with this disease in individuals [3]. In laboratory scale, postbiotics have the ability to prevent the inflammatory and immune effects of peptides derived from incomplete digestion of gliadin protein in Caco2 cell line. Multiple studies have shown that postbiotics derived from *Lactobacillus paracasei* CBA L74 have the ability to reduce the entry of peptides derived from incomplete digestion of gliadin protein into Caco2 cells and play an effective role in inhibiting or reducing the activation of the inflammatory response and autophagy pathway associated with gliadin protein [5, 10]. Activation of the autophagy pathway plays an important role in intestinal homeostasis [2]. Postbiotic HM0539 can also reduce the damage to intestinal mucus induced by tumor necrosis factor alpha by stimulating mucin production [1]. A study on the role of lactate, butyrate, and polysaccharide A postbiotics from *Bacteroides fragilis* bacteria in celiac disease showed that these postbiotics can modulate the immune response to gliadin proteins in the body. These researchers also reported that *B. fragilis* postbiotics can reduce the production of inflammatory mediators interleukin 15 and interferon gamma [11].

The bacterium *Lactobacillus rhamnosus* GG (LGG) is known as a probiotic strain because it exhibits resistance to bile and stomach acid, as well as good adhesive properties, allowing it to attach to the intestinal epithelial layer and exert potential effects. It has been shown that postbiotics derived from *L. rhamnosus* GG can have protective effects on intestinal mucus by producing a biofilm layer, and these compounds can also inhibit the inflammatory process mediated by NF-κB. This not only helps maintain the structural integrity of intestinal epithelial cells but also prevents tissue damage through apoptosis. In a study conducted in 2023 on the anti-inflammatory effects of *Lactobacillus rhamnosus* GG postbiotics, researchers found that peptides derived from incomplete digestion of gliadin protein (P31-43) induce a response in intestinal epithelial cells through the mTOR signaling pathway. Phosphorylation of the NF-κB pathway was also observed as another effect of these peptides. Treatment of Caco2 cell cultures with *Lactobacillus rhamnosus* GG postbiotics was able to reduce the activation of the mTOR signaling pathway and prevent phosphorylation of NF-κB, thereby reducing inflammatory chain reactions. Protein staining for LC3II also showed a decrease in the presence of P31-43 peptides, which could be reversed by postbiotics. The results of this study, along with other studies, confirm that postbiotics can inhibit the inflammatory process caused by peptides derived from incomplete digestion of gliadin protein and improve the quality of life for individuals with celiac disease [6].

History of Diagnosis and Identification of Celiac Disease

Two types of sensitivity to the consumption of gluten in wheat have been reported: gluten sensitivity with celiac disease and non-celiac gluten sensitivity [3]. The description of celiac disease and gluten sensitivity resulting from the consumption of wheat gluten is examined from various perspectives. One of the oldest views is a description proposed by the Greek physician, Aretaeus, which states that individuals with celiac disease actually suffer from continuous disruptions in the digestive processes related to digestion and absorption of food, leading to malabsorption of nutrients. Aretaeus also stated that this disorder improves with the avoidance of food consumption for a certain period each day. Therefore, it can be inferred from the statements of this Greek physician that the main cause of digestive disorders resulting from celiac disease is nutritional [12]. Samuel Jones Gee described another description of celiac disease in 1888 under the title "coeliac infection". He stated that this disease is a chronic malabsorption of food with symptoms of diarrhea and malabsorption that can occur at any age, but its occurrence is more common among young people [13]. In the following years, many specialists were seeking the cause and etiology of this disease, but among them, the descriptions of Dr. Willem Dicke in the 1930s are closer to today's comprehensive description. He described a diet consisting of vegetables and fruits called the banana and faconi diet for improving the symptoms of celiac disease, but at that time, he did not realize the connection between consuming wheat and the onset of symptoms of celiac disease. After various observations and examining the effects of diets, the toxic nature of wheat for individuals with celiac disease was recognized by Dr. Willem Dicke, and a wheat-free diet was recommended for patients. After this finding, various researchers also described the negative consequences of consuming a wheat-based diet for celiac patients and confirmed the findings of this Dutch pediatrician [13]. The first general term related to celiac disease was introduced in 1970 by Acta Paediatrica, which described this disease as a chronic condition that leads to flattening of the intestinal mucosal surface and sensitivity to wheat gluten protein. It was concluded that the consumption of gluten protein exacerbates the symptoms of this disease and adherence to a gluten-free diet improves the course of this disease [14, 15] (Figure 1).

The Role of Gluten Structure in CD-Related Inflammation

What happens in celiac disease is actually a series of inflammatory reactions triggered by wheat gluten protein [2, 3]. Wheat gluten contains a high amount of the amino acids glutamine and proline. Proline has the ability to form a more compact B-turn structure compared to α-helix. This compact structure allows the amino acids to be closely packed together in a continuous and tight structure, making it difficult for digestive enzymes to fully digest the protein [3]. The protease enzymes located in the pancreas and stomach do not have the ability to fully digest this protein [3]. In addition to the compact structure of gluten protein hindering its complete digestion, the human digestive system also lacks the necessary enzymes for complete digestion of gluten protein. Endoprotease is a serine peptidase that is necessary for the complete digestion of prolamins, including gluten proteins. Since the human digestive system lacks this enzyme, prolamins such as gluten proteins are not fully digested in the human digestive system, and therefore, large peptides resulting from incomplete digestion of these proteins can progress through the gastrointestinal tract without further alteration [2, 16]. In general, the sequence of consecutive proline and glutamine amino acids in gluten protein is the main cause of inadequate digestion of this protein in mammalian digestive systems, including humans. Findings from studies on the inflammatory properties of gluten protein and its gliadin fraction suggest that peptides resulting from incomplete digestion of these proteins are immunogenic or toxic. If they activate immune cells along the inflammatory pathway, they are considered immunogenic. If they activate immune cells associated with cellular immunity, they are considered toxic [2, 3].

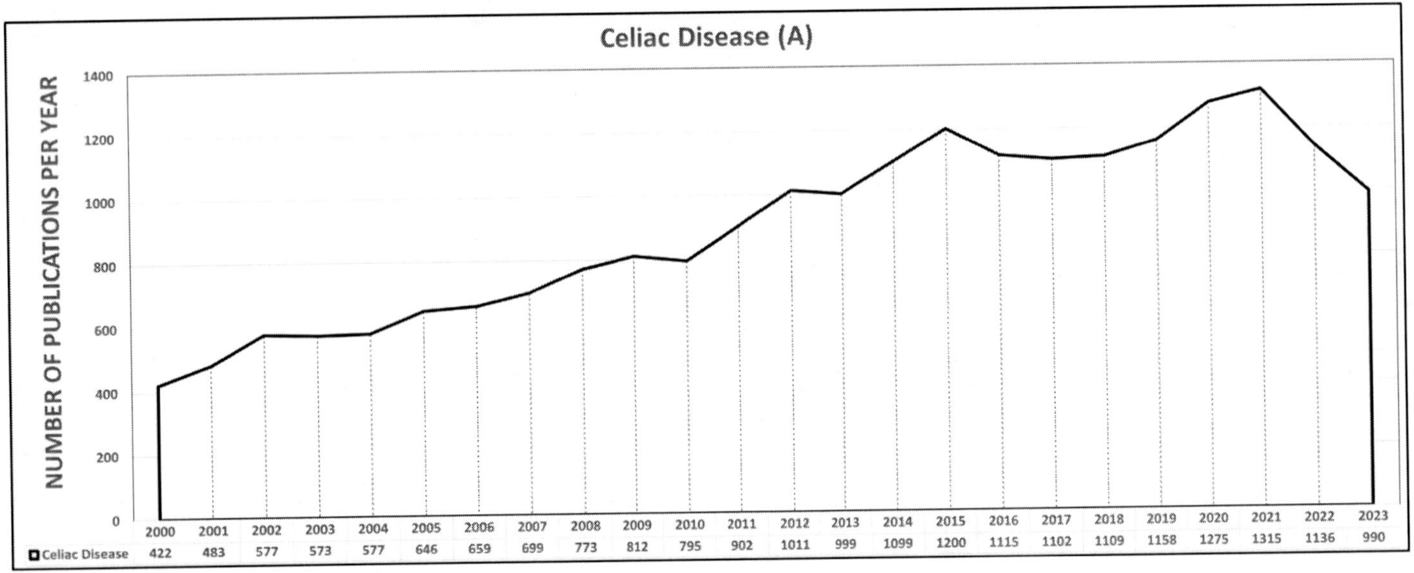

Figure 1. (Continued).

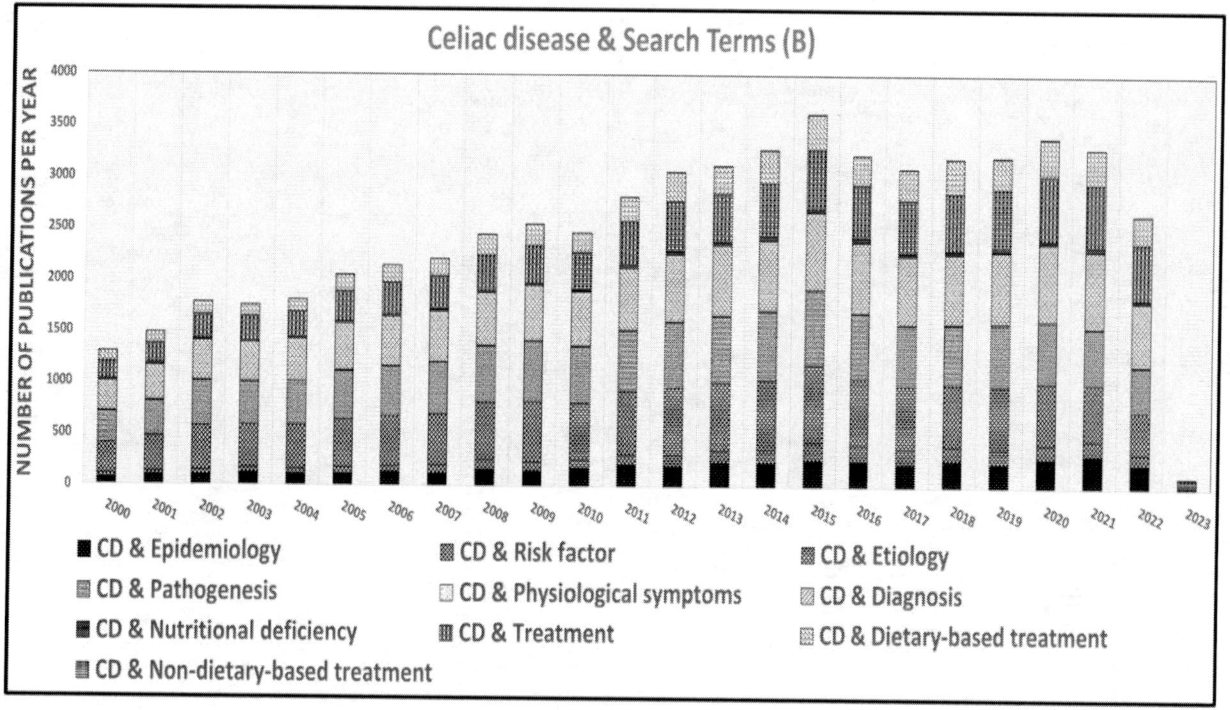

Figure 1. Illustrates the increase in the number of papers reporting research regarded celiac disease. Comparison between the number of publications; on top the search of celiac disease (A), and below the search of the association between celiac disease and search terms ('Epidemiology'; 'Etiology'; 'Pathogenesis'; 'Physiological symptoms'; 'Diagnosis'; 'Nutritional deficiency'; 'Treatment'; 'Dietary-based treatment'; and 'Non-dietary-based treatment') (B) in PubMed 2023.

The gliadin fraction of wheat gluten protein is an important factor in the development of complications related to celiac disease and most studies have been conducted on this protein. Recent studies have shown that large peptides derived from proteolysis of gluten protein and its gliadin fraction lead to activation of the inflammatory pathway associated with the production of cytokines and inflammatory mediators such as interleukin 15, which mediates the expression of mRNA associated with pro-apoptotic intestinal cells [2, 3]. Peptides derived from incomplete digestion of gliadin protein, after being produced, penetrate the lower layers through the small intestine mucosa [1, 3, 17]. The toxic gliadin peptide A, known as P31-43, is actually responsible for several different metabolic effects, including activation of the signaling pathway associated with the epidermal growth factor receptor [5, 18].

The Inflammation Mechanism in Celiac Disease

mTOR is a serine-threonine protein kinase and essentially a highly conserved signaling pathway that regulates cellular responses such as protein synthesis, inflammation, proliferation, cellular growth and metabolism, autophagy, and apoptosis in the presence of nutrients and growth factors, which in turn leads to maintaining cellular integrity and intestinal homeostasis. mTOR can be stimulated by peptides derived from incomplete digestion of gliadin protein [5, 6]. This, along with the activation of the nuclear transcription factor NF-κβ pathway, leads to excessive production of inflammatory mediators and cytokines in various parts of the intestines of celiac patients [6, 19]. Preserving some vital cellular functions including autophagy is essential for the body's metabolic system [5]. Autophagy is a vital process in regulating and maintaining cellular homeostasis, which is a kind of recycling of protein function, cytoplasmic components, and damaged organelles [6]. Initiating autophagy processes when cells are exposed to various pathogens is necessary for cell survival [5, 20]. If autophagy and its pathway are disrupted, neurological damage, microbial infections, and various chronic diseases may occur. Inflammatory responses following microbial infections or the presence of antigens can be prevented by activating the autophagy pathway. This action occurs by preventing the production of inflammatory mediators, including cytokines [6]. Activation of the mTOR signaling pathway by peptides derived from incomplete digestion of gliadin protein leads to inhibition of the autophagy pathway, exacerbating the accumulation of inflammatory mediators and damaging factors to intestinal homeostasis [5, 6]. LC3II protein is also an essential component of the autophagy pathway, and its presence is necessary for the formation of autophagosomes. The production of this protein is also suppressed by the presence of gliadin peptides [5]. Therefore, mTOR is a potential therapeutic target in the treatment of chronic inflammatory bowel diseases, including celiac disease, cancers, and microbial infections [6, 21]. One of the most common and well-known theories that explains the immunopathogenesis and inflammatory response in celiac disease is the dual signaling model. This model is based on an initial innate immune response and subsequent adaptive immune response in the presence of specific antigens [3, 22].

Interestingly, studies have shown that the induction of the inflammatory pathway by peptides derived from incomplete digestion of gliadin protein can delay vesicular trafficking. Other effects of these peptides include induction of actin remodeling, increased expression of epidermal growth factor receptor, and activation of signal-regulated kinase [6]. Wheat gluten, as an environmental factor in this disease, affects the genetic predisposing factors such as HLA-DQ2/8 loci and tissue transglutaminase 2 enzyme activity [2, 5]. In celiac disease, in addition to the involvement of cellular immune system mediated by T cells, which is stimulated in the presence of peptides derived from incomplete digestion of gliadin protein, the immune system including circulating antibodies (humoral immune system) also contributes to the progression of the inflammatory pathway by producing autoantibodies such as endomysial antibodies, tissue transglutaminase antibodies, and deamidated gliadin peptide antibodies. The presence of these antibodies is indicative of the diagnosis of chronic enteropathy or celiac disease [1, 23]. The interaction of peptides derived from incomplete digestion of gliadin protein with intestinal epithelial cells leads to their penetration into the mucosal layers of the intestine and interaction with tissue transglutaminase 2 enzyme in the lamina propria region [2]. Tissue transglutaminase 2 enzyme is an enzyme that converts residual neutral and polar amino acids to glutamic acid with a negative charge. In the submucosal region, peptides derived from incomplete digestion of gliadin protein are deamidated by tissue transglutaminase 2 enzyme, resulting in an increase in negatively charged amino acids in the peptides. As a result of this action, the affinity of these peptides to bind to human leukocyte antigens such as HLA-DQ2 and HLA-DQ8 molecules, which are located on the surface of antigen-presenting cells or human dendritic cells, increases [1-3]. Human dendritic cells present gluten antigens to T cells, resulting in an increase in CD^{4+} T cell numbers and the production of inflammatory mediators such as interleukins and interferon gamma [1-3]. It has been shown that the formation of a parallel beta structure, which can occur depending on the concentration of peptides derived from incomplete digestion of gliadin protein, is functionally and pathogenically similar to amyloid proteins. One way to prevent inflammation caused by peptides derived from incomplete digestion of gliadin protein is the production of molecules that bind to these peptides and prevent the action of tissue transglutaminase 2 enzyme in producing negatively charged peptides. This allows these peptides to be expelled from the body without penetrating the lamina propria and interacting with dendritic cells [2]. Studies have shown that interferon gamma and interleukins 4 and 10 are the dominant inflammatory mediators in the blood of untreated celiac patients. Tumor necrosis factor alpha is also expressed and produced in large amounts by lymphocytes located in the epithelial region of the intestine. Additionally, interleukins 15 and 21 are also of great importance in the pathogenesis of celiac disease, as it has been shown that these inflammatory mediators are produced by T cells located in the lamina propria region [3]. This inflammatory pathway ultimately leads to the destruction of epithelial cells in the intestinal mucosa by activating CD8+ cytotoxic T cells, which in turn is associated with the acute and chronic symptoms of celiac disease [2, 3]. In order for CD^{4+} T cells to recognize peptides derived from gluten protein digestion, these peptides must have epitopes associated with CD^{4+} T cells.

Therefore, various studies have shown that different proteins have epitopes associated with CD^{4+} T cells, including HMW and LMW glutenins, gamma, alpha and omega gliadins, hordein, avonin, and secalin. Epitopes associated with CD^{4+} T cells in gliadin peptides are resistant to hydrolysis by intestinal protease enzymes, allowing them to induce their own immune response. An interesting point to note is that CD^{4+} T cells in healthy individuals, like CD^{4+} T cells in celiac patients, do not have the ability to recognize gluten protein antigens. This means that celiac patients have CD^{4+} T cells sensitive to gluten protein, indicating that genetics play a very important and complex role in the etiology of celiac disease [3].

The Long-Term Impact, Effects and Challenges of Following and Not Following a Gluten-Free Diet on the Healing Process of Celiac Patients

In the treatment process of celiac patients, nutrition specialists play a key role. In fact, long-term adherence to gluten-free diets is the most accessible way to prevent the onset of celiac disease symptoms [1, 6]. Therefore, these specialists are the mainstay of celiac disease treatment [3]. Celiac patients are at risk of malnutrition due to dietary restrictions, which can lead to deficiencies in essential nutrients [24, 25]. Adherence to a gluten-free diet is the only effective therapeutic approach for managing inflammation in celiac patients. The diet of a celiac patient should be free of any food containing gluten, as even consuming a small amount of 50 milligrams per day of gluten protein can be immunogenic for celiac patients. The production of gluten-free products is supervised by two organizations, the Food and Agricultural Organization and the Codex Alimentarius Commission. These organizations continuously monitor the level of prolamin in gluten-free products and have stated that the gluten content in such products should not exceed 20 parts per million. Despite all the supervision and care, lifelong adherence to a gluten-free diet is very difficult and burdensome for celiac patients. Various dimensions of problems can make it challenging for celiac patients, including low nutritional value of gluten-free products, higher cost of these meals, insufficient availability, and lack of sufficient diversity in formulation and composition. Therefore, finding alternative treatments to improve the quality of life for celiac patients has been the focus of researchers [3]. Recently, a treatment method that has attracted researchers' attention relies on the interactions and metabolites derived from the gut microbiome. Many studies have concluded that celiac disease leads to dysbiosis, which has been demonstrated by comparing the microbiota of patients and control groups before and after adherence to a gluten-free diet [1]. Nowadays, attention to novel treatments such as probiotics and postbiotics for the treatment of celiac autoimmune disorders has gained more attention than ever before.

Probiotics

Probiotics refer to living microorganisms that have been shown to have positive impacts on human health when supplied in sufficient quantities. These bacteria work by maintaining the balance of the gut microbiome, so preventing dysbiosis of the gut microbiota and enhancing immune function [26]. In relation to this matter, there is ongoing research on probiotic bacteria, with a focus on their potential use as adjunctive therapies for a range of intestinal disorders, particularly CD (27). The majority of probiotic bacteria are classified under the genera Lactobacillus and Bifidobacterium. The United States Food and Drug Administration (USFDA) has designated them as

"Generally Recognized As Safe" (GRAS) [28]. Nevertheless, several studies have shown that many strains of Bacillus also exhibit the fundamental attributes of probiotics. These attributes include the ability to withstand antibiotics, as well as tolerate acidic environments, bile salts, and sodium chloride. Additionally, these strains are capable of producing a diverse range of antimicrobial peptides that possess a larger spectrum of inhibitory effects [29]. Probiotic options, such as *Bacillus* sp., and *Lactobacillus* sp. which are derived from various sources, are mostly used because to their inherent safety and cost-effectiveness [30]. Both of these species are often seen in high quantities throughout the upper gastrointestinal tracts of both human beings and animals. De Angelis et al. (2021) conducted a study in which they developed a formulation of commercial enzymes using a microbial consortium consisting of *Lactobacillus plantarum*, *L. paracasei*, *Bacillus subtilis*, *B. pumilus*, and *B. megaterium*. The researchers observed that this formulation exhibited the ability to hydrolyze gluten into peptides that are both non-immunogenic and non-toxic under gastrointestinal circumstances. The aforementioned results indicate that both microbial consortia possess the ability to detoxify immunogenic gluten peptides, suggesting their potential use in enhancing the intestinal digestion of individuals with CD and gluten sensitivity [27].

Probiotics have been shown to possess therapeutic properties that contribute to preventing and treating several medical problems. These ailments include inflammatory bowel disease (Crohn's disease and ulcerative colitis), autoimmune disorders (rheumatoid arthritis), celiac disease, lactose intolerance, irritable bowel syndrome, vaginal infections (candida or thrush), and atopic dermatitis [31, 32]. The use of probiotics has been shown to contribute to the reduction of both diarrhea and allergies. The use of probiotics derived from dairy and meats has been seen to result in a reduction in low-density lipoprotein (LDL) levels, the eradication of bacteria responsible for tooth decay, and a mitigation of the detrimental impacts associated with gingivitis. Probiotics have the ability to activate, alter, and control several aspects of the host's immunological response, gastrointestinal hormone secretion, and brain-behavior through means of bidirectional neuronal transmission [33, 34]. Probiotics possess physiological properties that enhance the overall well-being of the host environment, have regulatory effects on microbial populations, and show potential in addressing issues related to obesity and overweight conditions [35]. Several instances have been documented when patients diagnosed with severe acute pancreatitis were given probiotic prophylaxis, resulting in a notable exacerbation of adverse effects produced by the probiotics [36, 37]. Hence, the precise processes behind the health-enhancing properties of probiotics remain uncertain. Nevertheless, it is important to do an investigation into the membrane and extracellular proteins/enzymes, as well as other biomolecules, present in probiotics [38, 39]. The bacteria under consideration have the capacity to synthesize a wide range of substances, including exopolysaccharides, secreted low-calorie sweetening molecules, antibacterial compounds, bacteriocins, enzymes, organic acids, and nutraceuticals [40]. The field of probiotics is now seeing significant development potential, making it an increasingly important area of focus for food makers. Due to the consumption of viable probiotic bacterial cultures, it serves to augment the composition of the intestinal microbiota. The significance and efficacy of probiotics in the broader market will be contingent upon the efficiency of the specific probiotic strain or cultures used. Food items that include probiotics and prebiotics have an impact on the functioning of the foods, leading to the improvement of the microflora that supports gastrointestinal health [41].

In recent times, there has been a notable emphasis among researchers on the examination of gliadin-cleaving proteolytic activity derived from probiotic strains. *Lactobacilli* and *Bifidobacterium* are recognized as crucial components of the gut microbiota, having advantageous impacts on human well-being and being extensively used in the development of probiotic formulations. The use of probiotics containing gluten-degrading bacteria in therapy is a potential novel approach for the adjunctive management of individuals with celiac disease [42]. The *Bifidobacterium* species exhibited significant gluten protein digestion, resulting in decreased cytotoxicity and less pro-inflammatory reactions [43]. The probiotic mixture, consisting of two strains of *Lactobacilli* and three strains of *Bifidobacteria*, exhibits the ability to hydrolyze gliadin peptides and provide protection to intestinal cells against the detrimental effects of toxic pro-inflammatory peptides [44]. In their study, Heeney et al. observed that the presence of probiotic *Lactobacilli* at low levels yielded inconclusive results in the microbiomes of both adult and pediatric populations exhibiting active CD [45]. Nevertheless, several papers have shown the beneficial effects of probiotics in animal models exhibiting some characteristics of CD. These studies have indicated that probiotics have the potential to have a favorable impact on the pathophysiology of the illness via diverse pathways.

Akobeng et al. (2020) documented that the introduction of probiotics to the gluten-free diet (GFD) has been considered as an alternative therapeutic method due to the microbial imbalances that arise as a result of following a

GFD [46]. Probiotics are known to have a significant impact on the restoration and regulation of the gut microbiota. Undoubtedly, the makeup of gut microbiota has a significant role in shaping the range of gastrointestinal symptoms seen in individuals with CD [47]. Marasco et al. (2020) conducted a study which indicated that the use of probiotics in individuals with CD has the potential to influence the composition and functionality of the microbiota. This modulation of the microbiota might potentially lead to a delay in the onset of CD or possibly serve as a preventative measure. In the aforementioned study, it was observed that the introduction of probiotic strains derived from *Bifidobacterium* and *Lactobacilli* resulted in the restoration of gut microbiota and the pre-digestion of gluten peptides within the intestinal lumen. This process led to a reduction in inflammation associated with gluten consumption, as well as improvements in intestinal permeability, cytokine levels, and antibody production. These results provide insights into potential strategies for enhancing symptom management and increasing the overall quality of life in patients undergoing treatment with probiotics and a gluten-free diet [48].

Prebiotics

Prebiotics may be described as a substrate that is specifically used by bacteria residing inside the host in order to provide a health advantage. This advantage is often achieved by promoting the growth and activity of certain beneficial microbial groups, primarily Bifidobacterium and Lactobacillus, within the gastrointestinal tract. Instances of compounds found in various foods include garlic, onions, artichokes, and other similar examples. Consuming sufficient quantities of these dietary sources may be crucial in order to get the advantageous "bifidogenic" impact. An additional option involves the use of a prebiotic supplement in order to get optimal levels. Furthermore, it should be noted that prebiotics exhibit resistance to hydrolysis via digestive enzymes and possess limited absorption capabilities inside the upper gastrointestinal tract. As a result, they are able to traverse to the large intestine, where they effectively encourage the development of certain microbes [49]. Various substances have undergone testing to ascertain their efficacy as prebiotics. The most prevalent prebiotics are fructo-oligosaccharides (FOS), galacto-oligosaccharides (GOS), and trans-galacto-oligosaccharides (TOS). The gut microbiota engages in the fermentation process of prebiotics, resulting in the production of short-chain fatty acids (SCFAs), such as lactic acid, butyric acid, and propionic acid [50].

In their study, Drabinska et al. (2018) observed a significant rise in the population of Bifidobacterium in the gastrointestinal tract of children diagnosed with celiac disease when administered oligofructose-enriched inulin, a kind of prebiotic. The researchers found no evidence of any negative consequences resulting from this intervention. The present study focuses on exploring the potential causal relationship between gut dysbiosis and CD, but the precise underlying mechanism remains uncertain [51]. Research is also centered on the use of a diet low in fermentable oligo-, di-, monosaccharides, and polyols (FODMAPs), including short-chain polysaccharides such as fructans, lactose, mannitol, sorbitol, and others. The digestion of these sugars poses challenges, leading to fermentation inside the gastrointestinal tract and subsequent flatulence. Moreover, these sugars have been associated with the manifestation of some symptoms of irritable bowel syndrome (IBS) [52]. The low FODMAP diet has been shown to have potential benefits for individuals with celiac disease, particularly those with functional irritable bowel syndrome-like symptoms [53]. However, the specific molecular mechanism behind these benefits has yet to be fully understood.

Chen et al. (2017) conducted a study to investigate the potential mechanism of action of prebiotics on the Caco-2 intestinal epithelial cell line. They used a prebiotic mix consisting of fructooligosaccharides (FOS), galactooligosaccharides (GOS), inulin, and anthocyanins, which were co-incubated with Salmonella typhimurium. Furthermore, the researchers examined post-infectious models of irritable bowel syndrome (IBS) in C57BL/6 mice. The findings of the research indicate that the prebiotic mix had a notable impact on reducing the production of pro-inflammatory cytokines in both infected Caco-2 cells and post-infectious models of irritable bowel syndrome [54]. Marasco et al. conducted a comprehensive review that encompassed randomized controlled trials, cross-sectional studies, and prominent literature reviews. Their findings indicate that the incorporation of inulin as prebiotics in a gluten-free diet has the potential to promote the proliferation of beneficial bacterial strains, specifically Bifidobacterium and Lactobacillus [48]. The authors also noted that the majority of research conducted on patients with CD used inulin as the prebiotic of interest. Consequently, exploring the potential effects of other prebiotics in the context of CD is an intriguing avenue for further investigation.

Synbiotics

Synbiotics refer to the amalgamation of probiotics and prebiotics. Synbiotics are composed of probiotics, which are advantageous microorganisms, and prebiotics, which are non-digestible substances that enhance the proliferation of helpful bacteria. The inclusion of a prebiotic in a product promotes the development of the desired probiotic. One example of synbiotic food items is fermented dairy products, such as yogurt. The most often seen synbiotics consist of fructooligosaccharides (FOS) in combination with *Bifidobacteria*, inulins paired with *Lactobacillus*, and a combination of *Bifidobacteria* and *Lactobacilli* supplemented with FOS [55]. According to the findings of Wilms et al., the implementation of synbiotic dietary methods has the potential to enhance the functionality of the intestinal barrier. According to the findings, a study involving 20 healthy adult participants revealed that the administration of synbiotic supplements, namely Ecologic® 82S combined with a daily dosage of 10 g Fructooligosaccharides P6 (FOS P6), resulted in a significant rise in stool frequency over a period of two weeks. The study assessed the impact of synbiotics on intestinal permeability, immunological function, and gastrointestinal symptoms in both baseline and indomethacin-induced stressful settings. The results indicated that the administration of synbiotics did not significantly alter intestinal permeability, immune function, or gastrointestinal symptoms in either the basal or indomethacin-induced circumstances [56].

In their study, Demiroren et al. observed a reduction in anti-tTG levels in children who exhibited possible CD after receiving a 20-day dosage of synbiotics including a multi-strain of Lactobacillus and Bifidobacterium. This drop was in comparison to a control group that did not get the synbiotic supplementation [57].

Ugural and Akyol (2022) critically examined the potential contribution of pseudocereals, including amaranth, quinoa, and buckwheat, in symbiotic formulations aimed at addressing dysbiosis and chronic illnesses characterized by inflammation, such as CD [58]. The authors conducted a comprehensive analysis of current studies conducted in this emerging field. The researchers reported the observation of favorable substrate properties for probiotic bacteria when utilizing cultures or naturally fermented pseudocereals. They found that pseudocereals lead to an increased abundance of *Peptoclostridium, Prevotellaceae, Lactobacillus, Bifidobacterium, Enterococcus,* and *Eubacteriaceae*. Additionally, the researchers noted an augmentation in the synthesis of short-chain fatty acids, which can be attributed to the prebiotic effects of these substances. The available literature on the prebiotic benefits of amaranth, a pseudocereal known for its high protein content (13.56 g/100 g), is currently minimal. A notable experiment in this particular field has been documented by Gullon et al. This investigation included the inoculation of in vitro digested amaranth and quinoa grains into fecal samples obtained from people who were in good health. Following the incubation period, many microbiota species were identified, including *Faecalibacterium prausnitzii*, *Roseburia intestinalis*, *Atopobium*, *Lactobacillus–Enterococcus*, *Bacteroides–Prevotella*, *Bifidobacterium* spp., *Clostridium coccoides–Eubacterium rectale*, and Furthermore, an augmentation in bacterial diversity was seen, accompanied by an elevation in the levels of short-chain fatty acids like acetate, propionate, and butyrate. The study's findings indicated that quinoa and amaranth have potential prebiotic action [59].

Postbiotics

Postbiotics refer to the substances that are produced by live bacteria or released after their breakdown, such as short-chain fatty acids (SCFAs), lactic acid, bioactive peptides, and several other metabolites. Furthermore, this concept may be expanded to include protein molecules, hydrogen peroxide (H_2O_2), bacteriocins, organic acids, exopolysaccharides, and enzymes [60-63]. The administration of sufficient quantities of postbiotics has been shown to contribute to the enhancement of the host's overall well-being. However, the precise processes behind the observed improvements remain incompletely elucidated so far. The use of postbiotics, as opposed to probiotics, offers distinct benefits in terms of enhanced stability and safety. Postbiotics are devoid of viable bacteria, hence eliminating the potential for microbial infection and transfer [18, 64, 65].

Postbiotics have been utilized *in vitro* tests using Caco-2 cells to assess their potential in mitigating the detrimental impacts of gliadin and gliadin peptides on Caco-2 cells. In their study, Sarno et al. (2014) demonstrated the potential of postbiotics CBA L74, namely the supernatant derived from *Lactobacillus paracasei*, to mitigate the ingress of gliadin peptides into Caco-2 cells [66]. Conte et al. conducted a recent study examining the advantageous postbiotic impact of *Lactobacillus paracasei* CBA L74 on both Caco-2 cells and CD organoids *in vitro*. These cells and organoids were stimulated with pepsin-trypsin gliadin (PTG) digest or the cytotoxic 13-mer gliadin peptide. The administration of the postbiotic substance effectively inhibited the activation of the inflammatory response caused by gliadin. This was determined by assessing the levels of activation markers NF-κB and ERK phosphorylation, as well as the activation of mTOR signaling. Additionally, the postbiotic demonstrated the ability to counteract the decrease of the autophagy pathway created by gliadin. Therefore, the administration of postbiotics derived from *Lactobacillus paracasei* CBA L74 resulted in a reduction of the inflammatory response generated by gliadin, while also promoting autophagy, a process that plays a crucial role in maintaining intestinal homeostasis [67]. Freire et al. utilized an *in vitro* model of organoids derived from persons without celiac disease and those with celiac disease to investigate the pathophysiology of CD, as described in another article. This research also examined the impacts of three postbiotics, namely butyrate, lactate, and polysaccharide A derived from *B. fragilis*. It was discovered that these molecules had the ability to regulate the gut reactions to gluten. The researchers demonstrated a rise in paracellular permeability that was already evident in the initial state in celiac disease organoids. Specifically, the restoration of the barrier function in celiac disease may be achieved by the administration of butyrate and polysaccharide A, which leads to an upregulation of the tight junction sealing molecule known as claudin-18. Similarly, when the CD organoids were exposed to gliadin, there was an immunological response triggered, characterized by the production of IL-15 and IFN gamma. However, the presence of butyrate and lactate resulted in a reduction of this immune activation [68].

Conclusion

Numerous research studies have shown a strong correlation between probiotics, prebiotics, synbiotics, and postbiotics in connection to intestinal microbiota and immune response in the context of CD. Exploring this interplay within the broader framework of "biotics" is a promising avenue for further investigation in the field. Instead of using other non-dietary approaches, the use of "Pro-Pre-Syn-Post" biotics may serve as a suitable and biologically safe supplemental dietary intervention for individuals with CD. The comprehensive molecular processes underlying the activities of these "biotics" are now in their early stages and require more fundamental investigation. It was hypothesized that the future use of metabolomics will provide valuable insights into the understanding of the molecular processes behind these "biotics" as a potential dietary intervention for CD, either in conjunction with the gluten-free diet or in other therapeutic approaches.

Disclaimer

None.

References

[1] Conte M, Porpora M, Nigro F, Nigro R, Budelli AL, Barone MV, Nanayakkara, M Pro-Pre and Postbiotic in Celiac Disease. *Applied Sciences*. 2021;11(17):8185.

[2] Wagh SK, Lammers KM, Padul MV, Rodriguez-Herrera A, Dodero VI. Celiac Disease and Possible Dietary Interventions: From Enzymes and Probiotics to Postbiotics and Viruses. *International journal of molecular sciences*. 2022;23(19).

[3] Abbasi A, Bazzaz S, A. Ibrahim S, Hekmatdoost A, Hosseini H, Sabahi S, Sheykhsaran, E., Rahbar Saadat, Y., Asghari Ozma, M., & Lahouty, M. A Critical Review on the Gluten-Induced Enteropathy/Celiac Disease: Gluten-Targeted Dietary and Non-Dietary Therapeutic Approaches. *Food Reviews International.* 2023:1-41.

[4] Levescot A, Malamut G, Cerf-Bensussan N. Immunopathogenesis and environmental triggers in coeliac disease. *Gut.* 2022;71(11):2337-49.

[5] Conte M, Nigro F, Porpora M, Bellomo C, Furone F, Budelli AL, Nigro, R, Barone MV, & Nanayakkara M. Gliadin Peptide P31-43 Induces mTOR/NFkβ Activation and Reduces Autophagy: The Role of Lactobacillus paracasei CBA L Postbiotc. *International journal of molecular sciences*. 2022;23(7).

[6] Furone F, Bellomo C, Carpinelli M, Nicoletti M, Hewa-Munasinghege FN, Mordaa M, Roberta Mandile, Maria Vittoria Barone, Merlin Nanayakkara. The protective role of Lactobacillus rhamnosus GG postbiotic on the alteration of autophagy and inflammation pathways induced by gliadin in intestinal models. *Frontiers in Medicine*. 2023;10.

[7] Caminero A, Galipeau HJ, McCarville JL, Johnston CW, Bernier SP, Russell AK, Jury, J., Herran AR, Casqueiro J, Tye-Din JA, Surette MG, Magarvey NA, Schuppan D, & Verdu EF. Duodenal Bacteria From Patients With Celiac Disease and Healthy Subjects Distinctly Affect Gluten Breakdown and Immunogenicity. *Gastroenterology.* 2016;151(4):670-83.

[8] Helmerhorst EJ, Wei G. Experimental Strategy to Discover Microbes with Gluten-degrading Enzyme Activities. *Proceedings of SPIE--the International Society for Optical Engineering*. 2014;9112.

[9] Huibregtse IL, Marietta EV, Rashtak S, Koning F, Rottiers P, David CS, Sander JH van Deventer, Joseph A Murray. Induction of antigen-specific tolerance by oral administration of Lactococcus lactis delivered immunodominant DQ8-restricted

gliadin peptide in sensitized nonobese diabetic Abo Dq8 transgenic mice. *Journal of immunology* (Baltimore, Md : 1950). 2009;183(4):2390-6.

[10] Cuomo M, Nanayakkara M, Sarno M, Ferrara K, Discepolo V, Ponticelli D, Nigro F, Spagnardi M, Nigro R, Troncone R, Auricchio S, & Barone MV. Lactobacillus paracasei CBA-L74 and its postbiotic inhibit endocytosis in Caco-2 cells. *Digestive and Liver Disease*. 2013;45:e282.

[11] Freire R, Ingano L, Serena G, Cetinbas M, Anselmo A, Sapone A, Sadreyev RI, Fasano A, & Senger S. Human gut derived-organoids provide model to study gluten response and effects of microbiota-derived molecules in celiac disease. *Scientific reports*. 2019;9(1):7029.

[12] Dowd B, Walker-Smith J. Samuel Gee, Aretaeus, and the coeliac affection. *British medical journal*. 1974;2(5909):45-7.

[13] Yan D, Holt PR. Willem Dicke. Brilliant clinical observer and translational investigator. Discoverer of the toxic cause of celiac disease. *Clinical and translational science*. 2009;2(6):446-8.

[14] Weijers H, Lindquist B, Anderson C, Rey J, Shmerling D, Visakorpi J, et al. Diagnostic criteria in coeliac disease. *Acta Paediatr Scand*. 1970;59:461-3.

[15] Abbasi A, Sanej KD, Moradi S, Bazzaz S, Esmaeili A, Ghafourian K, Sahar Sabahi, Masoud Lahouty, Sousan Akrami, Ramin Aslani, Hedayat Hosseini. *Bioactive Compounds and Biological Activities of Allium sativum L. Bioactive Compounds in the Storage Organs of Plant*s: Springer; 2023. p. 1-40.

[16] Abbasi A, Bazzaz S, Da Cruz AG, Khorshidian N, Saadat YR, Sabahi S, Ozma MA, Lahouty M, Aslani R, & Mortazavian AM. A Critical Review on Akkermansia muciniphila: Functional Mechanisms, Technological Challenges, and Safety Issues. *Probiotics and Antimicrobial Proteins*. 2023:1-23.

[17] Sabahi S, Mortazavi SA, Nassiri M, Ghazvini K, Shahidi F, Abbasi A. Production of functional ice cream fortified by immunoglobulin Y against Escherichia coli O157: H7 and Helicobacter pylori. *Biointerface Research in Applied Chemistry*. 2022;13(2):188-98.

[18] Abbasi A, Aghebati-Maleki L, Homayouni-Rad A. The promising biological role of postbiotics derived from probiotic Lactobacillus species in reproductive health. *Critical Reviews in Food Science and Nutrition*. 2022;62(32):8829-41.

[19] Abbasi A, Hajipour N, Hasannezhad P, Baghbanzadeh A, Aghebati-Maleki L. Potential in vivo delivery routes of postbiotics. *Critical Reviews in Food Science and Nutrition*. 2022;62(12):3345-69.

[20] Sabahi S, Homayouni Rad A, Aghebati-Maleki L, Sangtarash N, Ozma MA, Karimi A, Hosseini H, & Abbasi A. Postbiotics as the new frontier in food and pharmaceutical research. *Critical Reviews in Food Science and Nutrition*. 2022:1-28.

[21] Abbasi A, Rad AH, Maleki LA, Kafil HS, Baghbanzadeh A. Cytotoxic Potentials of Cell-Free Supernatant Derived from Lactobacillus casei CRL431 on HCT-116 and HT-29 Human Colon *Cancer Cell Lines*. 2022.

[22] Ozma MA, Abbasi A, Akrami S, Lahouty M, Shahbazi N, Ganbarov K, Pasquale Pagliano, Sahar Sabahi, Şükran Köse, Mehdi Yousefi, Sounkalo Dao, Mohammad Asgharzadeh, Hedayat Hosseini, Hossein Samadi Kafil. Postbiotics as the key

mediators of the gut microbiota-host interactions. *Le infezioni in medicina [Infections in medicine].* 2022;30(2):180.

[23] Rad AH, Aghebati-Maleki L, Kafil HS, Abbasi A. Molecular mechanisms of postbiotics in colorectal cancer prevention and treatment. *Critical reviews in food science and nutrition*. 2021;61(11):1787-803.

[24] Deora V, Aylward N, Sokoro A, El-Matary W. Serum Vitamins and Minerals at Diagnosis and Follow-up in Children With Celiac Disease. *Journal of Pediatric Gastroenterology and Nutrition*. 2017;65(2):185-9.

[25] Amar A. Vitamin A deficiency in coeliac disease. *British Journal of Ophthalmology.* 2000;84(9):1075.

[26] Abbasi A, Aghebati-Maleki A, Yousefi M, Aghebati-Maleki L. Probiotic intervention as a potential therapeutic for managing gestational disorders and improving pregnancy outcomes. *Journal of reproductive immunology.* 2021;143:103244.

[27] De Angelis M, Siragusa S, Vacca M, Di Cagno R, Cristofori F, Schwarm M, Pelzer S, Flügel M, Speckmann B, Francavilla R, & Gobbetti M. Selection of gut-resistant bacteria and construction of microbial consortia for improving gluten digestion under simulated gastrointestinal conditions. *Nutrients.* 2021;13(3):992.

[28] Rubio R, Jofré A, Martín B, Aymerich T, Garriga M. Characterization of lactic acid bacteria isolated from infant faeces as potential probiotic starter cultures for fermented sausages. *Food microbiology.* 2014;38:303-11.

[29] Khochamit N, Siripornadulsil S, Sukon P, Siripornadulsil W. Antibacterial activity and genotypic–phenotypic characteristics of bacteriocin-producing Bacillus subtilis KKU213: potential as a probiotic strain. *Microbiological Research*. 2015;170:36-50.

[30] Swain MR, Anandharaj M, Ray RC, Rani RP. Fermented fruits and vegetables of Asia: a potential source of probiotics. *Biotechnology research international.* 2014;2014.

[31] Francavilla R, Cristofori F, Tripaldi ME, Indrio F. Intervention for dysbiosis in children born by C-section. *Annals of Nutrition and Metabolism.* 2018;73(Suppl. 3):33-9.

[32] Homayouni Rad A, Aghebati Maleki L, Samadi Kafil H, Abbasi A. Postbiotics: A novel strategy in food allergy treatment. *Critical reviews in food science and nutrition.* 2021;61(3):492-9.

[33] Scott KP, Jean-Michel A, Midtvedt T, van Hemert S. Manipulating the gut microbiota to maintain health and treat disease. *Microbial ecology in health and disease*. 2015;26(1):25877.

[34] Homayouni-rad A, Aghebati-Maleki L, Samadi-Kafil H, Abbasi A, Khani N. Postbiotics as a safe alternative to live probiotic bacteria in the food and pharmaceutical industries. *HBI_Journals*. 2021;26:132-57.

[35] Kobyliak N, Conte C, Cammarota G, Haley AP, Styriak I, Gaspar L, Fusek J, Rodrigo L, & Kruzliak P. Probiotics in prevention and treatment of obesity: a critical view. *Nutrition & metabolism.* 2016;13(1):1-13.

[36] Besselink MG, van Santvoort HC, Buskens E, Boermeester MA, van Goor H, Timmerman HM, Nieuwenhuijs VB, Bollen TL, Van Ramshorst B, Witteman BJ,

Rosman C, Ploeg RJ, Brink MA, Schaapherder AF, Dejong CH, Wahab PJ, Van Laarhoven CJ, Van Der Harst E, Van Eijck CH, Gooszen HG. Probiotic prophylaxis in predicted severe acute pancreatitis: a randomised, double-blind, placebo-controlled trial. *The Lancet*. 2008;371(9613):651-9.

[37] Rad AH, Maleki LA, Kafil HS, Zavoshti HF, Abbasi A. Postbiotics as promising tools for cancer adjuvant therapy. *Advanced Pharmaceutical Bulletin*. 2021;11(1):1.

[38] Abbasi A, Sheykhsaran E, Kafil HS. *Postbiotics: science, technology and applications:* Bentham Science Publishers; 2021.

[39] Rad AH, Abbasi A, Kafil HS, Ganbarov K. Potential pharmaceutical and food applications of postbiotics: a review. *Current pharmaceutical biotechnology*. 2020;21(15):1576-87.

[40] Capozzi V, Russo P, Dueñas MT, López P, Spano G. Lactic acid bacteria producing B-group vitamins: a great potential for functional cereals products. *Applied microbiology and biotechnology*. 2012;96:1383-94.

[41] Terpou A, Papadaki A, Lappa IK, Kachrimanidou V, Bosnea LA, Kopsahelis N. Probiotics in food systems: Significance and emerging strategies towards improved viability and delivery of enhanced beneficial value. *Nutrients*. 2019;11(7):1591.

[42] Cristofori F, Francavilla R, Capobianco D, Dargenio VN, Filardo S, Mastromarino P. Bacterial-based strategies to hydrolyze gluten peptides and protect intestinal mucosa. *Frontiers in immunology*. 2020;11:567801.

[43] De Almeida NEC, Esteves FG, dos Santos-Pinto JRA, Peres de Paula C, da Cunha AF, Malavazi I, Palma MS, & Rodrigues-Filho E. Digestion of intact gluten proteins by Bifidobacterium species: Reduction of cytotoxicity and proinflammatory responses. *Journal of agricultural and food chemistry*. 2020;68(15):4485-92.

[44] Giorgi A, Cerrone R, Capobianco D, Filardo S, Mancini P, Zanni F, Fanelli S, Mastromarino P, & Mosca L. A probiotic preparation hydrolyzes gliadin and protects intestinal cells from the toxicity of pro-inflammatory peptides. *Nutrients*. 2020;12(2):495.

[45] Heeney DD, Gareau MG, Marco ML. Intestinal Lactobacillus in health and disease, a driver or just along for the ride? *Current opinion in biotechnology*. 2018;49:140-7.

[46] Akobeng AK, Singh P, Kumar M, Al Khodor S. Role of the gut microbiota in the pathogenesis of coeliac disease and potential therapeutic implications. *European journal of nutrition*. 2020;59:3369-90.

[47] Di Biase AR, Marasco G, Ravaioli F, Dajti E, Colecchia L, Righi B, D'Amico V, Festi D, Iughetti L, & Colecchia A. Gut microbiota signatures and clinical manifestations in celiac disease children at onset: A pilot study. *Journal of Gastroenterology and Hepatology*. 2021;36(2):446-54.

[48] Marasco G, Cirota GG, Rossini B, Lungaro L, Di Biase AR, Colecchia A, Volta U, De Giorgio R, Festi D, & Caio G. Probiotics, prebiotics and other dietary supplements for gut microbiota modulation in celiac disease patients. *Nutrients*. 2020;12(9):2674.

[49] Gibson GR, Roberfroid MB. Dietary modulation of the human colonic microbiota: introducing the concept of prebiotics. *The Journal of nutrition*. 1995;125(6):1401-12.

[50] Rad AH, Maleki LA, Kafil HS, Zavoshti HF, Abbasi A. Postbiotics as novel health-promoting ingredients in functional foods. *Health promotion perspectives*. 2020;10(1):3-4.

[51] Drabińska N, Jarocka-Cyrta E, Markiewicz LH, Krupa-Kozak U. The effect of oligofructose-enriched inulin on faecal bacterial counts and microbiota-associated characteristics in celiac disease children following a gluten-free diet: Results of a randomized, placebo-controlled trial. *Nutrients*. 2018;10(2):201.

[52] Magge S, Lembo A. Low-FODMAP diet for treatment of irritable bowel syndrome. *Gastroenterology & hepatology*. 2012;8(11):739.

[53] Testa A, Imperatore N, Rispo A, Rea M, Tortora R, Nardone OM, Lucci L, Accarino G, Caporaso N, & Castiglione F. Beyond irritable bowel syndrome: the efficacy of the low fodmap diet for improving symptoms in inflammatory bowel diseases and celiac disease. *Digestive Diseases*. 2018;36(4):271-80.

[54] Chen Q, Ren Y, Lu J, Bartlett M, Chen L, Zhang Y, Guo X, & Liu C. A novel prebiotic blend product prevents irritable bowel syndrome in mice by improving gut microbiota and modulating immune response. *Nutrients*. 2017;9(12):1341.

[55] Markowiak P, Śliżewska K. Effects of probiotics, prebiotics, and synbiotics on human health. *Nutrients*. 2017;9(9):1021.

[56] Wilms E, Gerritsen J, Smidt H, Besseling-van der Vaart I, Rijkers GT, Garcia Fuentes A, Masclee AM and Troost FJ. Effects of supplementation of the synbiotic Ecologic® 825/FOS P6 on intestinal barrier function in healthy humans: A randomized controlled trial. *PLoS One*. 2016;11(12):e0167775.

[57] Demiroren K. Can a synbiotic supplementation contribute to decreasing anti-tissue transglutaminase levels in children with potential celiac disease? *Pediatric Gastroenterology, Hepatology & Nutrition*. 2020;23(4):397.

[58] Ugural A, Akyol A. Can pseudocereals modulate microbiota by functioning as probiotics or prebiotics? *Critical Reviews in Food Science and Nutrition*. 2022;62(7):1725-39.

[59] Gullón B, Gullón P, Tavaria FK, Yáñez R. Assessment of the prebiotic effect of quinoa and amaranth in the human intestinal ecosystem. *Food & Function*. 2016;7(9):3782-8.

[60] Abbasi A, Sabahi S, Bazzaz S, Tajani AG, Lahouty M, Aslani R, Hedayat Hosseini. An edible coating utilizing Malva sylvestris seed polysaccharide mucilage and postbiotic from Saccharomyces cerevisiae var. boulardii for the preservation of lamb meat. *International Journal of Biological Macromolecules*. 2023;246:125660.

[61] Hosseini H, Abbasi A, Sabahi S, Akrami S, Yousefi-Avarvand A. Assessing the Potential Biological Activities of Postbiotics Derived from Saccharomyces cerevisiae: An In Vitro Study. *Probiotics and Antimicrobial Proteins*. 2023:1-17.

[62] Abbasi A, Rad AH, Maleki LA, Kafil HS, Baghbanzadeh A. Antigenotoxicity and Cytotoxic Potentials of Cell-Free Supernatants Derived from Saccharomyces cerevisiae var. boulardii on HT-29 Human Colon Cancer Cell Lines. *Probiotics and Antimicrobial Proteins*. 2023:1-13.

[63] Abbasi A, Sanej KD, Mohammadi A, Moradi S, Nayeri BD, Bazzaz S, et al. *The Role of Postbiotics in Food Safety Promotion*.

[64] Abbasi A, Saadat TR, Saadat YR. Microbial exopolysaccharides–β-glucans–as promising postbiotic candidates in vaccine adjuvants. *International Journal of Biological Macromolecules*. 2022.

[65] Abbasi A, Rad AH, Ghasempour Z, Sabahi S, Kafil HS, Hasannezhad P, Yalda Rahbar Saadat, Nayyer Shahbazi. The biological activities of postbiotics in gastrointestinal disorders. *Critical Reviews in Food Science and Nutrition*. 2022;62(22):5983-6004.

[66] Sarno M, Lania G, Cuomo M, Nigro F, Passannanti F, Budelli A, Francesca Fasano, Riccardo Troncone, Salvatore Auricchio, Maria Vittoria Barone, Roberto Nigro, Merlin Nanayakkara. Lactobacillus paracasei CBA L74 interferes with gliadin peptides entrance in Caco-2 cells. *International Journal of food sciences and nutrition*. 2014;65(8):953-9.

[67] Conte M, Nigro F, Porpora M, Bellomo C, Furone F, Budelli AL, Roberto Nigro, Maria Vittoria Barone, Merlin Nanayakkara. Gliadin peptide P31-43 induces mTOR/NFkβ activation and reduces autophagy: The role of lactobacillus paracasei CBA L74 postbiotc. *International Journal of Molecular Sciences*. 2022;23(7):3655.

[68] Freire R, Ingano L, Serena G, Cetinbas M, Anselmo A, Sapone A, Ruslan I Sadreyev, Alessio Fasano, Stefania Senger. Human gut derived-organoids provide model to study gluten response and effects of microbiota-derived molecules in celiac disease. *Scientific reports*. 2019;9(1):7029.

Chapter 6

Targeted Delivery of Postbiotics: Oral, Intradermal and Intravenous Models

Masoud Lahouty[1], MSc
Reza Akbari[1], PhD
Mahdi Asghari Ozma[2], PhD
Amin Abbasi[3], PhD
and Lida Lotfollahi Hagghi[1,*], PhD
[1]Department of Microbiology, Faculty of Medicine,
Urmia University of Medical Sciences, Urmia, Iran
[2]Department of Microbiology, Faculty of Medicine,
Tabriz University of Medical Sciences, Tabriz, Iran
[3]Department of Food Science and Technology, National Nutrition and Food Technology Research Institute, Faculty of Nutrition Science and Food Technology,
Shahid Beheshti University of Medical Sciences, Tehran, Iran

Abstract

Among the natural chemical substances with significant medicinal value are bioactive micro- and macromolecules (postbiotics) produced by beneficial microorganisms in the gut. A novel treatment approach is now being developed that places a focus on the microbiome's small-molecular-weight biomolecules, which provide the host with a number of physiological health advantages. Many postbiotics have been identified, and because of their distinct pharmacokinetic characteristics in terms of adjustable dose and different delivery methods, they hold promise as potential medicinal agents since they exhibit both

* Corresponding Author's Email: lotfollahi.l@umsu.ac.ir.

In: Exploring Microbiotics in Health and Disease
Editor: Edward L. Stillman
ISBN: 978-8-89113-410-2

preventative and therapeutic effects on the host. Yet, major obstacles still stand in the way of postbiotic administration *in vivo*. The current body of scientific literature supports utilizing targeted delivery systems based on nanoparticles as a novel and secure method for the delivery or/and release of postbiotics in a variety of (oral, intradermal, and intravenous) in vivo models due to their attractive characteristics in regards to low toxicity, high biodegradability, biocompatibility, and considerable capacity for carrying both hydrophobic and hydrophilic postbiotics. If postbiotics are to be widely used as therapeutic approaches, they must undergo considerable research and randomized double-blind clinical studies because they are still in the early stages of development. This manuscript gives a comprehensive overview of the latest developments in the field of drug delivery and discusses the primary in vivo pathways for the targeted delivery of postbiotics.

Keywords: delivery routes, health benefits, nanoparticles, postbiotic, probiotic.

Introduction

With around 70% of the immune system in the human body being located in the digestive tract, it serves as the body's main immunological organ [1]. The intestine's surface area is between 300 and 400 sq. cm, and it is coated with a thick layer of live bacteria. Particularly, this surface is covered in around 10^{14} bacteria from more than 500 species [2]. Many biological functions in humans, including immunomodulation, neuronal activity, nutritional balance, and metabolic equilibrium, are considerably aided by the gut bacteria [3, 4]. Also, the host ensures a steady supply of dietary nutrients and offers a stable and ideal environment for the colonization, expansion, and functioning of commensal microbes. The ability of the gut microbiome to improve the host's health state has come to light thanks to technical advancements like genome sequencing (metagenomics) and gnotobiotic approaches, which utilize germ-free or gnotophoric species. The introduction of these techniques during the previous ten years has improved our comprehension of host-microbiome interactions. Dysbiosis, or abnormalities in the quantity, content, and function of the gut's microbes, has been linked to a variety of illnesses as their biological cause. Clinical studies' findings show that a variety of factors, including the mother's gut microbiota, the form of birth, the way that children are raised, inadequate use of various antibiotics and xenobiotics, a low-fiber diet, chronic illnesses, anxiety, and modified host genetics, are significant contributors to the loss of microbial heterogeneity and homeostatic function [5-7]. Future research will thus continue to focus on the objective of altering the gut microbiota as a practical and accessible way to advance human health.

In this context, recent research has shown that certain bioactive, non-viable compounds from gut microbial populations have a crucial role in modulating the control of the host's metabolic processes and state of health [8-10]. These bioactive compounds are crucial for supporting self- and other-beneficial organisms' growth, development, and reproduction as well as cell interaction and preservation from stressors due to their special chemical properties, which have drawn researchers to investigate their true potential [11-13]. The extensive use of bioactive chemicals in several domains of the pharmaceutical and food industries, medicine, veterinary science, etc. has been investigated due to their special properties in regard to clinical, technical, and economic considerations [14, 15]. The current thinking is that bioactive compounds (postbiotics) produced from the healthy microbiome in the gut can be used as a potential technique in personalized therapy to restore gut eubiosis and alleviate symptoms in patients with microbial infections [16, 17]. Despite the fact that bioactive substances have the innate ability to produce favorable impacts in *in vitro* models, it is essential to design various effective delivery approaches for their use *in vivo*. These approaches will allow the bioactive elements to pass through biological barriers, arrive at the desired site, and exert their therapeutic action. Researchers are always exploring for novel natural-source substances that can be used as adjuvant therapies or as a substitute to prescription medications. Robotics, high-throughput chemistry, and computer-based instrumentation systems have produced an outstanding trend for the reasonably priced evaluation and screening of a wide range of bioactive compounds. Bioactive compounds' operational success or failure can be easily evaluated *in vitro*, however validating them for use in *in vivo* studies can be quite difficult. The effectiveness of bioactive compounds can only be assessed in *in vivo* studies if they reach their intended action location in the body [18]. Here, a key difficulty that may have a large beneficial impact on how well bioactive compounds operate is the focused distribution approach. Nanoparticles were originally studied for their potential use in advancing targeted delivery systems after they were discovered and recognized as an efficient delivery technique. Bioactive chemicals must be effectively transported to the target place before being broken down by the body's digestive systems. For use in targeted delivery systems, a variety of biodegradable nanoparticles, including lysosomes, lipids, and non-digestible prebiotic components, are being researched. Hence, this manuscript provides an overview of the latest developments in the field of drug delivery and discusses the primary *in vivo* pathways for the targeted delivery of postbiotics.

In Vivo Delivery of Postbiotics

Although biomolecules produced from microorganisms are well known for their therapeutic properties, it is crucial to create and develop efficient *in vivo* delivery methods that allow biomolecules to penetrate the intended tissues and carry out their beneficial activity in the host's body [11, 19]. The *in vivo* transport of biomolecules is mostly determined by their particular molecular mechanism and target location inside the host body. For instance, to achieve high performance within the body, it is possible to provide traditional anti-diabetic drugs intravenously or/and directly to the target region (pancreatic tissue). A bioactive molecule's water solubility and membrane penetration inside the host are two essential characteristics that define its bioavailability and bio-accessibility. In this context, the United States Pharmacopeia (USP) developed the Biopharmaceutics Classification System (BCS), which classifies treatments into four classes based on membrane permeability and water solubility [20, 21]. One of BCS's primary goals is to predict a medicinal compound's effectiveness *in vivo* by *in vitro* studies of its water solubility and membrane permeability [22, 23].

A medicinal compound's optimal performance might be attained by successfully introducing it into the recipient. Yet, by choosing the right targeted administration methods, the bioavailability of such treatments might be enhanced. It is essential to transport therapeutic biological molecules to the targeted site until they are decomposed through the pharmacokinetics' pathways since most therapeutic biomolecules have chemical elements that are more unstable than manufactured drugs [24, 25]. Several drug delivery techniques, such as nanoparticle encapsulation, have been used by researchers in recent years to increase the potency of these therapeutic molecules. The finest delivery methods for therapeutic biomolecules must take into account characteristics such as high performance, safety (reduced potential cellular toxicity), and other crucial elements. This is because lipid-based nanoparticles have a suitable safety profile compared to other types of carbon nanotubes and metallic nanoparticles, making them an effective delivery system for biomolecules *in vivo* [26, 27]. Oral, intradermal, and intravenous administration methods for biomolecules are the three that are used the most commonly.

Oral Delivery

There are several various methods of delivery that have been used with varying degrees of effectiveness, including transcutaneous [28], rectal [29], ocular [30], oral, vaginal [31], intranasal [32], inhalational [33], and buccal [34]. The oral route is the most suitable method for administering medicinal medicines among all of these [35]. The oral route offers certain well-known advantages, including the ability to trigger a mucosal antibody reaction, greater patient compliance, suitability for frequentative delivery of the therapeutic agent, and cheap cost of care. The limited bioavailability of numerous therapeutic biomolecules is a serious hurdle for extending the oral dose of biomolecules [36, 37]. Moreover, the poor chemical consistency of biological molecules under digestive tract conditions hinders their overall functions and lowers their bioavailability in recipient plasma levels. When it comes to therapeutic biomolecules (such postbiotic substances), preserving their activity throughout storage, delivery, and administration is crucial for improving the oral dose. They also need to be strong sufficient to avoid gastrointestinal first-pass metabolism and reach their site of action [38, 39]. Yet, certain biomolecules' systemically expansion may be associated with toxicity and negative outcomes, such as hypersensitivity reactions and immunogenic reactions such antibodies against with the biomolecules that cause increased clearance and performance loss [40, 41]. By delivering tailored biomolecules to their active areas, it may be possible to offset a significant portion of the negative consequences associated with systemic expansion. The main benefits of local biomolecule delivery by oral treatment include: (a) enhancing intestinal permeation, (b) requiring smaller doses, (c) delivering the biomolecules directly to the site where they are needed, (d) having a high local concentration of the biomolecules in their active sites, (e) lowering the risk of unfavorable systemic effects; (f) diminishing the formation of complexes with other metabolites in the gut, which significantly intervenes with their beneficial functions, (g) and preventing the degradation of the biomolecules by chemical and enzymatic intermediaries in the stomach and small intestine [42, 43]. Nanocarriers stand out among other delivery methods for their remarkable capacity to preserve therapeutic biomolecules by outpacing several metabolic degradation processes, which in turn increases the bioavailability of the therapeutic biomolecules [44, 45]. Aqueous solubility and membrane permeability are the two essential factors that greatly control a therapeutic biomolecule's bioavailability. Thus, these factors play a significant role in the creation of formulations for oral therapeutic biomolecules.

As previously said, the BCS classification divides the therapeutic compounds/biomolecules into distinct classes, where the combination of the therapeutic compounds' aqueous solubility and membrane permeability properties is really taken into account. Figure 1 displays the different kinds of biomolecules and medicinal chemicals according to the BCS categorization [46, 47].

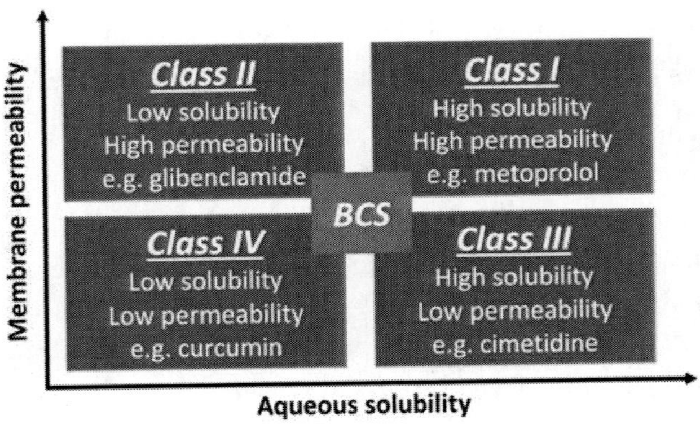

Figure 1. System of biopharmaceutics classification (BCS). Based on their water solubility and membrane permeability, this method classifies medicinal substances.

The class I category of the BCS classification includes medicines with high water solubility and membrane permeability. Moreover, the treatments in this class not only have a better bioavailability but also, in general, do not require a carrier system. The use of encapsulation is crucial for ensuring the excellent performance of these compounds, despite obstacles such low chemical stability or undesired solubility, particularly in food systems. The medicinal substances in the class II group have strong membrane permeability but limited water solubility. Due to their inherent properties that increase the solubility and safety profile, lipid-based nanocarriers are the most suitable delivery systems that can be used to enhance the cumulative bio-accessibility and biodistribution of the therapeutic compounds. Such therapeutics naturally exhibit lipophilic behavior [48, 49]. Although having somewhat reduced membrane permeability, the medicinal chemicals of the class III group have appropriate water solubility under digestive system conditions. In such cases, the components of mucoadhesive nanocarriers may help to improve the bioavailability by lengthening the period of contact between the therapeutic and the gastrointestinal epithelial cells. The establishment of intestinal tight junctions aids in the therapies' dissemination, which makes it easier to increase the therapeutic compound's efficiency. In terms of BCS classes, class IV therapies provide the greatest challenge due to their poor membrane permeability and limited aqueous solubility (e.g., curcumin or aluminum hydroxide). This class of medicinal substances requires a suitable carrier (for instance, carriers that are in the lipid mode or/and rich in surfactants) in addition to a mucoadhesive substance (chitosan), which could significantly improve the aqueous solubility characteristics and the interaction time with the intestines epithelial cells, respectively. Since nearly all delivery systems rely to some extent on one or more of these criteria to drive local release, the ability to deliver a therapeutic agent (such as postbiotics) to the gut relates to correspondence between the procedure of the delivery system, gut microbiome, transit time, and pH. These features are frequently altered in various gastrointestinal illnesses (such IBD), making it difficult to create delivery methods that ensure accurate administration to the colon. The most effective methods for delivering postbiotics to the colon will be reviewed in this section.

pH-Dependent Delivery Strategy

The pH of the stomach in a healthy individual ranges from 1 to 4, rising to 6 and 7.4 in the proximal and distal small intestines, respectively. The pH periodically falls and then increases in the colon between the ileum and the colon [50, 51]. Due to the fact that the aforementioned polymers are often insoluble at low pH levels but soluble at a slightly alkaline or neutral pH, the postbiotics are protected from adverse circumstances (acidic pH of the stomach) and are delivered specifically to the colon as a result. Nevertheless, intestinal pH levels are not always stable within a predetermined range. Diet, various disorders, etc., can all lead to major fluctuations in intestinal pH, and it can also significantly vary across people [52, 53]. This problem may result in the formulation including postbiotics prematurely dissolving in the small intestine, which would result in irreproducible colon delivery. Reduced colonic pH associated with several gastrointestinal illnesses might impair the dissolution of the postbiotic metabolites in the colonic fluid in addition to influencing the premature breakdown of the pH-dependent coating, which in turn results in less penetration. In this context, research on the enTRinsic™ capsules (inherently enteric capsules) showed that they increased the bioavailability of therapeutic agents in humans by ensuring no discharge in the stomach and quick releasing in the small intestine [54]. Pilot studies have shown that an alternative to colonic enema that uses targeted-release creation of an oral SCFA-based postbiotic and a pH-dependent release technique is beneficial for those with diverticulosis and Crohn's disease [55, 56]. The most popular pH-sensitive polymers/systems enabling oral pH-dependent administration are ColoPulse technology, Vcaps® Enteric and enTRinsic™ capsules, and methacrylic acid-based (also known as Eudragit®) polymers. For local delivery to the postbiotic small intestine, Puccetti et al. (2018) created a new indole-3-aldehyde-loaded gastro-resistant spray-dried microparticle. In this investigation, ethanol and NaOH solutions were used as solvent systems, and ethyl cellulose and Eudragit® L100 and S100 were used as wall materials. The study's findings back up using spray-drying to create gastro-resistant microparticles. The researchers came to the conclusion that the developed gastro-resistant composition of the 3-aldehyde-loaded microparticle, which allows for targeted distribution to the small intestine, will be useful to address new therapeutic uses for postbiotics [57].

Gut Microbiota-Triggered Release/Delivery Strategy

The commensal bacteria are present in great numbers in the gut, which is a complicated habitat. The majority of the various kinds of chemicals that enter the colon unabsorbed are fermented by this microbiota, providing it with its primary source of energy (prebiotics). The gut microbiota produces a variety of enzymes, including several polysaccharidases, to achieve this purpose [58]. By using the polysaccharides in the coating, this special property may be leveraged to produce colon-targeted delivery of postbiotics. Several polysaccharides have already been used as colon-targeted delivery methods due to their special properties, including chitosan, galactomannan, dextran, amylose, pectin, xanthan gum, and guar gum [59]. In addition to polysaccharides, the capability of several azo functional polymers for colon-targeted coating has been researched. The azoreductase enzymes produced either by gut microbiota cleave azo functional polymers [60]. Examples of commercially available gut microbiota-triggered release/delivery systems include the TARGIT® (an enteric-coated injection-molded starch capsule system), the COLAL® coating system, and COlon-targeted DElivery System (CODES™). Recently, a colon-targeted delivery method with two layers that includes an enteric coating on top of the core tablet's chitosan-based polymeric sub-coating for microenvironment acidification was developed. The method provides a controlled delivery by delaying the therapeutic agent's discharge in the stomach and small intestine while gradually releasing it in the colon with the help of chitosanase produced by the gut bacteria [61]. Recurrent diarrhea may contribute to the depletion of gut microbiota in various gastrointestinal illnesses, which may limit the targeted discharge of this form of the delivery system. In a recent study, probiotic microorganisms were co-administered with capsules that have an enteric outer layer and a guar gum core to overcome this barrier (Eudragit S100) [62].

Time-Dependent Release/Delivery Strategy

Time-dependent release techniques use patterns in gastrointestinal transit timings to time the discharge mechanism. The data that there is a significant difference in stomach evacuation periods across individuals, which makes the therapeutic agent's entrance time into the colon relatively unpredictable, may limit the utility of this approach. Patients with gastrointestinal disorders frequently exhibit elevated small intestine transit times and diarrhea, which might cause the therapeutic drug to be released prematurely and cleared quickly from the colon. Time-dependent delivery systems/technology include the Multimatrix® (MMX®) (Figure 2), and ChronoCap, Pulsincap (Figure 3).

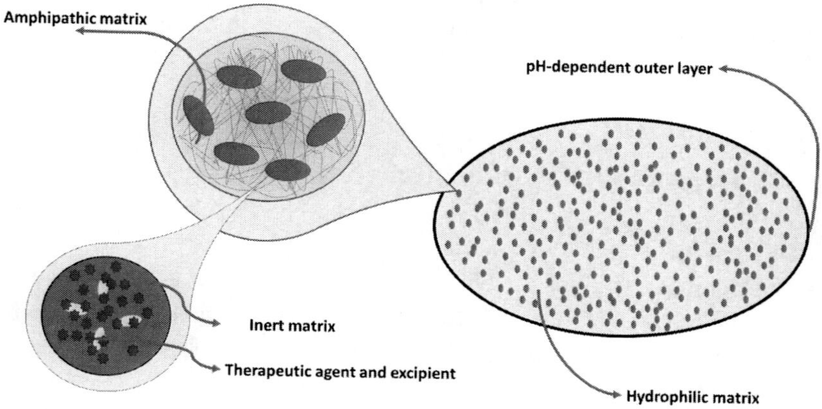

Figure 2. The Multimatrix (MMX) technology for targeted delivery/release.

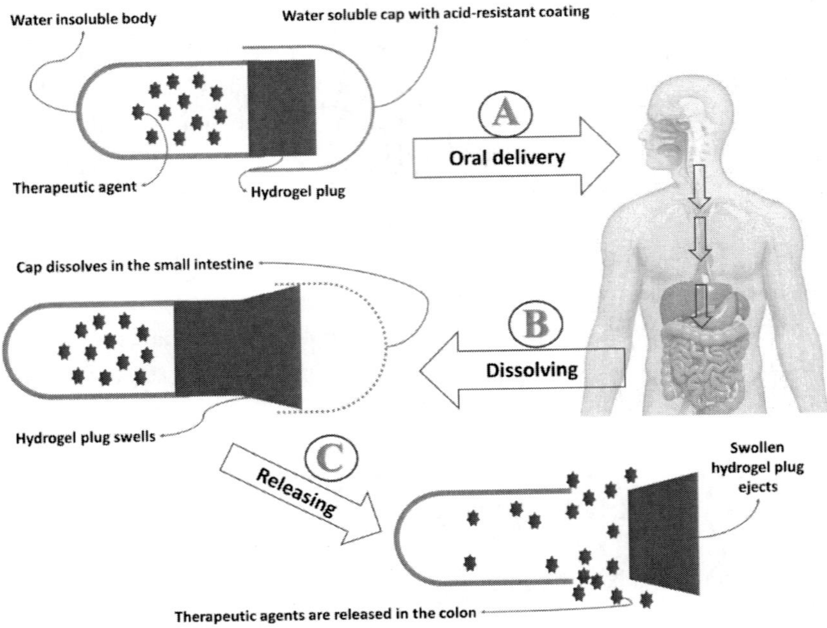

Figure 3. The Pulsincap system for time-dependent delivery/release.

In a 2017 study, Yu et al. evaluated the release characteristics of three distinct modified-release mesalamine compositions (locally acting intestinal therapeutic agents) and studied the direct assessment of therapeutic ingredient dissolving in the digestive system. In contrast to the substantial therapeutic agent concentrations in the colon, the MMX-based formulation exhibited negligible therapeutic agent concentrations in the small intestine and stomach [63].

Osmotic Pressure-Controlled Delivery Strategy

The OROS-CT technology is an illustration of an osmotic pressure-cntrolled delivery technique (Figure 4). This technique uses a firm gelatin capsule as the outer layer, which the small intestine can readily breakdown. Push-pull osmotic cells, which are often coated by an enteric coating, can range from 4-6 in each capsule. An osmotic push chamber and a therapeutic agent chamber are encircled by a semipermeable membrane on the inside face of the enteric coating. The therapeutic drug is forced out of the hole that is dug into the coating barrier when the enteric coating degrades and the push compartment expands as a result of water entering the device. The release procedure can also be carried out by OROS-CT units for a maximum of 24 hours.

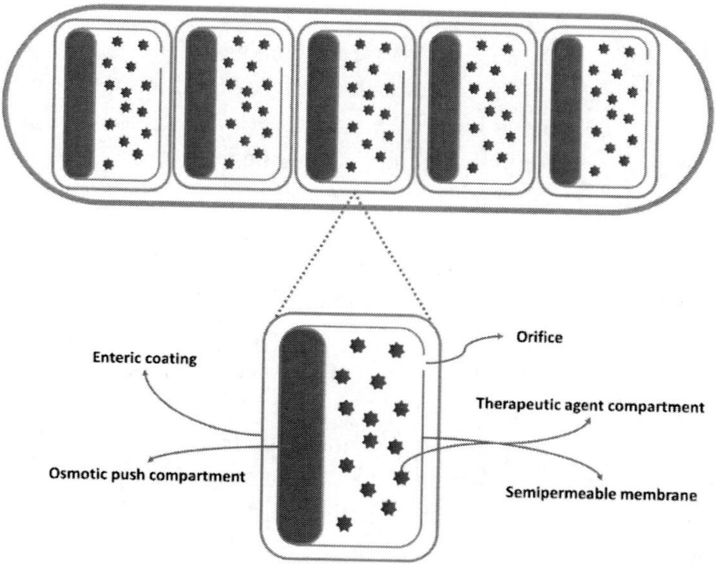

Figure 4. The OROS-CT system for osmotic pressure-controlled delivery.

Nanoparticle Delivery Strategy

Use of nanotechnology-based delivery techniques as vehicles for therapeutic compounds such as postbiotics is a relatively new strategy for colon-targeted release. The primary drawback of the delivery methods previously discussed is their reliance on the physiological and digestive circumstances of the host (such as the composition and variety of the host's intestinal microbiota), which can be drastically changed in various gastrointestinal illnesses. Using the differences between malignant cells or between normal and inflammatory mucosa, nanoparticle-based delivery techniques directed towards the intestines can target particular tumors or inflammations, respectively [64, 65]. By adding different substances to the membrane's outer edge or by changing the surface chemistry, it is easy to change the properties of lipid-based NPs. Several lipid-based NPs, including solid lipid NPs and liposomes, have been explored for oral colon-targeting because of its adaptability [66-70]. Anionic nano-delivery techniques have shown to selectively bind to inflamed regions, where there are plenty of positively charged proteins. In light of this, the creation of an anionic nanostructured lipid transporter loaded with postbiotics (with strong anti-inflammatory action) can be exploited as an unique targeted-delivery/release technique in future *in vivo* research.

In this context, the most often used techniques for encapsulating the therapeutic chemicals are carrier molecules based on lipids or polysaccharides. A polysaccharide coating on liposomes, one type of nanocarrier, significantly helps to encapsulate proteins or peptides within the lipid core [71]. Castoldi et al. (2017) looked into the therapeutic potential of vitamin-loaded liposomes for the topical treatment of lung bacterial infections caused by Pseudomonas aeruginosa. The developed vitamin-loaded liposomes used in this work had a negative surface charge, were nanosized and monodisperse, and had an entrapment effectiveness of about 23%. Comparing the delivery of the examined vitamin in liposomes to ethanolic solution revealed a notable improvement in the antibacterial activities. Moreover, vitamin-loaded liposomes appeared to be a viable anti-microbial treatment for lung chronic infections since they had no impact on the production of the proinflammatory cytokines [72]. The complicated metabolism of the gut microbiota results in the formation of certain vitamins as postbiotic molecules. These postbiotics have a low water solubility and must be dissolved in organic solvents like ethanol, which restricts their use *in vivo*. On the other hand, research findings showed that it was possible to effectively create a liposomal preparation of vitamin-based postbiotics with desired and powerful physicochemical characteristics for *in vivo* administration [73-75]. Another functional class of postbiotics is bacteriocin, which has been shown in scientific literature to have a crucial role in boosting host health status and food safety. Both organic and synthetic bacteriocins have been encapsulated using liposome nanoparticles. A further approach to overcoming challenges with bacteriocins' direct application to food items, such as reactions with food ingredients or proteolytic destruction, is the liposomal encapsulation of bacteriocins [76]. According to Benech et al. (2003), adding nisin directly to the cheese starting culture significantly altered the cheese's lipolysis and proteolysis characteristics, however adding nisin to a liposome prevented the cheese's proteolytic, rheological, and sensory qualities from being adversely affected (77). Moreover, da Silva Malheiros et al. (2010) used soybean phosphatidylcholines, a cheap and readily available raw material, to create liposome nanoparticles that contained nisin A. The created nisin-loaded liposomes displayed improved antibacterial characteristics and high encapsulation capability [78]. In order to compare the efficacy of the liposome-entrapped molecule and the free bacteriocin substance, these investigations on liposomes encapsulating postbiotics based on bacteriocin are advantageous. These encouraging study findings have increased interest in liposome-based research to increase food safety, shelf life, and usage.

Researchers in Scotland have created bilosomes, another new type of colloidal carrier system, for the first time by incorporating bile salts into the vesicular lipid bilayer membrane [79]. Bilosomes are bilayer membrane vesicles that contain bile salts like deoxycholate [80]. Bile salt content has a significant impact on the stability of bilosomes. In such a manner that their resistant and sensitive conditions, respectively, are closely related to the levels of 5 mM and 15–20 mM of bile salt [81]. The findings of the studies showed that bilosomes have promising potential for oral administration compared to other vesicular carriers and can have a more significant systemic impact than parenteral methods [82-84]. Moreover, physiological bile salts in the digestive system are more unstable than assimilation of bile salts into the lipid bilayer membrane of bilosomes, which can sustain the vesicles [80, 85, 86]. Nano-delivery techniques are a very promising and well-researched field, but before they can be used in clinical settings, more has to be learned about large-scale manufacturing possibilities, increased colon residency length, and safety evaluation of the techniques [87].

Moreover, some bioactive components of functional foods can transport medicinal chemicals efficiently. Due to their inherent capacity to protect the embedded biomolecules in the upper digestive process, prebiotics are one of the key dietary bioactive elements that have been used for the encapsulation of medicinal substances in this respect [23]. They are distinguished as functional dietary elements (raffinose, oligosaccharides, lactulose, stachyose, oligofructose, galactose, fructose, and inulin) that are not impacted by the host's digestive enzymes. But, they are used in the large colon through gut-colonized probiotics, which specifically encourage the development and growth of beneficial microorganisms and thus enhance the host's health [88, 89]. These strategies haven't been further explored, though, and need to be tested in more extensive placebo-controlled randomized clinical studies.

Intradermal Delivery

One of the most popular *in vivo* administration methods for postbiotics is intradermal distribution, which has a number of amazing advantages for the patient because it is not only a suitable approach but also non-invasive. The most reliable route for treating illnesses of the skin or/and tissues (such as infections caused by bacteria or fungi) is the intradermal administration technique because of its distinctive properties, such as the capacity to survive first-pass metabolism and avoid enzymatic destruction under digestive system circumstances [90-92]. A spore-generating probiotic Bacillus coagulans MTCC 5856's postbiotic metabolite, LactoSporin, was examined *in vitro* by Majeed et al. (2020) for its skin-protective effects. In this study, LactoSporin was evaluated for its possible antioxidant capacity by its ability to neutralize free radicals and reactive oxygen quenching behavior in human dermal fibroblast cells, preservation of fibroblasts from UV-triggered apoptosis and cell death through flow cytometry, and neutral red uptake assays, inhibition of collagenase, elastase, and hyaluronidase enzymes, and gene expression using polymerase chain reaction. The findings showed that LactoSporin, the postbiotic under investigation, has strong antioxidant effects, shielding skin cells from UV-triggered apoptosis and cell death, blocking elastase, collagenase, and hyaluronidase activity, and up-regulating the production of epidermal growth factor, transforming growth factor, and hyaluronan synthase [93]. Hence, the favorable findings from several studies support postbiotics' ability to protect skin and their capacity for widespread use in cosmetic preparations [93, 94]. Yet, the creation of a carrier system with postbiotic substances can lessen the effect of environmental conditions on the active ingredient, improve its performance, and offer a platform for large-scale industrial production.

It is well recognized that Microneedle (MN) arrays can increase the number of biomolecules suitable for intradermal delivery by penetrating the stratum corneum, which serves as the main barrier to topically applied substances, and creating a pathway for therapeutic substances to reach the skin's subcutaneous layers [95, 96]. MN arrays are minimally invasive devices that may penetrate the skin's tissue protective barrier to increase skin microcirculation and enable systemic administration through the intradermal pathway. MNs have lately received much research attention for their potential to transport biomolecules and serve as minimally invasive patient diagnostic tools. MNs are applied to the skin's surface and, using minute, pointed protrusions (ranging in height from 25 to 2000 μm), they painlessly puncture the stratum corneum to create microscopic aqueous holes that allow biomolecules to enter the skin's microcirculation [97]. The primary components used to create MNs include silicon, sugars, ceramics, metals, polymers and glass [98]. Because they enable comfortable intradermal sampling, monitoring, and biomolecule distribution without the need for highly trained staff, MNs can be employed as a unique form of a point-of-care tool [99].

Intravenous Delivery

It is common practice to provide medicinal substances intravenously to hasten the distribution of injectable biomolecules to the organs and tissues. The quick biotransformation of the biomolecule and likely quick elimination from the body are the primary benefits of intravenous biomolecule administration. There are a number of contemporary methods that have the potential to improve the efficiency of medicinal substances by prolonging their release into the body. Nanoparticles, among other materials, are suitable for transporting biomolecules *in vivo* in this respect. The efficiency of treatments using current molecules is substantially developed by the use of nanoparticles as biomolecules' carriers via the intravenous route for *in vivo* administration [100]. Using new micro- and macro-biomolecules of gut-microbial origin (postbiotics) that exhibit potent therapeutic action, such as organic acids, carbohydrates, nucleic acids, proteins, and peptides has enabled the development of innovative treatment strategies [14]. For intravenous distribution, Veloso et al. (2018) created a brand-new preparation for the antifungal Voriconazole. Their findings demonstrated that liposomal trapping of voriconazole might enhance the drug's fungicidal effects. The authors came to the conclusion that liposomal encapsulation offered a particular degree of preservation from premature metabolism, offering more effective blood concentrations of antimicrobials, allowing for closer and more specific infiltration and agglomeration into the body tissue more critically impacted by the pathogen [101, 102]. The capacity of the biomolecules' carrier to get past physiological barriers and the propriety of its bio-circulation have a considerable impact on the maximum efficiency of biomolecule delivery strategies employing nanoparticles. The efficiency of the intravenous administration channel depends on the delivery methods that are pulsed or/and pulsatile. Pulsatile delivery techniques are attracting a lot of interest because they provide spatial and temporal delivery, encourage patient compliance, and transport medicinal chemicals to their specific site of action at the right moment and in a suitable amount [103]. Several essential biological processes are regulated by the pulsed discharge of biomolecules at a specific time and place of action under the physiological circumstances of the body (37°C, pH

7.0) [104, 105]. From a therapeutic perspective, it would be crucial to design and create novel delivery equipment that will assist to achieve the targeted release of a defined quantity of a therapeutic at scheduled intervals of time, should we be successful in simulating the biological processes that living systems possess. The basic goal of biomolecule delivery research is to be able to deliver treatments to an individual with a pulsatile release profile. By planning the delivery of the therapeutic, the plasma peak is obtained at the optimal time. Moreover, the number of daily doses may be reduced. A variety of design/fabrication methods have been explored in the attainment of pulsatile release, depending on the restorative capability. These distribution methods might typically be categorized as osmotic, capsular, and reservoir delivery device types [106]. The pH, osmotic pressure, and regulated temperature are just a few of the characteristics that may be used to control delivery systems that are based on pulsatile release. Hydrogels are a prominent family of polymeric compounds that are widely used as key carriers in pulsatile delivery methods [107]. The hydrogels' three-dimensional (3D) hydrophilic polymer networks offer several distinctive qualities like swelling, hydrophilicity, and softness. Interior micro-/nanopores in hydrogels allow for the release of biomolecules into their surroundings [108-110]. Moreover, hydrogels are mechanically flexible and squishy, and these qualities can somewhat mimic the features of the body's soft living tissues [111]. Because of these special qualities, hydrogels are extremely useful in a variety of biomedical applications, such as the administration of medicinal substances, tissue engineering scaffolds, and tissue reinforcement [112]. Gels that reversibly vary their size in accordance with temperature changes are known as thermosensitive or thermoresponsive gels. These gels have the ability to contract at transient temperatures that are directly related to the linear polymer's Lower Critical Solution Temperature (LCST) behavior [113]. By placing hydrogel inside a rigid capsule, it is possible to create a compressed hydrogel tool using the hydrogels' size-alteration characteristics in reaction to temperature changes. Such adaptable size adjustment permits an on-off switchable medicinal discharge that is controlled by swelling/deswelling phases, with the swelling and shrinking occurring at temperatures below and above 32°C, respectively [114]. Moreover, pH-sensitive hydrogels might be used to deliver medicinal substances to different tissues and organs. Postbiotics with potent anticancer properties may be encapsulated into pH-sensitive nanoparticles, allowing for tailored delivery to various acidic tumor tissues [115, 116]. The hydrogels might be created and used to transfer biological postbiotic molecules to specific target tissues or organs, depending on the chemical characteristics and possible therapeutic significance of postbiotics.

Conclusion

The key problem and potential for the biomedical staff is the release of therapeutically useful bioactive molecules (postbiotics) produced from gut beneficial microorganisms. The preparation and the kind of *in vivo* administration pathways are primarily responsible for the efficacy of postbiotics in general. According to the BCS classification, the formulation of medicinal substances has to do with membrane permeability and aqueous solubility. As medicinal chemicals are often designed for oral delivery, it is crucial to take into account their water solubility and membrane permeability under digestive tract conditions. As a result, several strategies for efficient administration have been developed in this area, including formulations based on polysaccharides, prebiotics, and liposomes. In addition, researchers have proposed nanoparticle-based targeted delivery methods to realize the high therapeutic efficacy of bioactive compounds. MNs offer a simple and nearly painless intradermal administration method for pharmaceutical substances. The "poke with patch" approach used by MNs helps to circumvent first-pass metabolism, improving the effectiveness of the delivery of medicinal formulations. Due to the medicinal compound's quick removal from the circulation, the intravenous route is thought to be the most obstacle. In order to address these issues, hydrogels (as a major transporter in pulsatile delivery methods) offer regulated discharge in addition to greatly increased intravenous administration efficacy. *In vivo* administration of bioactive micro- and macro-molecules produced from gut beneficial microorganisms is still in the early stages of development and needs additional research and randomized double-blind clinical studies before being widely used as therapeutic approaches. Moreover, postbiotics' modes of distribution play a significant role in achieving the high efficiency of these potent medications. Although there are presently few postbiotic products on the market, long-term clinical studies with a significant number of samples should be used to prescribe postbiotic metabolites for the treatment of disorders.

Disclaimer

None.

References

[1] Wan ML, Ling K, El-Nezami H, Wang M. Influence of functional food components on gut health. *Critical reviews in food science and nutrition*. 2019;59(12):1927-36.

[2] Hsiao WW, Metz C, Singh DP, Roth J. The microbes of the intestine: an introduction to their metabolic and signaling capabilities. *Endocrinology and metabolism clinics of North America*. 2008;37(4):857-71.

[3] Cheng L, Qi C, Zhuang H, Fu T, Zhang X. gutMDisorder: a comprehensive database for dysbiosis of the gut microbiota in disorders and interventions. *Nucleic Acids Research*. 2020;48(D1):D554-D60.

[4] Abbasi A, Rad AH, Ghasempour Z, Sabahi S, Kafil HS, Hasannezhad P, Rahbar Saadat, Y., & Shahbazi, N. The biological activities of postbiotics in gastrointestinal disorders. *Critical Reviews in Food Science and Nutrition*. 2022;62(22):5983-6004.

[5] Muñoz-González C, Cueva C, Pozo-Bayon MA, Moreno-Arribas MV. Ability of human oral microbiota to produce wine odorant aglycones from odourless grape glycosidic aroma precursors. *Food chemistry*. 2015;187:112-9.

[6] Prato AP, Bartow-McKenney C, Hudspeth K, Mosconi M, Rossi V, Avanzini S, Faticato MG, Ceccherini, I, Lantieri F, Mattioli G, Larson D, Pavan W, Carlotta De Filippo, Monica Di Paola, Mavilio D and Cavalieri D. A metagenomics study on Hirschsprung's disease associated enterocolitis: biodiversity and gut microbial homeostasis depend on resection length and patient's clinical history. *Frontiers in pediatrics*. 2019;7:326.

[7] Rad A, Abbasi A, Javadi A, Pourjafar H, Javadi M, Khaleghi M. Comparing the microbial quality of traditional and industrial yoghurts. *Biointerface Research in Applied Chemistry*. 2020;10(4):6020-5.

[8] Chuah LO, Foo HL, Loh TC, Alitheen NBM, Yeap SK, Mutalib NEA, Abdul Rahim R, & Yusoff K. Postbiotic metabolites produced by Lactobacillus plantarum strains exert selective cytotoxicity effects on cancer cells. *BMC complementary and alternative medicine*. 2019;19(1):114.

[9] Gao J, Li Y, Wan Y, Hu T, Liu L, Yang S, Gong Z, Zeng Q, Wei Y, Yang W, Zeng Z, He X, Huang SH., & Cao H. A novel postbiotic from Lactobacillus rhamnosus GG with a beneficial effect on intestinal barrier function. *Frontiers in microbiology*. 2019;10:477.

[10] Bäuerl C, Coll-Marqués JM, Tarazona-González C, Pérez-Martínez G. Lactobacillus casei extracellular vesicles stimulate EGFR pathway likely due to the presence of proteins P40 and P75 bound to their surface. *Scientific reports*. 2020;10(1):1-12.

[11] Braga RM, Dourado MN, Araújo WL. Microbial interactions: ecology in a molecular perspective. *Brazilian journal of microbiology.* 2016;47:86-98.
[12] Netzker T, Fischer J, Weber J, Mattern DJ, König CC, Valiante V, Schroeckh V, & Brakhage, AA. Microbial communication leading to the activation of silent fungal secondary metabolite gene clusters. *Frontiers in microbiology.* 2015;6:299.
[13] Oleskin AV, Shenderov BA. Probiotics and psychobiotics: the role of microbial neurochemicals. *Probiotics and antimicrobial proteins.* 2019;11(4):1071-85.
[14] Rad A, Abbasi A, Kafil H, Ganbarov K. Potential Pharmaceutical and Food Applications of Postbiotics: A review. *Current pharmaceutical biotechnology.* 2020.
[15] Abbasi A, Sabahi S, Bazzaz S, Tajani AG, Lahouty M, Aslani R, Hosseini H. An edible coating utilizing Malva sylvestris seed polysaccharide mucilage and postbiotic from Saccharomyces cerevisiae var. boulardii for the preservation of lamb meat. *International Journal of Biological Macromolecules.* 2023;246:125660.
[16] Abramov V, Khlebnikov V, Kosarev I, Bairamova G, Vasilenko R, Suzina N, Machulin A, Sakulin V, Kulikova N, Vasilenko N, Karlyshev A, Uversky V, Chikindas ML, Melnikov V. Probiotic properties of Lactobacillus crispatus 2,029: homeostatic interaction with cervicovaginal epithelial cells and antagonistic activity to genitourinary pathogens. *Probiotics and antimicrobial proteins.* 2014;6(3-4):165-76.
[17] Reynés B, Palou M, Rodríguez AM, Palou A. Regulation of adaptive thermogenesis and browning by prebiotics and postbiotics. *Frontiers in physiology.* 2019;9:1908.
[18] Abbasi A, Sanej KD, Moradi S, Bazzaz S, Esmaeili A, Ghafourian K, Ali Esmaeili, Kiana Ghafourian, Sahar Sabahi, Masoud Lahouty, Sousan Akrami, Ramin Aslani, Hedayat Hosseini. Bioactive Compounds and Biological Activities of Allium sativum L. *Bioactive Compounds in the Storage Organs of Plants*: Springer; 2023. p. 1-40.
[19] Abbasi A, Hajipour N, Hasannezhad P, Baghbanzadeh A, Aghebati-Maleki L. Potential in vivo delivery routes of postbiotics. *Critical Reviews in Food Science and Nutrition.* 2022;62(12):3345-69.
[20] Cardot JM, Arieta AG, Paixao P, Tasevska I, Davit B. Implementing the biopharmaceutics classification system in drug development: reconciling similarities, differences, and shared challenges in the EMA and US-FDA-recommended approaches. *The AAPS journal.* 2016;18(4):1039-46.
[21] Abbasi A, Bazzaz S, Da Cruz AG, Khorshidian N, Saadat YR, Sabahi S, Ozma MA, Lahouty M, Aslani R, & Mortazavian AM. A Critical Review on Akkermansia muciniphila: Functional Mechanisms, Technological Challenges, and Safety Issues. *Probiotics and Antimicrobial Proteins.* 2023:1-23.
[22] Mehta MU, Uppoor RS, Conner DP, Seo P, Vaidyanathan J, Volpe DA, Stier E, Chilukuri D, Dorantes A, Ghosh T, Mandula H, Raines K, Dhanormchitphong P, Woodcock J, & Yu LX. Impact of the US FDA "Biopharmaceutics Classification System"(BCS) guidance on global drug development. *Molecular pharmaceutics.* 2017;14(12):4334-8.

[23] Mohanta D, Ghangal R, Solanki M, Patnaik S. Delivery of microbial metabolites for human health care: a review. *Environmental Chemistry Letters*. 2020:1-9.

[24] Yoshioka Y, Ochiya T. Extracellular vesicles as novel nanocarriers for therapeutic delivery. *Nucleic Acid Nanotheranostics*: Elsevier; 2019. p. 391-407.

[25] Cai X, Fang Z, Dou J, Yu A, Zhai G. Bioavailability of quercetin: problems and promises. *Current medicinal chemistry*. 2013;20(20):2572-82.

[26] Chuang SY, Lin CH, Huang TH, Fang JY. Lipid-based nanoparticles as a potential delivery approach in the treatment of rheumatoid arthritis. *Nanomaterials*. 2018;8(1):42.

[27] Khan I, Saeed K, Khan I. Nanoparticles: Properties, applications and toxicities. *Arabian Journal of Chemistry*. 2019;12(7):908-31.

[28] Banga AK, Chien YW. Hydrogel-based lontotherapeutic delivery devices for transdermal delivery of peptide/protein drugs. *Pharmaceutical research*. 1993;10(5):697-702.

[29] Mackay M, Phillips J, Hastewell J. Peptide drug delivery: colonic and rectal absorption. *Advanced drug delivery reviews*. 1997;28(2):253-73.

[30] Lee YC, Yalkowsky SH. Effect of formulation on the systemic absorption of insulin from enhancer-free ocular devices. *International journal of pharmaceutics*. 1999;185(2):199-204.

[31] Hussain A, Ahsan F. The vagina as a route for systemic drug delivery. *Journal of Controlled Release*. 2005;103(2):301-13.

[32] Maggio ET. Intravail™: highly effective intranasal delivery of peptide and protein drugs. *Expert Opinion on Drug Delivery*. 2006;3(4):529-39.

[33] O'Hagan D, Illum L. Absorption of peptides and proteins from the respiratory tract and the potential for development of locally administered vaccine. *Critical reviews in therapeutic drug carrier systems*. 1990;7(1):35-97.

[34] Sayani AP, Chien YW. Systemic delivery of peptides and proteins across absorptive mucosae. *Critical reviews in therapeutic drug carrier systems*. 1996;13(1-2):85-184.

[35] Shaji J, Patole V. Protein and peptide drug delivery: oral approaches. *Indian journal of pharmaceutical sciences*. 2008;70(3):269.

[36] Lin CH, Chen CH, Lin ZC, Fang JY. Recent advances in oral delivery of drugs and bioactive natural products using solid lipid nanoparticles as the carriers. *Journal of food and drug analysis*. 2017;25(2):219-34.

[37] Sabahi S, Homayouni Rad A, Aghebati-Maleki L, Sangtarash N, Ozma MA, Karimi A, Hosseini H, & Abbasi A. Postbiotics as the new frontier in food and pharmaceutical research. *Critical Reviews in Food Science and Nutrition*. 2022: 1-28.

[38] Jameel F, Hershenson S. *Formulation and process development strategies for manufacturing biopharmaceuticals*: John Wiley & Sons; 2010.

[39] Hosseini H, Abbasi A, Sabahi S, Akrami S, Yousefi-Avarvand A. Assessing the Potential Biological Activities of Postbiotics Derived from Saccharomyces cerevisiae: An *In Vitro* Study. *Probiotics and Antimicrobial Proteins*. 2023:1-17.

[40] Maurer JM, Hofman S, Schellekens RC, Tonnis WF, Dubois AO, Woerdenbag HJ, Hinrichs WLJ, Kosterink JGW, & Frijlink HW. Development and potential

application of an oral ColoPulse infliximab tablet with colon specific release: A feasibility study. *International journal of pharmaceutics.* 2016;505(1-2):175-86.

[41] Abbasi A, Bazzaz S, A. Ibrahim S, Hekmatdoost A, Hosseini H, Sabahi S, Sheykhsaran E, Rahbar Saadat Y, Asghari Ozma M, & Lahouty M. A Critical Review on the Gluten-Induced Enteropathy/Celiac Disease: Gluten-Targeted Dietary and Non-Dietary Therapeutic Approaches. *Food Reviews International.* 2023:1-41.

[42] Lautenschläger C, Schmidt C, Fischer D, Stallmach A. Drug delivery strategies in the therapy of inflammatory bowel disease. *Advanced drug delivery reviews.* 2014;71:58-76.

[43] Pattni BS, Torchilin VP. Targeted drug delivery systems: Strategies and challenges. *Targeted Drug Delivery: Concepts and Design:* Springer; 2015. p. 3-38.

[44] Dima C, Assadpour E, Dima S, Jafari SM. Bioactive-loaded nanocarriers for functional foods: from designing to bioavailability. *Current Opinion in Food Science.* 2020;33:21-9.

[45] Abbasi A, Rad AH, Maleki LA, Kafil HS, Baghbanzadeh A. Cytotoxic Potentials of Cell-Free Supernatant Derived from Lactobacillus casei CRL431 on HCT-116 and HT-29 *Human Colon Cancer Cell Lines*. 2022.

[46] Baki G, Chaudhari S, Gaudana R, Boddu SH. Selection of Excipients Based on the Biopharmaceutics Classification System of Drugs. *Excipient Applications in Formulation Design and Drug Delivery*: Springer; 2015. p. 351-83.

[47] Ozma MA, Abbasi A, Akrami S, Lahouty M, Shahbazi N, Ganbarov K, Pagliano P, Sabahi S, Köse Ş, Yousefi M, Dao S, Asgharzadeh M, Hosseini H, and Hossein Samadi Kafil. Postbiotics as the key mediators of the gut microbiota-host interactions. *Le infezioni in medicina. [Infections in medicine.]* 2022;30(2):180.

[48] Dolatabadi JEN, Omidi Y. Solid lipid-based nanocarriers as efficient targeted drug and gene delivery systems. *TrAC Trends in Analytical Chemistry*. 2016;77:100-8.

[49] Homayouni-rad A, Aghebati-Maleki L, Samadi-Kafil H, Abbasi A, Khani N. Postbiotics as a safe alternative to live probiotic bacteria in the food and pharmaceutical industries. *HBI_Journals.* 2021;26:132-57.

[50] Evans D, Pye G, Bramley R, Clark A, Dyson T, Hardcastle J. Measurement of gastrointestinal pH profiles in normal ambulant human subjects. *Gut.* 1988;29(8):1035-41.

[51] Rad AH, Aghebati-Maleki L, Kafil HS, Abbasi A. Molecular mechanisms of postbiotics in colorectal cancer prevention and treatment. *Critical reviews in food science and nutrition*. 2021;61(11):1787-803.

[52] Van den Mooter G. Colon drug delivery. *Expert opinion on drug delivery.* 2006;3(1):111-25.

[53] Homayouni Rad A, Aghebati Maleki L, Samadi Kafil H, Abbasi A. Postbiotics: A novel strategy in food allergy treatment. *Critical reviews in food science and nutrition.* 2021;61(3):492-9.

[54] Sager M, Grimm M, Aude P, Schick P, Merdivan S, Hasan M, Kromrey ML, Sivert A, Benameur H, Koziolek M, Tzvetkov MV, Weitschies W. *In vivo* characterization of enTRinsic™ drug delivery technology capsule after intake in

fed state: A cross-validation approach using salivary tracer technique in comparison to MRI. *Journal of Controlled Release*. 2019;313:24-32.

[55] Krokowicz L, Stojcev Z, Kaczmarek BF, Kociemba W, Kaczmarek E, Walkowiak J, Krokowicz P, Drews M, & Banasiewicz T. Microencapsulated sodium butyrate administered to patients with diverticulosis decreases incidence of diverticulitis—a prospective randomized study. *International Journal of Colorectal Disease*. 2014;29(3):387-93.

[56] Sabatino AD, Morera R, Ciccocioppo R, Cazzola P, Gotti S, Tinozzi F, Tinozzi S, Corazza G. Oral butyrate for mildly to moderately active Crohn's disease. *Alimentary pharmacology & therapeutics*. 2005;22(9):789-94.

[57] Puccetti M, Giovagnoli S, Zelante T, Romani L, Ricci M. Development of Novel Indole-3-Aldehyde–Loaded Gastro-Resistant Spray-Dried Microparticles for Postbiotic Small Intestine Local Delivery. *Journal of pharmaceutical sciences*. 2018;107(9):2341-53.

[58] Cummings J, Macfarlane G. The control and consequences of bacterial fermentation in the human colon. *Journal of Applied Bacteriology*. 1991;70(6):443-59.

[59] Hovgaard L, Brondsted H. Current applications of polysaccharides in colon targeting. *Critical Reviews™ in Therapeutic Drug Carrier Systems*. 1996;13(3-4).

[60] Hita V, Singh R, Jain SK. Colonic targeting of metronidazole using azo aromatic polymers: development and characterization. *Drug delivery*. 1997;4(1):19-22.

[61] Kim MS, Yeom DW, Kim SR, Yoon HY, Kim CH, Son HY, Kim JH, Lee S, and Choi YW. Development of a chitosan based double layer-coated tablet as a platform for colon-specific drug delivery. *Drug design, development and therapy*. 2017;11:45.

[62] Mohanta S, Singh SK, Kumar B, Gulati M, Kumar R, Yadav AK, Wadhwa S, Jyoti J, Som S, Dua K, Pandey NK. Efficacy of co-administration of modified apple polysaccharide and probiotics in guar gum-Eudragit S100 based mesalamine mini tablets: A novel approach in treating ulcerative colitis. *International journal of biological macromolecules*. 2019;126:427-35.

[63] Yu A, Baker JR, Fioritto AF, Wang Y, Luo R, Li S, Bo Wen, Michael Bly, Yasuhiro Tsume, Mark J Koenigsknecht, Xinyuan Zhang, Robert Lionberger, Gordon L Amidon, William L Hasler, Duxin Sun. Measurement of *in vivo* gastrointestinal release and dissolution of three locally acting mesalamine formulations in regions of the human gastrointestinal tract. *Molecular pharmaceutics*. 2017;14(2):345-58.

[64] Shen MY, Liu TI, Yu TW, Kv R, Chiang WH, Tsai YC, Hsin-Hung Chen, Sung-Chyr Lin, Hsin-Cheng Chiu. Hierarchically targetable polysaccharide-coated solid lipid nanoparticles as an oral chemo/thermotherapy delivery system for local treatment of colon cancer. *Biomaterials*. 2019;197:86-100.

[65] Cavalli R, Gasco MR, Chetoni P, Burgalassi S, Saettone MF. Solid lipid nanoparticles (SLN) as ocular delivery system for tobramycin. *International journal of pharmaceutics*. 2002;238(1-2):241-5.

[66] Amekyeh H, Billa N, Yuen KH, Chin SLS. A gastrointestinal transit study on amphotericin B-loaded solid lipid nanoparticles in rats. *Aaps Pharmscitech*. 2015;16(4):871-7.

[67] De Leo V, Milano F, Mancini E, Comparelli R, Giotta L, Nacci A, Francesco Longobardi, Antonella Garbetta, Angela Agostiano, Lucia Catucci. Encapsulation of curcumin-loaded liposomes for colonic drug delivery in a pH-responsive polymer cluster using a pH-driven and organic solvent-free process. *Molecules*. 2018;23(4):739.

[68] Hua S. Orally administered liposomal formulations for colon targeted drug delivery. *Frontiers in pharmacology*. 2014;5:138.

[69] Kosaraju SL. Colon targeted delivery systems: review of polysaccharides for encapsulation and delivery. *Critical reviews in food science and nutrition*. 2005;45(4):251-8.

[70] Zare M, Norouzi Roshan Z, Assadpour E, Jafari SM. Improving the cancer prevention/treatment role of carotenoids through various nano-delivery systems. *Critical Reviews in Food Science and Nutrition*. 2020:1-13.

[71] Ting Y, Jiang Y, Ho C-T, Huang Q. Common delivery systems for enhancing in vivo bioavailability and biological efficacy of nutraceuticals. *Journal of Functional Foods*. 2014;7:112-28.

[72] Castoldi A, Herr C, Niederstraßer J, Labouta HI, Melero A, Gordon S, Nicole Schneider-Daum, Robert Bals, Claus-Michael Lehr. Calcifediol-loaded liposomes for local treatment of pulmonary bacterial infections. *European Journal of Pharmaceutics and Biopharmaceutics*. 2017;118:62-7.

[73] Merz K, Sternberg B. Incorporation of vitamin D3-derivatives in liposomes of different lipid types. *Journal of Drug Targeting*. 1994;2(5):411-7.

[74] Zucker D, Marcus D, Barenholz Y, Goldblum A. Liposome drugs' loading efficiency: a working model based on loading conditions and drug's physicochemical properties. *Journal of controlled release*. 2009;139(1):73-80.

[75] Łukawski M, Dałek P, Borowik T, Foryś A, Langner M, Witkiewicz W, Magdalena Przybyło. New oral liposomal vitamin C formulation: properties and bioavailability. *Journal of liposome research*. 2020;30(3):227-34.

[76] Shukla S, Haldorai Y, Hwang SK, Bajpai VK, Huh YS, Han YK. Current demands for food-approved liposome nanoparticles in food and safety sector. *Frontiers in microbiology*. 2017;8:2398.

[77] Benech RO, Kheadr E, Lacroix C, Fliss I. Impact of nisin producing culture and liposome-encapsulated nisin on ripening of Lactobacillus added-Cheddar cheese. *Journal of dairy science*. 2003;86(6):1895-909.

[78] da Silva Malheiros P, Daroit DJ, Brandelli A. Food applications of liposome-encapsulated antimicrobial peptides. *Trends in Food Science & Technology*. 2010;21(6):284-92.

[79] El-Nabarawi MA, Shamma RN, Farouk F, Nasralla SM. Bilosomes as a novel carrier for the cutaneous delivery for dapsone as a potential treatment of acne: preparation, characterization and in vivo skin deposition assay. *Journal of Liposome Research*. 2020;30(1):1-11.

[80] Conacher M, Alexander J, Brewer JM. Oral immunisation with peptide and protein antigens by formulation in lipid vesicles incorporating bile salts (bilosomes). *Vaccine*. 2001;19(20-22):2965-74.

[81] Senior K. Bilosomes: the answer to oral vaccine delivery? *Drug discovery today*. 2001;20(6):1031-2.

[82] Mann JF, Scales HE, Shakir E, Alexander J, Carter KC, Mullen AB, & Ferro VA. Oral delivery of tetanus toxoid using vesicles containing bile salts (bilosomes) induces significant systemic and mucosal immunity. *Methods*. 2006;38(2):90-5.

[83] Shukla A, Khatri K, Gupta PN, Goyal AK, Mehta A, Vyas SP. Oral immunization against hepatitis B using bile salt stabilized vesicles (bilosomes). *Journal of Pharmacy & Pharmaceutical Sciences*. 2008;11(1):59-66.

[84] Singh P, Prabakaran D, Jain S, Mishra V, Jaganathan K, Vyas SP. Cholera toxin B subunit conjugated bile salt stabilized vesicles (bilosomes) for oral immunization. *International journal of pharmaceutics*. 2004;278(2):379-90.

[85] Schubert R, Jaroni H, Schoelmerich J, Schmidt K. Studies on the mechanism of bile salt-induced liposomal membrane damage. *Digestion*. 1983;28(3):181-90.

[86] Joseph Naguib M, Moustafa Kamel A, Thabet Negmeldin A, Elshafeey AH, Elsayed I. Molecular docking and statistical optimization of taurocholate-stabilized galactose anchored bilosomes for the enhancement of sofosbuvir absorption and hepatic relative targeting efficiency. *Drug Delivery*. 2020;27(1):996-1009.

[87] Vass P, Démuth B, Hirsch E, Nagy B, Andersen SK, Vigh T, Verreck G, Csontos I, Nagy ZK, & Marosi G. Drying technology strategies for colon-targeted oral delivery of biopharmaceuticals. *Journal of Controlled Release*. 2019;296:162-78.

[88] Rad AH, Maleki LA, Kafil HS, Zavoshti HF, Abbasi A. Postbiotics as novel health-promoting ingredients in functional foods. *Health promotion perspectives*. 2020;10(1):3-4.

[89] Tomasik P, Tomasik P. Probiotics, Non-Dairy Prebiotics and Postbiotics in Nutrition. *Applied Sciences*. 2020;10(4):1470.

[90] Hutin Y, Hauri A, Chiarello L, Catlin M, Stilwell B, Ghebrehiwet T, Garner J; Injection Safety Best Practices Development Group. Best infection control practices for intradermal, subcutaneous, and intramuscular needle injections. *Bulletin of the World Health Organization*. 2003;81:491-500.

[91] Sadik CD, Zillikens D. Skin-specific drug delivery: a rapid solution to skin diseases? *Journal of Investigative Dermatology*. 2013;133(9):2135-7.

[92] Yellepeddi VK, Donnelly R, Singh T. Nanotechnology-Based Applications for Transdermal Delivery of Therapeutics. *Novel Delivery Systems for Transdermal and Intradermal Drug Delivery*. 2015:125.

[93] Majeed M, Majeed S, Nagabhushanam K, Lawrence L, Arumugam S, Mundkur L. Skin Protective Activity of LactoSporin-the Extracellular Metabolite from Bacillus coagulans MTCC 5856. *Cosmetics*. 2020;7(4):76.

[94] Majeed M, Majeed S, Nagabhushanam K, Mundkur L, Rajalakshmi H, Shah K, Kirankumar Beede. Novel Topical Application of a Postbiotic, LactoSporin®, in Mild to Moderate Acne: A Randomized, Comparative Clinical Study to Evaluate its Efficacy, Tolerability and Safety. *Cosmetics*. 2020;7(3):70.

[95] Courtenay AJ, McAlister E, McCrudden MT, Vora L, Steiner L, Levin G, Levy-Nissenbaum E, Shterman N, Kearney MC, McCarthy HO, & Donnelly RF. Hydrogel-forming microneedle arrays as a therapeutic option for transdermal esketamine delivery. *Journal of Controlled Release*. 2020.

[96] Sabahi S, Abbasi A, Mortazavi SA. Characterization of cinnamon essential oil and its application in Malva sylvestris seed mucilage edible coating to the enhancement of the microbiological, physicochemical and sensory properties of lamb meat during storage. *Journal of Applied Microbiology*. 2022;133(2):488-502.

[97] Donnelly RF, Moffatt K, Alkilani AZ, Vicente-Pérez EM, Barry J, McCrudden MT, Woolfson AD. Hydrogel-forming microneedle arrays can be effectively inserted in skin by self-application: a pilot study centred on pharmacist intervention and a patient information leaflet. *Pharmaceutical research*. 2014;31(8):1989-99.

[98] Xie L, Zeng H, Sun J, Qian W. Engineering Microneedles for Therapy and Diagnosis: A Survey. *Micromachines*. 2020;11(3):271.

[99] Blicharz TM, Gong P, Bunner BM, Chu LL, Leonard KM, Wakefield JA, Williams RE, Dadgar M, Tagliabue CA, El Khaja R, Marlin SL, Haghgooie R, Davis SP, Chickering DE, Bernstein H. Microneedle-based device for the one-step painless collection of capillary blood samples. *Nature biomedical engineering*. 2018;2(3):151-7.

[100] de la Torre P, Pérez-Lorenzo MJ, Alcázar-Garrido Á, Flores AI. Cell-Based Nanoparticles Delivery Systems for Targeted Cancer Therapy: Lessons from Anti-Angiogenesis Treatments. *Molecules*. 2020;25(3):715.

[101] Veloso DF, Benedetti NI, Ávila RI, Bastos TS, Silva TC, Silva MR, Aline C Batista, Marize C Valadares, Eliana M Lima. Intravenous delivery of a liposomal formulation of voriconazole improves drug pharmacokinetics, tissue distribution, and enhances antifungal activity. *Drug delivery*. 2018;25(1):1585-94.

[102] Abbasi A, Aghebati-Maleki L, Homayouni-Rad A. The promising biological role of postbiotics derived from probiotic Lactobacillus species in reproductive health. *Critical Reviews in Food Science and Nutrition*. 2022;62(32):8829-41.

[103] El-Hady SM, AbouGhaly MH, El-Ashmoony MM, Helmy HS, El-Gazayerly ON. Colon targeting of celecoxib nanomixed micelles using pulsatile drug delivery systems for the prevention of inflammatory bowel disease. *International Journal of Pharmaceutics*. 2020;576:118982.

[104] Patel VP, Desai TR, Matholiya CR, Chhayani R. *Pulsatile Drug Delivery System: A Review. Pharmatutor Pharmacy Infopedia,* Reference Id: Pharmatutor-Art-1060. 2015;2.

[105] Madhavi AV, Reddy DRB, Venugopal M, Srihari N, Chenniah P, Koteswarao P. Formulation and Evaluation of Pulsatile Drug Delivery System of Zafirlukast. *Journal of Drug Delivery and Therapeutics*. 2020;10(2):122-8.

[106] Amani N, Javar HA, Dorkoosh FA, Rouini MR, Amini M, Sharifzadeh M, Shahin Boumi. Preparation and Pulsatile Release Evaluation of Teriparatide-Loaded Multilayer Implant Composed of Polyanhydride-Hydrogel Layers Using Spin Coating for the Treatment of Osteoporosis. *Journal of Pharmaceutical Innovation*. 2020:1-22.

[107] Dreiss CA. Hydrogel design strategies for drug delivery. *Current Opinion in Colloid & Interface Science*. 2020.

[108] Fu J. Hydrogel properties and applications. *Journal of Materials Chemistry* B. 2019;7(10):1523-5.

[109] Martín C, Martín-Pacheco A, Naranjo A, Criado A, Merino S, Díez-Barra E, Antonia Herrero and Ester Vázquez. Graphene hybrid materials? The role of graphene materials in the final structure of hydrogels. *Nanoscale.* 2019;11(11):4822-30.

[110] Chai Q, Jiao Y, Yu X. Hydrogels for biomedical applications: their characteristics and the mechanisms behind them. *Gels.* 2017;3(1):6.

[111] Xue K, Wang X, Yong PW, Young DJ, Wu YL, Li Z, Xian Jun Loh. Hydrogels as Emerging Materials for Translational Biomedicine. *Advanced Therapeutics.* 2019;2(1):1800088.

[112] Yi J, Choe G, Park J, Lee JY. Graphene oxide-incorporated hydrogels for biomedical applications. *Polymer Journal.* 2020:1-15.

[113] Lee CH, Bae YC. Thermodynamic framework for switching the lower critical solution temperature of thermo-sensitive particle gels in aqueous solvent. *Polymer.* 2020:122428.

[114] James HP, John R, Alex A, Anoop K. Smart polymers for the controlled delivery of drugs–a concise overview. *Acta Pharmaceutica Sinica B.* 2014;4(2):120-7.

[115] Abbasi A, Rad AH, Maleki LA, Kafil HS, Baghbanzadeh A. Antigenotoxicity and Cytotoxic Potentials of Cell-Free Supernatants Derived from Saccharomyces cerevisiae var. boulardii on HT-29 Human Colon Cancer Cell Lines. *Probiotics and Antimicrobial Proteins.* 2023:1-13.

[116] Abbasi A, Saadat TR, Saadat YR. Microbial exopolysaccharides–β-glucans–as promising postbiotic candidates in vaccine adjuvants. *International Journal of Biological Macromolecules.* 2022.

Chapter 7

Postbiotics: Current Therapeutic Landscape and Future Horizons

Amin Abbasi[1,*], PhD
Hamideh Fathi Zavoshti[2], BSc
Sahar Sabahi[3], PhD
Kiana Ghafourian[4], Intern
Negar Ghotbi[5], Intern
Sara Arshadi[6], BSc
Negin Lohrasbi[6], BSc
and Hedayat Hosseini[1,†], PhD

[1]Department of Food Science and Technology,
National Nutrition and Food Technology Research Institute,
Faculty of Nutrition Science and Food Technology,
Shahid Beheshti University of Medical Sciences, Tehran, Iran
[2]Department of Food Hygiene and Aquatics, Faculty of Veterinary Medicine,
Tabriz University, Tabriz, Iran
[3]Department of Nutrition, School of Allied Medical Sciences,
Ahvaz Jundishapur University of Medical Sciences, Ahvaz, Iran
[4]Medical School, Shahid Beheshti University of Medical Sciences, Tehran, Iran
[5]Faculty of Medicine, Tehran Medical Sciences, Islamic Azad University, Tehran, Iran
[6]Department of Nutrition, Faculty of Nutrition Sciences and Food Technology,
National Nutrition and Food Technology Research Institute,
Shahid Beheshti University of Medical Sciences, Tehran, Iran

[*] Corresponding Author's Email: aminabasi.tbz.med.ac@gmail.com; abbasia@sbmu.ac.ir.
[†] Corresponding Author's Email: hedayat@sbmu.ac.ir.

In: Exploring Microbiotics in Health and Disease
Editor: Edward L. Stillman
ISBN: 978-8-89113-410-2

Abstract

In recent years, there has been an increase in the use of probiotics and prebiotics to modulate microbiota. Due to the increasing use of probiotics and prebiotics, it has attracted recent interest in studies about their metabolites, called postbiotics. Postbiotics refer to substances released or produced by microorganisms through metabolic activity that benefit the host, whether directly or indirectly. There have been discussions about the benefits and disadvantages of postbiotics in recent years and their ability to become a new alternative agent. The scientific literature confirms that these microbial-derived biomolecules can have different effects on health disorders and even can be used as a diagnostic or therapeutic tool with fewer side effects. The positive effects on human health observed in clinical trials could be linked to certain bioactivities. Although scientific evidence supports this, the exact mechanisms and pathways involved still require further research. Nevertheless, postbiotics show promise as a source of functional ingredients for developing biotechnological products in the nutraceutical industry. This chapter provides a clinical review of postbiotics described in the literature, including their mechanisms of action, characteristics, and potential therapeutic applications. Detailed pleiotropic effects of postbiotics, including neurologic disorders, endocrine and metabolic syndromes, gastrointestinal diseases, and other systemic disorders, will be discussed.

Keywords: gastrointestinal diseases, health, neurologic disorders, postbiotics

Introduction

The gastrointestinal tract (GIT) serves as the primary immune organ, constituting roughly 70% of the immune system in the human body [1]. The intestinal surface area is around 300 to 400 square centimeters and is colonized by abundant populations of live microorganisms. The aforementioned surface is inhabited by an estimated 1014 bacteria, including a diverse array of more than 500 distinct species [2]. The findings of clinical investigations have revealed that several factors, including the maternal gut microbiota composition, mode of delivery, caregiving practices during infancy, administration of antibiotics, consumption of a low-fiber diet, presence of chronic disorders, and anxiety, have significant implications for the maintenance of gut microbiota equilibrium [3, 4]. The presence of commensal bacteria in a well-functioning gastrointestinal tract is correlated with the host's cells, resulting in the activation and maturation of the immune responses inside the gut. This, in turn, plays a crucial role in maintaining homeostasis in the host organism. The terms 'dysbiosis' and 'eubiosis' are used in the context of elucidating the gut's state of health and microbial constitution. 'Dysbiosis' pertains to pathological circumstances, while 'eubiosis' characterizes advantageous microorganisms or probiotics [4-6]. Dysbiosis refers to a state characterized by the coexistence of pathogenic microorganisms and their harmful metabolites, which leads to a decline in the abundance of helpful microorganisms and a subsequent drop in immunological functionality. This compromised immune response renders the host vulnerable to a wide range of both infectious and non-infectious ailments [4]. One of the primary strategies used to achieve eubiosis is the restoration of gut microbial equilibrium by the ingestion of probiotics, either in the form of food or nutritional supplements [7]. Probiotics refer to non-pathogenic bacteria that, when taken in enough quantities, have been seen to elicit beneficial effects on the health of the host [8] and contain both yeast (e.g., *Kluyveromyces*, *Saccharomyces*, *Torulaspora*, and *Pichia*) and bacteria (e.g., *Lactobacillus*, *Bacillus*, and *Bifidobacterium*) genera [9, 10]. The mechanisms of action of probiotic cells, as determined by the International Scientific Association for Probiotics and Prebiotics (ISAPP) consensus panel, can be classified as strain-dependent, species-dependent, and prevalent among frequently studied probiotic genera. Strain-dependent mechanisms are infrequent and limited to a few strains within a specific species. Species-dependent mechanisms are commonly observed across most strains of a probiotic species, such as *Lactobacillus paracasei* or *Bifidobacterium infantis*. Additionally, certain mechanisms of action are prevalent among probiotic genera that are frequently investigated [11]. The therapeutic efficacy of probiotics has been substantiated in the treatment of a wide range of diseases, particularly intra- and extra-intestinal disorders including hepatic encephalopathy, Necrotizing Enterocolitis (NEC), Irritable Bowel Syndrome (IBS), acute infectious diarrhea, colorectal cancer, lactose intolerance, ulcerative colitis, and antibiotic-associated diarrhea [12-16].

Despite the presence of positive indicators, there is a lack of evidence from extensive long-term clinical studies with a substantial statistical sample to support the claim that the use of probiotic products improves the health status of individuals who were previously in good health [17]. The guidelines established by the Food and Agriculture Organization (FAO) and the World Health Organization (WHO) in 2002 [18], along with the findings from case report studies, have indicated that certain probiotic cells, such as *Streptococcus thermophilus*, *L. helveticus*, *L. buchneri*, *L. hilgardii*, *Bifidobacterium*, and *Bacillus*, when administered through different delivery systems like pharmaceuticals or foods, may potentially be associated with adverse side effects. These side effects include the presence of virulence factors, the transmission of resistance genes, metabolic disturbances, the production of biogenic amines, and the possibility of opportunistic infections. It is particularly important to consider these potential risks in pediatric populations and individuals with underlying medical conditions [17, 19-24].

In recent years, there has been a growing interest in addressing the challenges associated with the utilization of live probiotic cells in various domains, including clinical, technological, and economic aspects. As a result, alternative agents such as non-digestible fibers (prebiotics) and microbial-derived biomolecules (postbiotics) have emerged as potential solutions. These agents are employed with the aim of modulating the composition of the gut microbiome, thereby promoting a state of eubiosis and facilitating the establishment of homeostasis [25, 26]. There is a growing body of evidence indicating that the primary health-promoting effects of gut microbiota may be linked to their non-viable byproducts, known as postbiotics. These postbiotics have the ability to imitate the beneficial health effects of live parent cells by utilizing similar or different metabolic pathways [27, 28]. The term "postbiotic," despite being a recent development, has gained rapid acceptance in the field of food science, as well as in the domains of host health and nutrition. Consequently, there has been significant interest in their potential application as nutraceuticals, functional foods, and pharmaceuticals within the biotechnological, food, and pharmaceutical industries [11, 29, 30]. This chapter provides a clinical review of postbiotics described in the literature, including their mechanisms of action, characteristics, and potential therapeutic applications. Detailed pleiotropic effects of postbiotics, including neurologic disorders, endocrine and metabolic syndromes, gastrointestinal diseases, and other systemic disorders, will be discussed.

The Concept of Postbiotics

In recent years, most researchers have employed terms such as 'biogenic,' 'cell-free supernatant (CFS),' 'abiotic,' 'metabiotic,' 'pseudoprobiotic,' 'ghost probiotic,' and 'postbiotic' to describe the non-viable parts of probiotic cells. Among these, the term 'postbiotic' is the most used in the literature [31-

34]. The term 'postbiotic' is associated with inactive microbial cells, cellular components derived from these cells such as peptidoglycan-derived muropeptides, teichoic acids, endo- and exo-polysaccharides, and cell-surface proteins, as well as cell metabolites including Short-Chain Fatty Acids (SCFAs), enzymes, bacteriocins, and organic acids. These substances are produced by live probiotic cells during the fermentation process, in response to gut conditions, or released after cell lysis caused by physical and/or chemical inactivation. When administered in sufficient quantities, postbiotics provide various physiological health benefits to the host [35, 36].

Main Action Mechanisms

Postbiotics refer to a sophisticated formulation that encompasses several bioactive chemicals, each with diverse modes of action. The precise mechanisms via which postbiotics confer their beneficial effects and their significance in relation to human health remain largely ambiguous in the majority of cases. These processes have the potential to manifest either alone or in combination, and in some instances, they may exhibit similarities to established probiotic modes of action [37, 38]. There are two primary pathways via which postbiotics have the potential to enhance clinical outcomes: immune system regulation and the enhancement of intestinal barrier function.

Local and systemic immunomodulation often takes place via the stimulation of different cytokines and immune modulators, as well as the interaction between microorganism-associated molecular patterns and particular immune cell receptors, such as C-type lectins and toll-like receptors (TLR) [39-41]. Postbiotics may include many immunomodulatory microbial metabolites, such as branched chain fatty acids, histamine, and short-chain fatty acids (SCFA). Additionally, cell wall components including muramic acid and peptidoglycans may also be present in postbiotics, exerting an impact on diverse immunological responses [42, 43].

The enhancement of intestinal barrier function may be achieved by using exopolysaccharides, which include those derived from *Bifidobacterium* spp. Certain species of *Bifidobacterium* have also shown the ability to enhance the functionality of tight junctions [44]. Moreover, when present in enough quantities, short-chain fatty acids have the capacity to alter barrier function and provide protection against the disruption caused by lipopolysaccharides. Furthermore, postbiotics have the potential to regulate the composition and function of the gut microbiome. For instance, the antimicrobial effect of lactic acid and bacteriocins can be observed directly [45, 46]. Additionally, the modulation of the microbiome can occur indirectly through mechanisms such as the transportation of lactic acid, which is subsequently consumed by microorganisms in the microbiome. This consumption leads to the production of short-chain fatty acids and butyrate, both of which play beneficial roles [47]. Postbiotic preparations have the potential to exhibit antagonistic effects against intestinal infections by the delivery of antimicrobial substances, including metabolites and bacteriocins. These chemicals have the ability to hinder biofilm development and deactivate certain bacteria [48].

Health Effects of Postbiotics: Experimental and Clinical Pieces of Evidence

Evidence of Health Effects in Gastrointestinal Disorders

Acute diarrhea poses a substantial threat to the health and well-being of children in poor nations, leading to increased rates of illness and death [49]. Among the several pathogens responsible for severe episodes of diarrhea, rotavirus is the predominant culprit, accounting for between 29% to 45% of these instances [50]. The presence of acute gastroenteritis has been seen to result in significant changes to the composition and structure of the intestinal microbiome [51]. Enteric bacterial infections have a significant impact on the richness and diversity of the gut microbiome, leading to a prolonged decrease that may last for up to 14 weeks after the infection [52]. Comparable alterations are seen in cases of viral diarrhea [53]. Children diagnosed with a condition known as "failure to thrive" have more pronounced changes in their microbiome composition. Additionally, these children experience a prolonged recovery period after episodes of diarrheal sickness, compared to their counterparts without this condition [54]. Postbiotics have the potential to ameliorate these modifications and maintain a harmonious microbiome during and after episodes of diarrheal diseases. Previous research has shown the efficacy of live *Lactobacillus* in combating viral diarrhea [55, 56]. Additionally, investigations have provided evidence that heat-treated *Lactobacillus* LB may expedite the recovery process, decrease morbidity rates, and shorten the time of hospitalization [57, 58]. In addition, rigorously conducted trials have shown that the administration of heat-treated

Lactobacillus paracasei is effective in mitigating the occurrence of diarrhea. This intervention has been found to considerably decrease the frequency of diarrhea episodes when compared to a placebo [59]. Antibiotics have the potential to modify the composition of the intestinal microbiome, hence resulting in the occurrence of antibiotic-associated diarrhea. The usefulness of probiotics in treating diarrhea is well-documented, and they have been recommended as a potential treatment for antibiotic-associated diarrhea. However, there is a concern that the viability of probiotics may be reduced by the use of antibiotics [60]. Exploratory research has shown that the administration of heat-treated *Lactobacillus* LB, a kind of postbiotic, may potentially mitigate the likelihood of antibiotic-associated diarrhea in patients undergoing antibiotic treatment. The study revealed a significant decrease in the incidence of diarrhea among those taking antibiotics who were assigned to the heat-treated *Lactobacillus* LB group [60].

Chronic diarrhea is often attributed to chronic functional diarrhea and chronic parasite and bacterial infections in underdeveloped nations [61, 62]. Conversely, in industrialized nations, irritable bowel syndrome (IBS) emerges as the predominant cause, affecting around 15% of people [63]. The standard course of treatment often involves the use of antibiotics and antimotility medications; nevertheless, their efficacy might be limited and they may give rise to undesirable side effects [64]. Postbiotics may potentially serve as a viable alternative. According to a recent randomized-controlled trial, the administration of heat-treated *Lactobacillus* LB demonstrated a substantial improvement in chronic diarrhea and associated clinical symptoms when compared to the use of live lactobacilli [65]. The study demonstrated that the non-viable strain of *B. bifidum* MIMBb75 exhibited significant efficacy in alleviating symptoms associated with irritable bowel syndrome (IBS) as compared to the placebo group [66]. In a similar vein, the administration of inactivated *Lactobacillus* LB, together with a fermented culture medium, demonstrated a substantial reduction in the frequency of weekly bowel movements. Additionally, this intervention exhibited improvements in abdominal discomfort, bloating, and overall quality of life among those diagnosed with irritable bowel syndrome (IBS) [67-69].

Postbiotics have the potential to enhance the effectiveness of conventional treatment methods for *Helicobacter pylori* infections [70]. *In vitro* studies have shown the inhibitory effect of Lactobacilli on the attachment of *H. pylori* to stomach epithelial cells [71]. In addition, it has been shown that the discarded culture supernatant of *L. acidophilus* LB exhibits a reduction in the viability of *H. pylori*, both *in vitro* and *in vivo*, irrespective of variations in pH and lactic acid concentrations [72]. In an open-label, prospective, randomized experiment, patients who tested positive for *H. pylori* were given heat-stabilized *L. acidophilus* LB in addition to the conventional therapy. The study provided evidence that the addition of *L. acidophilus* to the usual treatment regimen resulted in a considerable improvement in eradication rates when compared to the use of conventional therapy alone [73].

Evidence of Health Effects in Immunity and Allergies

Research has shown that the presence of viable Lactobacillus species may enhance immunological function, increase health-related quality of life (HRQoL), and regulate allergic reactions [74]. This phenomenon might perhaps be attributed to its capacity to shift the immune system's balance from T helper 2 (Th2) responses towards T helper 1 (Th1) responses [75, 76]. This phenomenon may provide advantages in countries that have adopted Westernized practices, since the implementation of effective public hygiene measures and the decreased prevalence of illnesses contribute to a diminished occurrence of this reaction, hence increasing the susceptibility to allergy development [77]. A compromised immune system also heightens susceptibility to pathogenic infections and has the potential to diminish health-related quality of life. Moreover, there exists a body of well-regulated clinical research indicating that the use of heat-treated *L. plantarum* (HK-LP) might potentially enhance immune function associated with Th-1 response. In comparison to a placebo, the HK-LP group exhibited a higher shift in Con A-induced proliferation and Th1: Th2 ratio, together with a more pronounced improvement in health-related quality of life (HRQoL) [78]. Moreover, previous studies have shown the efficacy and safety of administering live *L. paracasei* 33 (LP33) in enhancing the quality of life (QoL) among individuals suffering from perennial allergic rhinitis generated by house-dust mite allergens [79]. A second randomized-controlled experiment demonstrated that the effectiveness of heat-treated LP33 was comparable to that of the live form. This was shown as patients who received either the live or heat-treated LP33 had better quality of life ratings in terms of frequency and degree of bother, in comparison to those who received the placebo [80]. Additionally, previous studies have shown that the inactivated form of *Lactobacillus* LB and non-pathogenic Escherichia coli may effectively regulate the allergic immune response associated with grass pollen allergies. These effects are mostly mediated by Th1-dominated responses [81]. The long-term management of allergic rhinitis necessitates considering therapeutic options that provide effectiveness, safety, affordability, and convenient storage. In this regard, postbiotics may present themselves as a favorable choice [82]. There is also a suggestion that postbiotics may have the ability to enhance the management of food allergies [83, 84].

Evidence of Health Effects in Upper Respiratory Tract Infections

The use of three specific postbiotic strains, namely *Pediococcus acidilactici*, *L. plantarum*, and *L. pentosus*, has garnered support from both animal and clinical studies in the context of mitigating upper respiratory tract infections (URTI) [85]. The stimulation of type 1 interferon production by heat-treated *L. plantarum* L-137 in mice has been shown to enhance protection against the influenza virus [86]. This phenomenon has also been reported in people [87]. There exists a suggestion that higher degrees of psychological stress are associated with an increased susceptibility to acute respiratory disease 65. Based on robust clinical data, it has been shown that regular consumption of heat-treated *L. plantarum* L-137 (HK L-137) might potentially reduce the occurrence of URTI in individuals who are psychologically stressed, by potentially enhancing immune function. The results of the 12-week randomized-controlled research indicated that the incidence of URTI was considerably lower in the group administered with HK L-137 compared to the control group. Furthermore, a noteworthy inverse relationship was seen between the duration of HK L-137 consumption and the occurrence, duration, severity, and medication duration of upper respiratory tract infections. The development of peripheral blood mononuclear cells generated by concanavalin A was shown to be considerably higher in the group treated with HK L-137 compared to the control group [88]. This implies that the intake of HK L-137 has the ability to decrease the incidence of upper respiratory tract infections. Likewise, other research has examined the feasibility of mitigating respiratory tract infections in pediatric populations. In two rigorously conducted studies including children aged 12–48 months, it was shown that the administration of *L. paracasei* CBA L74 resulted in a decrease in the incidence of tracheitis, laryngitis, and pharyngitis [89]. Moreover, a randomized-controlled study conducted on pre-school children revealed that the consumption of fermented foods containing *Pediococcus acidilactici* K15 resulted in the enhancement of anti-infectious immune systems. Additionally, it was observed that the salivary secretory IgA levels were maintained in all participants, particularly in those who consumed fewer fermented foods. The primary objective of this study was to investigate the preventive effects of *Pediococcus acidilactici* K15 on respiratory tract infections in children. The research, which spanned a length of four months, also observed that children who consumed little amounts of fermented food saw a substantial reduction in fever duration when administered K15, as opposed to those who were given a placebo [90]. The decline in salivary IgA levels seen with advancing age implies that older individuals may exhibit heightened vulnerability to upper respiratory tract infections [7, 91]. The research findings indicate that the consumption of *L. pentosus* b240 has been associated with an elevation in salivary IgA levels [92, 93]. Furthermore, a rigorously conducted experiment has provided evidence that the intake of b240 greatly lowers the occurrence of common colds among senior individuals. This effect is believed to be attributed to the enhancement of mucosal immunity, hence potentially enhancing resistance against infections. The present investigation revealed that the frequencies of common cold occurrence were comparatively reduced, whereas overall health perceptions, as assessed by the SF-36 w, exhibited a dose-dependent rise [94, 95].

Evidence of Health Effects in Stress and Neurological Circumstances

Research has shown that the gut-brain axis plays a vital role in the maintenance of gastrointestinal homeostasis and brain function [96, 97]. The connection between the gastrointestinal tract and the brain is influenced by the intestinal microbiome through several channels, including immunological, endocrine, and neurological mechanisms. Existing research indicates that the gut microbiome has a notable influence on brain function, hence impacting aspects such as mood, cognition, and behavior [98]. Research studies have shown that probiotics may influence the control of the hypothalamic-pituitary-adrenal axis via the modulation of the hippocampus. Additionally, they have been found to alleviate pain and behavioral changes generated by stress. Furthermore, probiotics are capable of transmitting signals to the brain through the afferent vagal nerve, leading to the alleviation of mood abnormalities. Ongoing research is being conducted to examine the impacts of heat-treated microorganisms. Empirical evidence from rigorously conducted clinical trials indicates that the sustained use of *L. gasseri* CP2305 has the potential to enhance the psychological well-being, sleep patterns, and gut microbiota composition in otherwise healthy adult individuals exposed to stressful circumstances. The research, which lasted for a duration of 24 weeks, used a randomized-controlled design and included students who were in the process of preparing for national medical exams. The administration of CP2305 on a daily basis was shown to have a substantial impact on reducing anxiety levels, sleep disturbance, and salivary chromogranin A levels when compared to the administration of a placebo. The administration of CP2305 shown a mitigating effect on the decrease of *Bifidobacterium* spp. caused by stress, as well as the increase of *Streptococcus* spp. produced by stress [99]. Postbiotics have been shown to possess several applications in the context of different illnesses connected to the nervous system. For instance, previous studies have shown evidence in murine models that regular consumption of plasmalogens, a constituent of postbiotics, may effectively impede memory decline via the inhibition of glial activation [100]. In addition, a rigorously conducted investigation shown that the administration of plasmalogen may lead to enhancements in cognitive performance among individuals diagnosed with moderate Alzheimer's disease [101]. Possible applications include novel strategies for treating depression, since there is evidence suggesting a correlation between changes in the gut microbiota and the occurrence of depression [102]. In addition, there is evidence suggesting a connection between the development of multiple sclerosis and changes in the microbiome. These abnormalities include a decrease in bacteria that produce short-chain fatty acids, which may provide a promising target for postbiotic interventions.

Evidence of Health Effects in Cardiac and Vascular Disorders

The occurrence of oxidative damage has been shown to be associated with the development of inflammation and cardiovascular disease. The presence of molecules with antioxidant characteristics in postbiotic preparations may have the ability to mitigate this phenomenon. The presence of inflammation and endothelial dysfunction in individuals with chronic kidney disease (CKD) has been linked with cardiac injury. Nevertheless, there is evidence suggesting that postbiotic preparations might serve as a preventive measure against cardiac damage related to CKD. Additional evidence indicates that bacterial metabolites and components have the potential to inhibit or decelerate the advancement of chronic kidney disease and hypertension [103].

Evidence of Health Effects in Metabolic Syndrome

Metabolic syndrome is defined by the presence of many comorbidities that increase the likelihood of developing cardiovascular diseases and type 2 diabetes mellitus. The emergence of disorders associated with obesity may be attributed to the composition and activity of the gut microbiome. The manipulation of the gut microbiota via the use of postbiotics has been associated with encouraging weight loss [104]. Additionally, research conducted on rats revealed that the administration of *B. longum* resulted in a decrease in cholesterol levels [105]. Additionally, it has been shown that muramyl dipeptide, which is a constituent of bacterial cell walls, has the ability to regulate the release of GLP-1. This, in turn, leads to an enhancement in insulin sensitivity and an improvement in glucose tolerance [106]. The administration of live *Akkermansia muciniphila* in mouse models resulted in a reduction in obesity, glucose intolerance, insulin resistance, steatosis, and intestinal permeability, as reported in previous studies [107, 108]. Later on, it was shown that the process of pasteurization amplifies its impact on obesity, insulin resistance, and glucose tolerance [109]. The findings of a randomized-controlled trial including persons who are overweight or obese and have insulin resistance indicate that the administration of pasteurized *A. muciniphila* leads to a reduction in liver dysfunction and inflammatory blood marker levels. Notably, this intervention does not have a significant impact on the overall composition of the gut microbiome. The research conducted over a period of three months discovered that the administration of pasteurized *A. muciniphila* was shown to be both safe and well-tolerated. Furthermore, it was seen that the intervention resulted in improvements in insulin sensitivity, as well as reductions in insulinemia, plasma total cholesterol, and body weight, as compared to the placebo group. Additionally, it was observed that the intervention led to a decrease in fat mass and hip circumference when compared to the initial measurements [110].

Conclusion

Postbiotics have shown potential benefits in many places, such as the liver. The gut-liver axis refers to the reciprocal interaction between the gastrointestinal tract, its microbial community, and the liver. The portal vein transports substances obtained from the gastrointestinal tract to the liver, while the liver reciprocates by releasing bile and antibodies into the intestine. The maintenance of gut-liver axis balance is dependent on the presence of a healthy microbiome. Liver cirrhosis is characterized by a significantly modified microbiota and impaired integrity of the intestinal barrier. There is a growing body of data suggesting that metabolites generated by microorganisms, such as trimethylamine, short-chain fatty acids, and ethanol, play a pathogenic role in the development of non-alcoholic fatty liver disease. Postbiotics are becoming recognized as a promising novel therapeutic approach for the treatment of liver illnesses. However, more investigation is required to substantiate their efficacy and establish their potential benefits [111]. The field of probiotic genome editing has previously been established and has the potential to be combined with postbiotics in order to change the precursor bacteria, hence creating novel postbiotic therapies. Moreover, the progress in microbiome metagenomic mapping might provide additional clarity on the interactions between commensal microorganisms and the intestinal environment, hence enhancing the substantiation of postbiotics. The potential use of customized microbiome phenotyping for disease prevention is a concept that has promise, but with a considerable distance to traverse before becoming a reality. Enhancing comprehension of the possible therapeutic advantages and maybe facilitating tailored postbiotic treatment can be achieved by investigating the interaction mechanisms between postbiotics and commensal microbes [112].

Consequently, Postbiotics possess a commendable level of safety and stability, allowing for convenient storage and transit over extended periods. Moreover, their administration with antibiotic therapy does not compromise their effectiveness, making them an attractive substitute for probiotics. There is an increasing body of data supporting the therapeutic advantages of postbiotics in the treatment and control of widely common illnesses such as gastrointestinal, dermatological, and neurological problems, as well as respiratory infections and metabolic syndrome. Postbiotics provide a promising treatment strategy for the aforementioned illnesses and may serve as a potentially safer substitute for probiotics, especially in susceptible groups like pediatric patients. Further validation of the therapeutic advantages of postbiotics necessitates the conduction of supplementary randomized, placebo-controlled clinical studies.

Disclaimer

None.

References

[1] Denev, P, Kratchanova, M, Ciz, M, Lojek, A, Vasicek, O, Nedelcheva, P, Blazheva, D, Toshkova, R, Gardeva, E, Yossifova, L, Hyrsl, P, & Vojtek, L. Biological activities of selected polyphenol-rich fruits related to immunity and gastrointestinal health. *Food Chemistry*. 2014;157:37-44.

[2] Hsiao WWL, Metz C, Singh DP, Roth J. The microbes of the intestine: an introduction to their metabolic and signaling capabilities. *Endocrinol Metab Clin North Am*. 2008;37(4):857-71.

[3] Muñoz-González C, Cueva C, Ángeles Pozo-Bayón M, Victoria Moreno-Arribas M. Ability of human oral microbiota to produce wine odorant aglycones from odourless grape glycosidic aroma precursors. *Food Chemistry*. 2015;187:112-9.

[4] Moludi J, Alizadeh M, Lotfi Yagin N, Pasdar Y, Nachvak SM, Abdollahzad H, & Sadeghpour Tabaei, A. New insights on atherosclerosis: A cross-talk between endocannabinoid systems with gut microbiota. *J Cardiovasc Thorac Res*. 2018;10(3):129-37.

[5] Khan N, Mendonca L, Dhariwal A, Fontes G, Menzies D, Xia J, Divangahi, M, & King, IL. Intestinal dysbiosis compromises alveolar macrophage immunity to Mycobacterium tuberculosis. *Mucosal immunology*. 2019;12(3):772.

[6] Ozma MA, Abbasi A, Ahangarzadeh Rezaee M, Hosseini H, Hosseinzadeh N, Sabahi S, Noori, SMA, Sepordeh, S, Khodadadi, E, Lahouty, M, & Kafil, HS. A critical review on the nutritional and medicinal profiles of garlic's (Allium sativum L.) bioactive compounds. *Food Reviews International*. 2022:1-38.

[7] Abbasi A, Aghebati-Maleki A, Yousefi M, Aghebati-Maleki L. Probiotic intervention as a potential therapeutic for managing gestational disorders and improving pregnancy outcomes. *Journal of reproductive immunology*. 2021;143: 103244.

[8] Haghshenas B, Haghshenas M, Nami Y, Khosroushahi AY, Abdullah N, Barzegari A, Rosli, R, & Hejazi, MS. Probiotic assessment of Lactobacillus plantarum 15HN and Enterococcus mundtii 50H isolated from traditional dairies microbiota. *Advanced pharmaceutical bulletin*. 2016;6(1):37.

[9] Saber A, Alipour B, Faghfoori Z, Yari Khosroushahi A. Cellular and molecular effects of yeast probiotics on cancer. *Critical reviews in microbiology*. 2017;43(1):96-115.

[10] Rad A, Abbasi A, Javadi A, Pourjafar H, Javadi M, Khaleghi M. Comparing the microbial quality of traditional and industrial yoghurts. *Biointerface Research in Applied Chemistry*. 2020;10(4):6020-5.

[11] Cuevas-González P, Liceaga A, Aguilar-Toalá J. Postbiotics and Paraprobiotics: From concepts to applications. *Food Research International*. 2020:109502.

[12] Vaghef-Mehrabany E, Vaghef-Mehrabany L, Asghari-Jafarabadi M, Homayouni-Rad A, Issazadeh K, Alipour B. Effects of probiotic supplementation on lipid profile of women with rheumatoid arthritis: a randomized placebo-controlled clinical trial. *Health Promotion Perspectives*. 2017;7(2):95.

[13] Mohamadshahi M, Veissi M, Haidari F, Shahbazian H, Kaydani G-A, Mohammadi F. *Effects of probiotic yogurt consumption on inflammatory biomarkers in patients with type 2 diabetes*. BioImpacts: BI. 2014;4(2):83.

[14] Maia LP, Levi YLdAS, do Prado RL, Santinoni CdS, Marsicano JA. Effects of probiotic therapy on serum inflammatory markers: A systematic review and meta-analysis. *Journal of Functional Foods*. 2019;54:466-78.

[15] Jamalkandi SA, Ahmadi A, Ahrari I, Salimian J, Karimi M, Ghanei M. Oral and nasal probiotic administration for the prevention and alleviation of allergic diseases, asthma and chronic obstructive pulmonary disease. *Nutrition Research Reviews*. 2020:1-16.

[16] Karimi N, Jabbari V, Nazemi A, Ganbarov K, Karimi N, Tanomand A, Karimi, S, Abbasi, A, Yousefi, B, Khodadadi, E, & Kafil, HS. Thymol, cardamom and Lactobacillus plantarum nanoparticles as a functional candy with high protection against Streptococcus mutans and tooth decay. *Microbial Pathogenesis*. 2020:104481.

[17] Cohen PA. Probiotic safety—no guarantees. *JAMA internal medicine*. 2018;178(12):1577-8.

[18] Joint F. WH*O working group report on drafting guidelines for the evaluation of probiotics in food*. London, Ontario, Canada. 2002;30.

[19] Piqué N, Berlanga M, Miñana-Galbis D. Health benefits of heat-killed (Tyndallized) probiotics: An overview. *International journal of molecular sciences*. 2019;20(10):2534.

[20] Appel-da-Silva MC, Narvaez GA, Perez LR, Drehmer L, Lewgoy J. *Saccharomyces cerevisiae var. boulardii fungemia* following probiotic treatment. *Medical mycology case reports*. 2017;18:15-7.

[21] Doron S, Snydman DR. Risk and safety of probiotics. *Clinical Infectious Diseases*. 2015;60(suppl_2):S129-S34.

[22] Gezginc Y, Akyol I, Kuley E, Özogul F. Biogenic amines formation in Streptococcus thermophilus isolated from home-made natural yogurt. *Food chemistry*. 2013;138(1):655-62.

[23] Taylor AL, Dunstan JA, Prescott SL. Probiotic supplementation for the first 6 months of life fails to reduce the risk of atopic dermatitis and increases the risk of allergen sensitization in high-risk children: a randomized controlled trial. *Journal of Allergy and Clinical Immunology*. 2007;119(1):184-91.

[24] Ordóñez JL, Troncoso AM, García-Parrilla MDC, Callejón RM. Recent trends in the determination of biogenic amines in fermented beverages–A review. *Analytica chimica acta*. 2016;939:10-25.

[25] Rad AH, Maleki LA, Kafil HS, Zavoshti HF, Abbasi A. Postbiotics as novel health-promoting ingredients in functional foods. *Health Promotion Perspectives*. 2020;10(1):3.

[26] Sabahi S, Abbasi A, Mortazavi SA. Characterization of cinnamon essential oil and its application in Malva sylvestris seed mucilage edible coating to the enhancement of the microbiological, physicochemical and sensory properties of lamb meat during storage. *Journal of Applied Microbiology*. 2022;133(2):488-502.

[27] Guéniche A, Bastien P, Ovigne JM, Kermici M, Courchay G, Chevalier V, Breton, L, & Castiel-Higounenc, I. Bifidobacterium longum lysate, a new ingredient for reactive skin. *Experimental dermatology*. 2010;19(8):e1-e8.

[28] Abbasi A, Rad AH, Ghasempour Z, Sabahi S, Kafil HS, Hasannezhad P, Rahbar Saadat, Y, & Shahbazi, N. The biological activities of postbiotics in gastrointestinal disorders. *Critical Reviews in Food Science and Nutrition*. 2022;62(22):5983-6004.

[29] Rad A, Abbasi A, Kafil H, Ganbarov K. Potential Pharmaceutical and Food Applications of Postbiotics: A review. *Current pharmaceutical biotechnology*. 2020.

[30] Homayouni Rad A, Samadi Kafil H, Fathi Zavoshti H, Shahbazi N, Abbasi A. Therapeutically Effects of Functional Postbiotic Foods. *Clinical Excellence*. 2020;10(2):33-52.

[31] de Almada CN, Almada CN, Martinez RC, Sant'Ana AS. Paraprobiotics: evidences on their ability to modify biological responses, inactivation methods and perspectives on their application in foods. *Trends in food science & technology*. 2016;58:96-114.

[32] Aguilar-Toalá J, Garcia-Varela R, Garcia H, Mata-Haro V, González-Córdova A, Vallejo-Cordoba B, & Hernández-Mendoza, A. Postbiotics: An evolving term within the functional foods field. *Trends in Food Science & Technology*. 2018;75:105-14.

[33] Homayouni Rad A, Aghebati Maleki L, Samadi Kafil H, Abbasi A. Postbiotics: A novel strategy in food allergy treatment. *Critical Reviews in Food Science and Nutrition*. 2020:1-8.

[34] Barros CP, Guimarães JT, Esmerino EA, Duarte MCK, Silva MC, Silva R, Ferreira, BM, Sant'Ana, AS, Freitas, MQ, & Cruz, AG. Paraprobiotics and postbiotics: Concepts and potential applications in dairy products. *Current Opinion in Food Science*. 2020;32:1-8.

[35] Cicenia A, Scirocco A, Carabotti M, Pallotta L, Marignani M, Severi C. Postbiotic activities of lactobacilli-derived factors. *Journal of clinical gastroenterology*. 2014;48:S18-S22.

[36] Rai AK, Pandey A, Sahoo D. Biotechnological potential of yeasts in functional food industry. *Trends in food science & technology*. 2018.

[37] Salminen S, Collado MC, Endo A, Hill C, Lebeer S, Quigley EM, Sanders, ME, Shamir, R, Swann, JR, Szajewska, H, & Vinderola, G. The International Scientific Association of Probiotics and Prebiotics (ISAPP) consensus statement on the definition and scope of postbiotics. *Nature Reviews Gastroenterology & Hepatology*. 2021;18(9):649-67.

[38] Abbasi A, Sabahi S, Bazzaz S, Tajani AG, Lahouty M, Aslani R, & Hosseini, H. An edible coating utilizing Malva sylvestris seed polysaccharide mucilage and postbiotic from *Saccharomyces cerevisiae var. boulardii* for the preservation of

lamb meat. *International Journal of Biological Macromolecules*. 2023;246: 125660.

[39] Lebeer S, Vanderleyden J, De Keersmaecker SC. Host interactions of probiotic bacterial surface molecules: comparison with commensals and pathogens. *Nature Reviews Microbiology*. 2010;8(3):171-84.

[40] Sheykhsaran E, Abbasi A, Ebrahimzadeh Leylabadlo H, Sadeghi J, Mehri S, Naeimi Mazraeh F, Feizi, H, & Bannazadeh Baghi, H. Gut microbiota and obesity: an overview of microbiota to microbial-based therapies. *Postgraduate medical journal*. 2023;99(1171):384-402.

[41] Abbasi A, Rad AH, Maleki LA, Kafil HS, Baghbanzadeh A. Antigenotoxicity and Cytotoxic Potentials of Cell-Free Supernatants Derived from *Saccharomyces cerevisiae var. boulardii* on HT-29 Human Colon Cancer Cell Lines. *Probiotics and Antimicrobial Proteins*. 2023:1-13.

[42] Thomas CM, Hong T, Van Pijkeren JP, Hemarajata P, Trinh DV, Hu W, Britton, RA, Kalkum, M, & Versalovic, J. Histamine derived from probiotic *Lactobacillus reuteri* suppresses TNF via modulation of PKA and ERK signaling. *PloS one*. 2012;7(2):e31951.

[43] Abbasi A, Sanej KD, Moradi S, Bazzaz S, Esmaeili A, Ghafourian K, et al. *Bioactive Compounds and Biological Activities of Allium sativum L. Bioactive Compounds in the Storage Organs of Plants*: Springer; 2023. p. 1-40.

[44] Abbasi A, Hajipour N, Hasannezhad P, Baghbanzadeh A, Aghebati-Maleki L. Potential *in vivo* delivery routes of postbiotics. *Critical Reviews in Food Science and Nutrition*. 2022;62(12):3345-69.

[45] Sun Z, Harris HM, McCann A, Guo C, Argimón S, Zhang W, Yang, X, Jeffery, IB, Cooney, JC, Kagawa, TF, Liu, W, Song, Y, Salvetti, E, Wrobel, A, Rasinkangas, P, Parkhill, J, Rea, MC, O'Sullivan, O, Ritari, J, … O'Toole, PW. Expanding the biotechnology potential of lactobacilli through comparative genomics of 213 strains and associated genera. *Nature communications*. 2015;6(1):8322.

[46] Abbasi A, Bazzaz S, A. Ibrahim S, Hekmatdoost A, Hosseini H, Sabahi S, Sheykhsaran, E, Rahbar Saadat, Y, Asghari Ozma, M, & Lahouty, M. A Critical Review on the Gluten-Induced Enteropathy/Celiac Disease: Gluten-Targeted Dietary and Non-Dietary Therapeutic Approaches. *Food Reviews International*. 2023:1-41.

[47] Laverde Gomez JA, Mukhopadhya I, Duncan SH, Louis P, Shaw S, Collie-Duguid E, Crost, E, Juge, N, & Flint, HJ. Formate cross-feeding and cooperative metabolic interactions revealed by transcriptomics in co-cultures of acetogenic and amylolytic human colonic bacteria. *Environmental microbiology*. 2019;21(1):259-71.

[48] Hernández-Granados MJ, Franco-Robles E. Postbiotics in human health: Possible new functional ingredients? *Food Research International*. 2020;137:109660.

[49] Ozma MA, Moaddab SR, Hosseini H, Khodadadi E, Ghotaslou R, Asgharzadeh M, Abbasi, A, Kamounah, FS, Aghebati Maleki, L, Ganbarov, K, & Samadi Kafil, H. A critical review of novel antibiotic resistance prevention approaches with a focus on postbiotics. *Critical Reviews in Food Science and Nutrition*. 2023:1-19.

[50] Parashar UD, Gibson CJ, Bresee JS, Glass RI. Rotavirus and severe childhood diarrhea. *Emerging infectious diseases*. 2006;12(2):304.

[51] Pop M, Walker AW, Paulson J, Lindsay B, Antonio M, Hossain MA, Oundo, J, Tamboura, B, Mai, V, Astrovskaya, I, Bravo, H, Rance, R, Stares, M, Levine, MM, Panchalingam, S, Kotloff, K, Ikumapayi, UN, Ebruke, C, Adeyemi, M, … Stine, O. Diarrhea in young children from low-income countries leads to large-scale alterations in intestinal microbiota composition. *Genome biology*. 2014;15(6):1-12.

[52] Singh P, Teal TK, Marsh TL, Tiedje JM, Mosci R, Jernigan K, Zell, A, Newton, DW, Salimnia, H, Lephart, P, Sundin, D, Khalife, W, Britton, RA, Rudrik, JT, & Manning, SD. Intestinal microbial communities associated with acute enteric infections and disease recovery. *Microbiome*. 2015;3(1):1-12.

[53] Ma C, Wu X, Nawaz M, Li J, Yu P, Moore JE, & Xu, J. Molecular characterization of fecal microbiota in patients with viral diarrhea. *Current microbiology*. 2011;63(3):259-66.

[54] Rouhani S, Griffin NW, Yori PP, Gehrig JL, Olortegui MP, Salas MS, Trigoso, DR, Moulton, LH, Houpt, ER, Barratt, MJ, Koser, MN, Gordon, JI. Diarrhea as a potential cause and consequence of reduced gut microbial diversity among undernourished children in Peru. *Clinical Infectious Diseases*. 2020;71(4):989-99.

[55] Collinson S, Deans A, Padua-Zamora A, Gregorio GV, Li C, Dans LF, Allen, SJ. Probiotics for treating acute infectious diarrhea. *Cochrane Database of Systematic Reviews*. 2020(12).

[56] Sabahi S, Homayouni Rad A, Aghebati-Maleki L, Sangtarash N, Ozma MA, Karimi A, Hosseini, H, & Abbasi, A. Postbiotics as the new frontier in food and pharmaceutical research. *Critical Reviews in Food Science and Nutrition*. 2022:1-28.

[57] Salazar-Lindo E, Figueroa-Quintanilla D, Caciano MI, Reto-Valiente V, Chauviere G, Colin P. Effectiveness and safety of Lactobacillus LB in the treatment of mild acute diarrhea in children. *Journal of pediatric gastroenterology and nutrition*. 2007;44(5):571-6.

[58] Liévin-Le Moal V, Sarrazin-Davila LE, Servin AL. An experimental study and a randomized, double-blind, placebo-controlled clinical trial to evaluate the antisecretory activity of Lactobacillus acidophilus strain LB against nonrotavirus diarrhea. *Pediatrics*. 2007;120(4):e795-e803.

[59] Corsello G, Carta M, Marinello R, Picca M, De Marco G, Micillo M, Ferrara, D, Vigneri, P, Cecere, G, Ferri, P, Roggero, P, Bedogni, G, Mosca, F, Paparo, L, Nocerino, R, & Berni Canani, R. Preventive effect of cow's milk fermented with *Lactobacillus paracasei* CBA L74 on common infectious diseases in children: a multicenter randomized controlled trial. *Nutrients*. 2017;9(7):669.

[60] Mosca A, Abreu Y Abreu AT, Gwee KA, Ianiro G, Tack J, Nguyen TVH, & Hill, C. The clinical evidence for postbiotics as microbial therapeutics. *Gut Microbes*. 2022;14(1):2117508.

[61] Altuntaş B, Gül H, Yarali N, Ertan U. Etiology of chronic diarrhea. *The Indian Journal of Pediatrics*. 1999;66:657-61.

[62] Sabahi S, Mortazavi SA, Nassiri M, Ghazvini K, Shahidi F, Abbasi A. Production of functional ice cream fortified by immunoglobulin Y against *Escherichia coli* O157: H7 and Helicobacter pylori. *Biointerface Research in Applied Chemistry*. 2022;13(2):188-98.

[63] Lovell RM, Ford AC. Prevalence of gastro-esophageal reflux-type symptoms in individuals with irritable bowel syndrome in the community: a meta-analysis. *Official journal of the American College of Gastroenterology| ACG*. 2012;107 (12):1793-801.

[64] Ozma MA, Abbasi A, Sabahi S. Characterization of postbiotics derived from *Lactobacillus paracasei* ATCC 55544 and its application in *Malva sylvestris* seed mucilage edible coating to the improvement of the microbiological, and sensory properties of lamb meat during storage. *Biointerface Res Appl Chem*. 2022;13.

[65] Xiao S-D, De Zhang Z, Lu H, Jiang SH, Liu HY, Wang GS, Xu, GM, Zhang, ZB, Lin, GJ, & Wang, GL. Multicenter, randomized, controlled trial of heat-killed Lactobacillus acidophilus LB in patients with chronic diarrhea. *Advances in therapy*. 2003;20:253-60.

[66] Andresen V, Gschossmann J, Layer P. Heat-inactivated Bifidobacterium bifidum MIMBb75 (SYN-HI-001) in the treatment of irritable bowel syndrome: a multicentre, randomised, double-blind, placebo-controlled clinical trial. *The lancet Gastroenterology & hepatology*. 2020;5(7):658-66.

[67] Tarrerias A, Costil V, Vicari F, Letard J, Adenis-Lamarre P, Aisene A, Batistelli, D, Bonnaud, G, Carpentier, S, Dalbiès, P, Ecuer, S, Etienne, J, Fantoli, M, Grunberg, B, Lannoy, P, Lapuelle, J, Margulies, A, Neumeier, M, Rouillon, JM, … Canard, JM. The effect of inactivated *Lactobacillus LB* fermented culture medium on symptom severity: observational investigation in 297 patients with diarrhea-predominant irritable bowel syndrome. *Digestive Diseases*. 2011;29(6): 588-91.

[68] Somi MH, Tanhaei A, Abbasi A, Moaddab SY, Leylabadlo HE. Fecal Microbiota Transplantation in Liver Diseases and Recent Developments. *Journal of Shahid Sadoughi University of Medical Sciences*. 2022.

[69] Abbasi A, Rad AH, Maleki LA, Kafil HS, Baghbanzadeh A. *Cytotoxic Potentials of Cell-Free Supernatant Derived from Lactobacillus casei CRL431 on HCT-116 and HT-29 Human Colon Cancer Cell Lines*. 2022.

[70] Ozma MA, Abbasi A, Akrami S, Lahouty M, Shahbazi N, Ganbarov K, Pagliano, P, Sabahi, S, Kose, S, Yousefi, M, Dao, S, Asgharzadeh, M, Hosseini, H, Kafil, HS. Postbiotics as the key mediators of the gut microbiota-host interactions. *Le infezioni in medicina*. 2022;30(2):180.

[71] Homayouni-rad A, Aghebati-Maleki L, Samadi-Kafil H, Abbasi A, Khani N. Postbiotics as a safe alternative to live probiotic bacteria in the food and pharmaceutical industries. *HBI_Journals*. 2021;26:132-57.

[72] Coconnier M-H, Lievin V, Hemery E, Servin AL. Antagonistic activity against Helicobacter infection *in vitro* and *in vivo* by the human Lactobacillus acidophilus strain LB. *Applied and Environmental Microbiology*. 1998;64(11): 4573-80.

[73] Canducci F, Armuzzi A, Cremonini F, Cammarota G, Bartolozzi F, Pola P, Gasbarrini, G, & Gasbarrini, A. A lyophilized and inactivated culture of *Lactobacillus acidophilus* increases *Helicobacter pylori* eradication rates. *Alimentary pharmacology & therapeutics*. 2000;14(12):1625-9.

[74] Hosseini H, Abbasi A, Sabahi S, Akrami S, Yousefi-Avarvand A. Assessing the Potential Biological Activities of Postbiotics Derived from Saccharomyces cerevisiae: An *In Vitro* Study. *Probiotics and Antimicrobial Proteins*. 2023:1-17.

[75] Mohamadzadeh M, Olson S, Kalina WV, Ruthel G, Demmin GL, Warfield KL, Bavari, S, & Klaenhammer, TR. *Lactobacilli* activate human dendritic cells that skew T cells toward T helper 1 polarization. *Proceedings of the National Academy of Sciences*. 2005;102(8): 2880-5.

[76] Abbasi A, Saadat TR, Saadat YR. Microbial exopolysaccharides–β-glucans–as promising postbiotic candidates in vaccine adjuvants. *International Journal of Biological Macromolecules*. 2022.

[77] Yazdanbakhsh M, Kremsner PG, Van Ree R. Allergy, parasites, and the hygiene hypothesis. *Science*. 2002;296(5567):490-4.

[78] Hirose Y, Murosaki S, Yamamoto Y, Yoshikai Y, Tsuru T. Daily intake of heat-killed *Lactobacillus plantarum* L-137 augments acquired immunity in healthy adults. *The Journal of nutrition*. 2006;136(12):3069-73.

[79] Wang MF, Lin HC, Wang YY, Hsu CH. Treatment of perennial allergic rhinitis with lactic acid bacteria. *Pediatric Allergy and Immunology*. 2004;15(2):152-8.

[80] Peng GC, Hsu CH. The efficacy and safety of heat-killed *Lactobacillus paracasei* for treatment of perennial allergic rhinitis induced by house-dust mite. *Pediatric allergy and immunology*. 2005;16(5):433-8.

[81] Rasche C, Wolfram C, Wahls M, Worm M. Differential immunomodulating effects of inactivated probiotic bacteria on the allergic immune response. *Acta dermato-venereologica*. 2007;87(4):305-11.

[82] Rad AH, Aghebati-Maleki L, Kafil HS, Abbasi A. Molecular mechanisms of postbiotics in colorectal cancer prevention and treatment. *Critical reviews in food science and nutrition*. 2021;61(11):1787-803.

[83] Homayouni Rad A, Aghebati Maleki L, Samadi Kafil H, Abbasi A. Postbiotics: A novel strategy in food allergy treatment. *Critical reviews in food science and nutrition*. 2021;61(3):492-9.

[84] Sheykhsaran E, Abbasi A, Baghi HB, Ghotaslou R, Sharifi Y, Sefidan FY, et al. *Staphylococcus* aureus: A bacterial candidate for multiple sclerosis incidence and progression. *Reviews and Research in Medical Microbiology*. 2022;33(4):212-20.

[85] Abbasi A, Sheykhsaran E, Kafil HS. *Postbiotics: science, technology and applications:* Bentham Science Publishers; 2021.

[86] Maeda N, Nakamura R, Hirose Y, Murosaki S, Yamamoto Y, Kase T, & Yoshikai, Y. Oral administration of heat-killed *Lactobacillus plantarum* L-137 enhances protection against influenza virus infection by stimulation of type I interferon production in mice. *International immunopharmacology*. 2009;9(9): 1122-5.

[87] Arimori Y, Nakamura R, Hirose Y, Murosaki S, Yamamoto Y, Shidara O, Ichikawa, H, & Yoshikai, Y. Daily intake of heat-killed *Lactobacillus plantarum* L-137 enhances type I interferon production in healthy humans and pigs. *Immunopharmacology and immunotoxicology*. 2012;34(6):937-43.

[88] Hirose Y, Yamamoto Y, Yoshikai Y, Murosaki S. Oral intake of heat-killed *Lactobacillus plantarum* L-137 decreases the incidence of upper respiratory tract infection in healthy subjects with high levels of psychological stress. *Journal of nutritional science*. 2013;2:e39.

[89] Nocerino R, Paparo L, Terrin G, Pezzella V, Amoroso A, Cosenza L, Cecere, G, De Marco, G, Micillo, M, Albano, F, Nugnes, R, Ferri, P, Ciccarelli, G, Giaccio,

G, Spadaro, R, Maddalena, Y, Berni Canani, F, & Berni Canani, R. Cow's milk and rice fermented with *Lactobacillus paracasei* CBA L74 prevent infectious diseases in children: a randomized controlled trial. *Clinical Nutrition.* 2017;36(1):118-25.

[90] Hishiki H, Kawashima T, Tsuji NM, Ikari N, Takemura R, Kido H, & Shimojo, N. A double-blind, randomized, placebo-controlled trial of heat-killed *Pediococcus acidilactici* K15 for prevention of respiratory tract infections among preschool children. *Nutrients*. 2020;12(7):1989.

[91] Miletic I, Schiffman S, Miletic V, Sattely-Miller E. Salivary IgA secretion rate in young and elderly persons. *Physiology & behavior*. 1996;60(1):243-8.

[92] Kotani Y, Shinkai S, Okamatsu H, Toba M, Ogawa K, Yoshida H, Fukaya, T, Fujiwara, Y, Chaves, PH, Kakumoto, K, & Kohda, N. Oral intake of *Lactobacillus pentosus* strain b240 accelerates salivary immunoglobulin A secretion in the elderly: A randomized, placebo-controlled, double-blind trial. *Immunity & ageing*. 2010;7(1):1-11.

[93] Rad AH, Maleki LA, Kafil HS, Zavoshti HF, Abbasi A. Postbiotics as promising tools for cancer adjuvant therapy. *Advanced Pharmaceutical Bulletin*. 2021;11(1):1.

[94] Shinkai S, Toba M, Saito T, Sato I, Tsubouchi M, Taira K, Kakumoto, K, Inamatsu, T, Yoshida, H, Fujiwara, Y, Fukaya, T, Matsumoto, T, Tateda, K, Yamaguchi, K, Kohda, N, & Kohno, S. Immunoprotective effects of oral intake of heat-killed *Lactobacillus pentosus* strain b240 in elderly adults: a randomised, double-blind, placebo-controlled trial. *British journal of nutrition*. 2013;109(10): 1856-65.

[95] Rad AH, Abbasi A, Kafil HS, Ganbarov K. Potential pharmaceutical and food applications of postbiotics: a review. *Current pharmaceutical biotechnology*. 2020;21(15):1576-87.

[96] Mayer EA. Gut feelings: the emerging biology of gut–brain communication. *Nature Reviews Neuroscience*. 2011;12(8):453-66.

[97] Abbasi A, Aghebati-Maleki L, Homayouni-Rad A. The promising biological role of postbiotics derived from probiotic *Lactobacillus* species in reproductive health. *Critical Reviews in Food Science and Nutrition*. 2022;62(32):8829-41.

[98] Cryan JF, Dinan TG. Mind-altering microorganisms: the impact of the gut microbiota on brain and behaviour. *Nature reviews neuroscience*. 2012;13(10): 701-12.

[99] Nishida K, Sawada D, Kuwano Y, Tanaka H, Rokutan K. Health benefits of Lactobacillus gasseri CP2305 tablets in young adults exposed to chronic stress: a randomized, double-blind, placebo-controlled study. *Nutrients*. 2019;11(8):1859.

[100] Hossain MS, Tajima A, Kotoura S, Katafuchi T. Oral ingestion of plasmalogens can attenuate the LPS-induced memory loss and microglial activation. *Biochemical and biophysical research communications*. 2018;496(4):1033-9.

[101] Fujino T, Yamada T, Asada T, Tsuboi Y, Wakana C, Mawatari S, & Kono, S. Efficacy and blood plasmalogen changes by oral administration of plasmalogen in patients with mild Alzheimer's disease and mild cognitive impairment: a

multicenter, randomized, double-blind, placebo-controlled trial. *EBioMedicine*. 2017;17:199-205.

[102] Flux M, Lowry CA. Finding intestinal fortitude: integrating the microbiome into a holistic view of depression mechanisms, treatment, and resilience. *Neurobiology of disease*. 2020;135:104578.

[103] Cosola C, Rocchetti MT, Cupisti A, Gesualdo L. Microbiota metabolites: Pivotal players of cardiovascular damage in chronic kidney disease. *Pharmacological Research*. 2018;130:132-42.

[104] Vallianou N, Stratigou T, Christodoulatos GS, Tsigalou C, Dalamaga M. Probiotics, prebiotics, synbiotics, postbiotics, and obesity: current evidence, controversies, and perspectives. *Current obesity reports*. 2020;9:179-92.

[105] Shin HS, Park SY, Lee DK, Kim SA, An HM, Kim JR, Kim, MJ, Cha, MG, Lee, SW, Kim, KJ, Lee, KO, & Ha, NJ. Hypocholesterolemic effect of sonication-killed *Bifidobacterium longum* isolated from healthy adult Koreans in high cholesterol fed rats. *Archives of pharmacal research*. 2010;33:1425-31.

[106] Williams L, Alshehri A, Robichaud B, Cudmore A, Gagnon J. The role of the bacterial muramyl dipeptide in the regulation of GLP-1 and glycemia. *International Journal of Molecular Sciences*. 2020;21(15):5252.

[107] Everard A, Plovier H, Rastelli M, Van Hul M, de Wouters d'Oplinter A, Geurts L, Druart, C, Robine, S, Delzenne, NM, Muccioli, GG, De Vos, WM, Luquet, S, Flamand, N, Di Marzo, V, & Cani, PD. Intestinal epithelial N-acylphosphatidylethanolamine phospholipase D links dietary fat to metabolic adaptations in obesity and steatosis. *Nature communications*. 2019;10(1):457.

[108] Abbasi A, Bazzaz S, Da Cruz AG, Khorshidian N, Saadat YR, Sabahi S, Ozma, MA, Lahouty, M, Aslani, R, & Mortazavian, AM. A Critical Review on *Akkermansia muciniphila*: Functional Mechanisms, Technological Challenges, and Safety Issues. *Probiotics and Antimicrobial Proteins*. 2023:1-23.

[109] Plovier H, Everard A, Druart C, Depommier C, Van Hul M, Geurts L, Chilloux, J, Ottman, N, Duparc, T, Lichtenstein, L, Myridakis, A, Delzenne, NM, Klievink, J, Bhattacharjee, A, Van Der Ark, KCH, Aalvink, S, Martinez, LO, Dumas, ME, Maiter, D, ... Cani, PD. A purified membrane protein from *Akkermansia muciniphila* or the pasteurized bacterium improves metabolism in obese and diabetic mice. *Nature medicine*. 2017;23(1):107-13.

[110] Depommier C, Everard A, Druart C, Plovier H, Van Hul M, Vieira-Silva S, Falony, G, Raes, J, Maiter, D, Delzenne, NM, De Barsy, M, Loumaye, A, Hermans, MP, Thissen, JP, De Vos, WM, & Cani, PD. Supplementation with *Akkermansia muciniphila* in overweight and obese human volunteers: a proof-of-concept exploratory study. *Nature medicine*. 2019;25(7):1096-103.

[111] Albillos A, De Gottardi A, Rescigno M. The gut-liver axis in liver disease: Pathophysiological basis for therapy. *Journal of hepatology*. 2020;72(3):558-77.

[112] Abbasi A, Sanej KD, Mohammadi A, Moradi S, Nayeri BD, Bazzaz S, et al. *The Role of Postbiotics in Food Safety Promotion*.

Chapter 8

A Proteomic Analysis of Postbiotics in Medical Bacteriology

Mahdi Asghari Ozma[1,*], PhD
Niloofar Fallahi Alileh[1], BSc
Sina Mahdavi[2], MSc
Amin Abbasi[3], PhD
Masoud Asghari Ozma[4], MSc
Masoud Lahouty[5], MSc
Javad Nezhadi[2], PhD
and Hossein Samadi Kafil[1], PhD

[1]Drug Applied Research Center, Tabriz University of Medical Sciences, Tabriz, Iran
[2]Department of Microbiology and Virology, Tabriz University of Medical Sciences, Tabriz, Iran
[3]Department of Food Science and Technology, National Nutrition and Food Technology Research Institute, Faculty of Nutrition Sciences and Food Technology, Shahid Beheshti University of Medical Sciences, Tehran, Iran
[4]Department of Food Science and Technology, Islamic Azad University, Tabriz Branch, Tabriz, Iran
[5]Department of Microbiology and Virology, Urmia University of Medical Sciences, Urmia, Iran

Abstract

The structure of bacteria consists of various macromolecules such as proteins, polysaccharides, phospholipids, and nucleic acids, which, in

* Corresponding Author's Email: asghariozma@gmail.com.

In: Exploring Microbiotics in Health and Disease
Editor: Edward L. Stillman
ISBN: 978-8-89113-410-2

addition to their role in forming their structure, play an essential role in maintaining their life and pathogenicity. To study these macromolecules, in addition to genomic methods, there are proteomic methods that provide information about the structural and functional proteins of bacteria, including wall proteins, secretion systems, toxins, biofilm formation mechanisms, and antibiotic resistance, which by knowing them, we can more comprehensively understand the pathogenic mechanisms of these microorganisms and deal with their damage more effectively. In addition to pathogenic bacteria, there are probiotic bacteria, which are live microorganisms that provide beneficial effects to the body when consumed in sufficient quantities. As a part of the structure of these microorganisms and also as a result of their activity, postbiotics are produced, which are responsible for the beneficial effects of probiotics and include various compounds, which the protein compounds are a large part of them, including enzymes such as peptidases, lipases, amylases, proteases, ureases, phenol oxidases, catalase, superoxide dismutase, as well as compounds such as bacteriocin, lactospins, and wall proteins, which, due to their specific chemical structure, safe properties, long shelf life, and various signaling molecules, have various properties, including antimicrobial, antidiabetic, anti-inflammatory, immune-modulating, anti-hypertensive and antioxidant activity, which has caused them to be used in various food and pharmaceutical industries nowadays for high-performance products and safe therapeutic properties.

Keywords: bacteriology, proteome, probiotic, postbiotic, proteomics

Introduction

Bacteria are microorganisms that thrive in warm, moist conditions and infect a variety of hosts, including people, animals, and plants [1]. These microorganisms can produce a wide range of macromolecules, including proteins, polysaccharides, phospholipids, and nucleic acids, which are required for the formation of their structure, survival within the host, and pathogenicity, and this pathogenicity has made bacterial infections a major public health concern [2, 3]. To research these macromolecules, which give detailed information about microbes, several approaches including genomics and proteomics are applied. Proteomics is concerned with proteins, which are more active macromolecules than nucleic acids. Genomics approaches investigate the discovery and expression of numerous genes in cells [4].

Proteomics is the comprehensive study of different structural and functional proteins of a cell, which can identify these macromolecules by several methods, including liquid chromatography-mass spectrometry (LC-MS), two-dimensional electrophoresis (2DE), or matrix laser ionization and absorption technique mass spectrometry (MALDI- TOF MS). These findings indicate that extensive information may be gathered by examining bacterial proteins, allowing for faster, easier, and more accurate detection of illnesses and more efficient therapy [5]. The current chapter focuses on the comprehensive investigation of various bacterial proteins, their effects on bacteria's ability to cause disease in host cells and their pathogenicity, as well as the study of their protein postbiotics to provide new insights about microorganisms and help us deal with them more effectively.

Proteomic Analysis of Bacterial Secretion Systems

Bacteria employ numerous methods, such as protein production, to avoid detection by the host's immune system and continue to develop. Through their numerous secretion systems, they secrete proteins from their cytoplasm to the host's body or the environment. These secreted proteins play a variety of tasks, including binding to host cells, cytotoxicity altering host cell function, and eventually boosting bacterial survival in the host. Bacteria have many secretion systems with varying shapes and activities that secrete various proteins. Sec and Tat are the most often employed secretion systems in gram-negative and gram-positive bacteria that release proteins into the cell, periplasm, or internal membrane, allowing harmful agents to enter the cell and cause infection [6, 7].

SecYEG proteins transport folded proteins, SecA protein has ATPase activity, SecB protein has chaperone activity and can connect to the preformed protein on one hand and the messenger peptidase enzyme in the periplasm on the other, and finally SecYEG proteins transport folded proteins [8, 9]. This secretion mechanism is found in both Gram-positive and Gram-negative bacteria to carry chemicals outside. The Tat pathway consists of TatA, TatB, and TatC protein parts, which are used to move proteins that have found proper folding, and is essential for pathogenic and non-pathogenic bacteria, gram-positive and gram-negative bacteria, including Yersinia pseudotuberculosis and Pseudomonas aeruginosa [10]. Bacteria employ seven distinct secretion mechanisms to move various macromolecules outside the cell. T1SS is found in both Gram-negative and Gram-positive bacteria and is made up of three protein components: ATP-binding cassette transporter (ABC), membrane fusion protein (MFP), and factor The outer membrane (OMF) is the total of these three components, which together constitute a channel via which secretory protein is discharged from the bacterial cell [11, 12]. This secretory pathway transports a variety of chemicals, including poisons and antibiotics, as well as lipase, protease, and protein enzymes that can cause holes in the host's cytoplasmic membrane. Ferritin is a protein found on the surface of bacteria that allows them to obtain the iron they requires [13].

The type two secretion system (T2SS) is made up of four proteins found in most gram-negative bacteria: inner membrane platform, outer membrane secretin, cytoplasmic ATPase, and pseudopilus, as well as folded molecules such as phosphatase, lipase, protease, and carbohydrate. secretes that are efficient in the pathogenesis of bacteria. Pseudomonas aeruginosa secretes exotoxin A via the type 2 secretion system, which harms host cell protein synthesis [14]. The type three secretion system (T3SS), also known as needle-like injectisomes, is present in many Gram-negative bacteria. This system is made up of three parts: the Basal Body, the Needle, and the Translocon, which allow bacterial proteins to enter the host cell and alter its many activities. This mechanism secretes protein molecules known as effector proteins, which are then injected directly into the target cell. This secretion system was discovered for the first time in the plague-causing bacteria Yersina pestis. This system does not require the presence of signal peptides, and its structure functions like a syringe, allowing the secreted protein to be sent straight over the membrane to the cytoplasm of the bacterium and the host cell enters its contents directly into them [15].

T4SS is found in both gram-negative and gram-positive bacteria and may transmit both DNA and protein molecules to other prokaryotes and eukaryotes. This mechanism can engage in conjugation, which results in the transfer of genomes across bacteria, due to the transfer of DNA. This secretion system was discovered for the first time in the *Agrobacterium thomphascens*, and it consists of numerous proteins, including VirB1, VirB2, and VirD4 [16]. Unlike other secretion systems, gram-negative bacteria's type 5 secretion system (T5SS) operates as an autotransporter and typically carries released bacterial toxins. This secretory system is split into various categories, the most significant of which are Va (Classical or Monomeric), Vb (Two-partner Secretory System or TPSS), and TAA (Trimeric Autotransporter Adhesins), and each of these systems is made up of distinct proteins. In *Escherichia coli*, for example, the most critical proteins in the production of Va are Bam A-E, which serve to transport chemicals and improve bacterial pathogenicity. TpsA and TpsB are the most important proteins in the structure of TPSS, and Bam protein is required for the creation of TAAs [17, 18]. SurA, SkpA, FkpA, and DegP are chaperone proteins that are connected to autotransporters to maintain folded proteins in Va so that this system can function well. One application of the type five secretion system in group Va is the secretion of IgA Protease or immunoglobulin A protease in *Neisseria meningitidis*, which disrupts the target cell's antibody and weakens the immune system, and TAAs bind to the target cell in the initiation of pathogenicity in *Bartonella*. In addition, infecting the host cell is beneficial [19].

T6SS (type six secretion system) was discovered in *Vibrio cholerae* and *Pseudomonas aeruginosa*. This system is made up of two pieces, a sheath, and a tube, as well as several protein components. Bacteria employ this secretion system not just to produce disease, but also to defend themselves against bigger bacteria that could assault them. In response to environmental challenges and stimuli, the expression of this secretory system and its active proteins rises, allowing bacteria to survive in harsh environments [20, 21]. Some bacteria, including *Mycobacteria*, have a rigid wall around them, which leads to high resistance to environmental stimuli and antibiotics [22]. However, the low permeability of the wall makes it difficult for bacteria to transport secreted macromolecules, so these bacteria use a special structure called secretion system type 7 (T7SS) to transport molecules [23]. This secretion system, termed ESX, was discovered for the first time in *Mycobacteria* and consists of five proteins: EccB, EccC, EccD, EccD, and MycP. Other bacteria, such as *Corynebacterium*, have a type seven secretion mechanism. Because of the specificity of this secretion system's expression in bacteria, it has been utilized as a therapeutic target for the manufacture of drugs and vaccines [24].

Proteomic Analysis of Bacterial Cell Wall

Bacteria require various virulence factors to adhere to the host cell, including surface layer proteins, cell protein coating, and the flagellum, which cause illness in the host cell via adhering. The surface layer is a two-dimensional structure that exists outside of the bacterial cell wall and covers the bacteria's exterior surface, allowing the bacteria to communicate with the outside environment [25, 26]. This structure is formed of protein or glycoprotein and serves numerous functions, including adhering bacteria to the host cell, antigenic alterations and shielding bacteria from environmental harm, and lastly boosting pathogenicity and allowing bacteria to proliferate and live [27, 28]. The surface layer protein consists of two proteins with weights of 45 kilodaltons named surface layer protein with high molecular weight (HMW-SLP) and 36 kilodaltons termed surface layer protein with low molecular weight (LMW-SLP) both of these proteins are derived from the same gene called SlpA and have distinct roles in the pathophysiology of bacteria that induce malabsorption of food in the gut [29, 30].

Flagellum is another protein surface structure generated from numerous proteins, including flagellin (FlaA, FlaB), cap (FliD), hook (FlgE), and basal body protein (FlgG). It allows bacteria to migrate among host cells, causing adhesion, colonization, and persistent infections in the host body, and anti-FlaA antibodies can be employed in the treatment of bacterial infections in the clinic. Bacteria are enclosed by a structure known as a cell envelope, which efficiently preserves the bacteria's form and protects it from osmotic pressure and other environmental pressures [31]. This complex structure, which comprises carbohydrates, lipids, and different proteins and is found within and on the surface of bacteria, regulates a variety of bacterial functions. The proteins that make up this structure perform a variety of functions, including cell membrane construction, transcription, translation, transfer, metabolism, energy production, messaging, and defense against the human immune system, as well as increasing the bacteria's survival and destructive effect on the host body [32].

To defend themselves against harsh circumstances, such as a shortage of nitrogen, phosphate, and carbon, certain bacteria produce a tough and resistant structure known as a spore through a process known as sporulation (Germination) become reactivated and restart pathogenic action [33]. The spore is made up of several parts. Its cover is made up of two layers and contains a variety of proteins, including CotC, CotE, SafA, and Spo4D, which are essential for the cover's function in protecting bacteria from the host's immune system and transporting essential substances that allow bacteria to survive in the host [34]. Gram-negative bacteria have an outside membrane that contains outer membrane proteins (OMPs) that play a role in bacterial host activities such as maintaining and delivering communications and may also operate as a pathogenic factor in bacterial attachment to host cells. These bacteria can also bypass the host's immune system via the proteins of the outer membrane, and by obtaining critical nutrients across this membrane, they can increase their survival in target cells. Gram-negative bacteria also have a unique protein structure known as outer membrane vesicles (OMV), which are formed from the outer membrane proteins and serve a variety of tasks such as attaching to the host cell, weakening the host's immune system, resistance to antibiotics, stress response, proteolytic activity, iron absorption, and, ultimately, bacterial survival in the host cell [35].

Proteomic Analysis of Biofilm Formation by Bacteria

Biofilm is a population of bacterial cells that cling to a surface in close contact and are surrounded by an exopolysaccharide matrix, protecting bacteria from harmful environmental conditions and the host's defense system, which eventually causes infections [36, 37]. In the host body, they become chronic [38]. When compared to planktonic or floating settings, bacteria activate several biofilm formation genes and manufacture critical functional proteins that eventually cause bacteria to cling to living or non-living surfaces and establish their cell communities. RpoSs, which is one of the key regulators of *E. coli* in response to environmental stress, is one of the most critical proteins involved in biofilm creation, and its removal promotes biofilm instability [39]. The flagellum is another key component, and the expression of its constituent proteins, as well as chemotactic proteins like CheA, rises during biofilm development. Bacteria in biofilms boost energy-producing proteins including succinate and thiokinase, indicating the existence of bacterial growth within biofilms [40].

Proteomic Analysis of the Occurrence of Antibiotic Resistance in Bacteria

Antibiotics have several applications in the treatment of bacterial illnesses. The advent of antibiotic resistance in bacteria resulted in new hurdles in dealing with and controlling these resistances. Antibiotic resistance in bacteria has resulted in a rise in bacterial pathogenicity and a hazard to society's health and cleanliness [41]. Bacteria develop antibiotic resistance through a variety of mechanisms, including the production of an efflux pump to expel drugs from the bacterium, lowering antibiotic permeability across the bacterial membrane, obtaining resistance genes, and utilizing particular metabolites. He suggested many proteins and antibacterial medication neutralization. Some antibiotics block the enzymes involved in the creation of peptidoglycan to exert their action, and beta-lactams and glycopeptides are part of this category of antibiotics that hinder cell wall synthesis [42, 43]. Bacteria deal with beta-lactams in a variety of ways, including the use of beta-lactamase enzyme, increased synthesis of efflux pumps that remove the antibiotic from the bacteria, and the production of penicillin-binding proteins (PBPs) that bind to antibiotics and reduce their affinity, one of which is the antibiotics' ineffectiveness against methicillin-resistant *Staphylococcus aureus* (MRSA) bacteria [44].

Some antibiotics disrupt protein synthesis in bacteria; for example, tetracycline causes bacterial dysfunction by preventing tRNA binding to the ribosome; and, of course, bacteria respond to these antibiotics by producing proteins such as ribosomal protective proteins (RPPs) and increasing the expression of efflux pumps. For example, tetracycline-resistant Escherichia coli increases the expression of OmpC, FimD, Tsx, and OmpW proteins while decreasing the expression of LamB protein, resulting in antibiotic resistance and increased bacterial viability in the infected cell [45]. Antibiotics also inhibit DNA synthesis; for example, *E. coli* resistant to nalidixic acid increases the production of OmpC, OmpT, OmpW, and TolC proteins while decreasing the output of FadL protein, resulting in bacterial resistance to this antibiotic. Increased expression of the efflux pump AcAB/TolC in *Salmonella Typhimurium* induces bacterial resistance to fluoroquinolones and chronic and persistent infection [46, 47].

Proteomic Analysis of Bacterial Toxins

To survive, bacteria create a variety of molecules, including harmful ones known as toxins. These are poisonous, immunogenic, and deadly hydrophilic molecules that are mostly proteins and influence cells by several processes. They first enter the target cell by attaching to the membrane receptor, then penetrate the cell, enter the cell, and finally destroy it [48]. Poisons or toxins are classified according to where they act; enterotoxins, which affect the digestive system, include enterotoxin B in *Staphylococcus aureus*, neurotoxins, which affect the nervous system, including *Clostridium botulinum* neurotoxin, and leukocidins, which affect leukocytes. They gave permission. Cytotoxin, which affects host cells and is found in bacteria such as Helicobacter pylori, and hemolysin, which affects red blood cells and is found in bacteria such as *S. aureus* in various forms such as alpha, beta, and gamma hemolysins. It causes harm to the host cell enhances the life of bacteria in the target cell and raises its pathogenicity [49].

The majority of the toxins are proteins with two active enzymes and binding portions, known as AB toxins. For example, *Clostridium botulinum* produces a protein toxin with enzymatic activity called neurotoxin, which causes botulism in the host, and is classified into seven serotypes A-G, the differences between which have been revealed by proteomic studies, which have provided comprehensive information about these microorganisms [50, 51]. Furthermore, the toxin discovered in *Bacillus anthracis*, the source of anthrax, is a protein toxin composed of three non-toxic protein components. Protective Antigen (PA), Edoema Factor (EF), and Lethal Factor (LF) interact to generate a poisonous molecule that eventually causes anthrax or anthrax in the patient. Another example is the *Clostridium tetani*, which secretes tetanospasmin, a hazardous toxic protein that blocks neurotransmitter activity and produces tetanus in the host. Different proteins from these bacteria work as efficient molecules in vaccine development in the treatment of this disease. The most effective method of preventing tetanus is to utilize a vaccine manufactured from the bacterium's neurotoxic, which enhances the body's immunity against infections [52, 53].

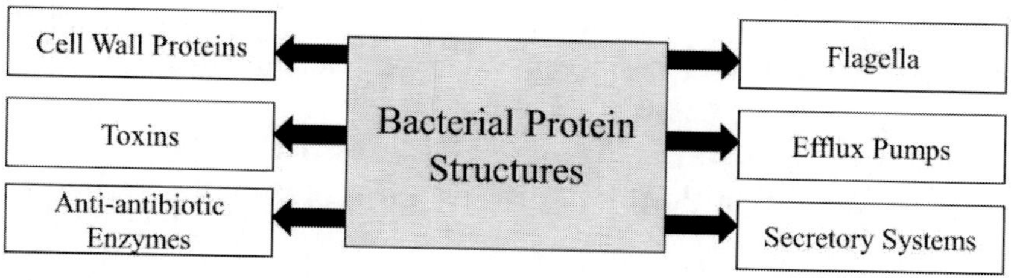

Figure 1. Bacterial protein structures.

Prebiotic, Probiotic, Synbiotic, Postbiotic, Hyperpostbiotic

Because changes in intestinal microbiota induce a variety of clinical disorders, the composition of intestinal microflora is crucial in human health. Probiotics are living bacteria that are helpful to host microbes when taken in adequate quantities [47]. Prebiotics feed probiotics while also providing health and physiological advantages to the host. Synbiotics are next-generation probiotics created from several probiotic and prebiotic formulations that work together to re-establish a healthy gut ecology [7, 54]. Postbiotics are soluble compounds or metabolic byproducts produced by probiotics or released after their lysis that enhance the host's health. Postbiotics are less dangerous than probiotics since they have no major negative effects [55]. Nutribiotics are probiotics that perform nutritional tasks such as the production of important nutrients such as vitamins and minerals and the conversion of precursors into bioactive metabolites. Pharmabiotics are probiotics that have been shown to have a pharmacological impact on health or illness [56, 57].

Antimicrobial medications that boost their efficacy when administered in combination, a phenomenon known as synergism, have long been sought by the medical and pharmaceutical worlds. Synergy in the use of other substances, such as the simultaneous use of plant extracts and medications, grew as a result of the simultaneous use of pharmaceuticals to boost their efficacy. With the introduction of probiotics, the synergistic use of antimicrobial compounds went even further, leading to the simultaneous use of postbiotics obtained from several probiotics [58, 59]. Because each postbiotic produced from a given probiotic has various effects, using postbiotics derived from several probiotics at the same time might reinforce these positive and diverse benefits of postbiotics, particularly in the area of antimicrobials and resistance prevention. enhance antibiotic; As a result, for the first time, we introduce the new name hyperpostbiotic for these molecules, which is a collection of postbiotics derived from two or more distinct probiotics that have several positive effects when combined [60].

Proteomic Analysis of Postbiotics Derived from Probiotics

Nutrients are one of the primary demands of human existence, and their ingestion promotes development and health. The gastrointestinal tract microbiota contains vital bacteria that, in addition to benefiting the body's health, are known as probiotics [54]. Postbiotics are metabolic byproducts produced by these bacteria. To be effective, probiotics must endure the rigorous conditions of production, storage, transport, preparation, and digestion. Postbiotics, on the other hand, have effectively surmounted these unfavorable circumstances and may be a viable alternative to probiotics [61]. Because of their unique chemical structure, safe qualities, extended shelf life, and many signaling molecules, postbiotics have anti-diabetic, anti-inflammatory, immunomodulating, anti-hypertensive, anti-aging, and reducing aberrant cell proliferation capabilities. Among its other good effects are the reduction of digestive and urinary issues, the reduction of heart illnesses, the strengthening of mental health, the maintenance of skin health, and the increase of antioxidant activity [12]. As a result, the research confirms that postbiotics can imitate the basic and clinical role of probiotics, and because of their unique characteristics, they can be used in the health system as pharmaceuticals and health preservers, and they have fewer risks and are safer to use than probiotics because they lack live bacteria [51].

Enzymatic Postbiotics

Enzymes are now utilized in a variety of applications, including food, the paper industry for bleaching paper pulp, agriculture, and the leather industry, and they are being employed in new industries, including medicinal applications, due to their low cost [62, 63]. Probiotics may create several enzymes that can be involved in a variety of biological processes, such as peptidases, lipases, amylases, proteases, ureases, phenol oxidases, and so on, and some of these enzymes are known as antioxidant proteins. Lactic acid bacteria can scavenge free radicals using antioxidant enzyme systems such as catalase (CAT), glutathione peroxidase (GPx), NADH oxidase, and superoxide dismutase (SOD), which convert free radicals into O_2 and hydrogen peroxide (H_2O_2) [64].

Superoxide dismutase activity has been demonstrated in postbiotics produced from *Lactococcus* and *Streptococcus thermophilus* strains as an antioxidant enzyme that aids in the prevention of free radical buildup in the host. *Lactobacillus casei* can produce catalase or superoxide dismutase, which causes an initial improvement in weight loss in Crohn's disease patients caused by trinitrobenzene sulfonic acid, and it also improves enzyme activities and reduces intestinal inflammation, according to a study. Furthermore, certain lactic acid bacteria, including *Bifidobacterium adolescentis*, *Bifidobacterium longum*, *Bifidobacterium infantis*, and *Bifidobacterium breve*, can breakdown hydrogen peroxide by releasing NADH peroxidase [65].

Bacteriocins

Bacteriocins are extracellular antimicrobial peptides that are synthesized as primary metabolites in ribosomes by phylogenetically different bacteria and archaea and are major factors in gut microbiota diversification [66, 67]. Probiotics may create a variety of bacteriocins, which block infections and the harm they cause and have gained popularity as natural biopreservatives because of their widespread usage in food processing and fermentation.

Bacteriocins are tiny cationic peptides of 30 to 60 amino acids generated by lactic acid bacteria that promote the leaking of important intracellular contents by forming holes in the cytoplasmic membranes [68]. Bacteriocins released by probiotics can combat antibiotic-resistant bacteria such as *Mycobacterium* TB and *Listeria monocytogenes* infections, in addition to their potential uses in food preservation. Furthermore, bacteriocins contribute to probiotics' anti-inflammatory properties. Plantaricin EF (PlnEFI), a class II bacteriocin generated by *Lactobacillus plantarum*, has demonstrated strong anti-inflammatory efficacy against TNBS-induced inflammatory bowel illness [69, 70].

The bacteria *Lactobacillus plantarum* reduces weight gain and inflammation in the liver and adipose tissue in diet-induced obese individuals. In the absence of apparent changes in gut microbiota, *Lactobacillus plantarum* bacteriocin plantaricin displays considerable effectiveness as a probiotic agent in lowering body weight and food consumption. Furthermore, following exposure to *Lactobacillus plantarum*, plasminogen activator inhibitor-1 (PAI-1) was dramatically decreased, which is implicated in the development of type 2 diabetes and obesity. These data suggest that PlnEF peptides can prevent cytokine-induced disruptions in epithelial barrier integrity, demonstrating that plantarisin has a direct modulatory action on intestinal epithelial cells [71].

Enveloping and Extracellular Components

Bacterial cell walls are made up of substances termed lipopolysaccharide in Gram-negatives and peptidoglycan in Gram-positive and Gram-negatives, which are continually secreted throughout bacterial cell development and death. Peptidoglycan is a stiff complex structure composed of sugar and amino acids that makes up 30 to 70% of the cell wall of gram-positive bacteria. It is composed of teichoic acids, polysaccharides, and proteins [25]. Teichoic acids are negatively charged molecules found solely in gram-positive bacteria. They are classified as wall teichoic acid and membrane lipo teichoic acid based on their attachment to peptidoglycan and cell membrane, respectively. Bacterial cell wall components have a role in both host signaling and adhesion. These are effective macromolecules involved in immune system activation and the production of numerous cytokines such as IL-1, IL-6, IL-8, IL-12, TNF, and IFN, the excessive release of which can result in pathophysiological responses such as septic shock, multiple organ failure, and so on [72]. Two peptidoglycan hydrolases from *Lactobacillus rhamnosus* bacteria, p75, and p40, are known to protect gut lining integrity and prevent programmed cell death. Lipoteichoic acid from bifidobacteria inhibits hepatocyte proliferation by reducing the regulatory activity of CD 25+ regulatory T lymphocytes and improving cellular immunity. It demonstrates anti-cancer effects [73, 74].

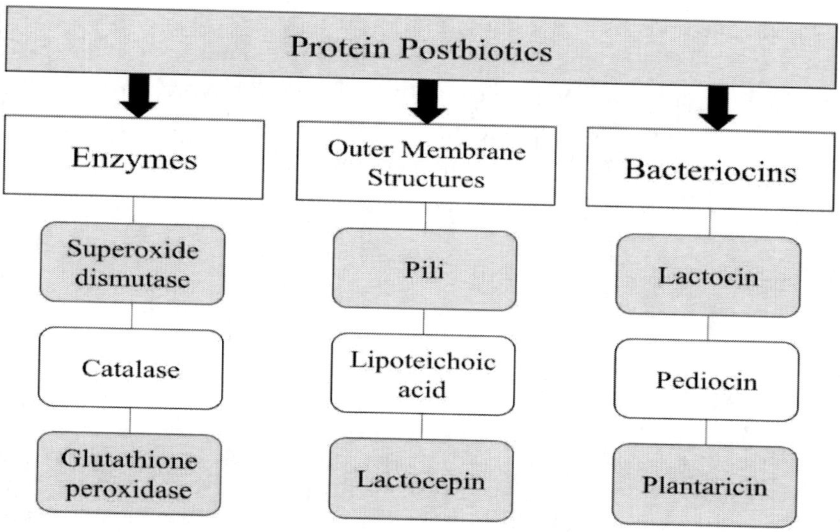

Figure 2. Proteinous postbiotics produced by lactic acid bacteria.

Pili is a structure made up of pilin proteins, which are long extracellular extensions on the cell surface that help in cell attachment to the intestinal wall and bacterial accumulation. These structures can also be used by bacteria to share genetic material during conjugation. This structure functions as a post-biotic and has a variety of uses, including the control of pro-inflammatory cytokines in baby immune system development. Lactospins are a kind of cell envelope proteinase that is mostly expressed by lactococci and lactobacilli. Lactococcal and lactobacilli lactospins are encoded by prtP, prtB, and prtH genes, which differ depending on the species or strain [75, 76]. Lactospins encoded by PrtP are well recognized for their caseinolytic characteristics, and they play a significant role in the dairy industry. Based on their caseinolytic substrate capabilities, PrtP-encoded lactospins are classified as PI or PIII-type proteinases. These proteins play a variety of activities, the most significant of which is anti-inflammatory activity in chronic inflammatory disorders [77, 78].

Conclusion

The science of proteomics is important in understanding more and more different microorganisms and their harmful and beneficial effects, which can be better understood by understanding the mechanisms of pathogen disease as well as the methods by which probiotics exert their beneficial effects on the host body. This strategy fought pathogenic microbes and increased the use of beneficial microbes for therapeutic purposes, but more comprehensive studies are needed in the future to identify the proteomic content of different microorganisms and clarify more aspects of this issue.

Disclaimer

None.

References

[1] Ozma MA, Khodadadi E, Rezaee MA, Kamounah FS, Asgharzadeh M, Ganbarov K, Aghazadeh M, Yousefi M, Pirzadeh T, Kafil HS. Induction of proteome changes involved in biofilm formation of Enterococcus faecalis in response to gentamicin. *Microbial Pathogenesis.* 2021;157:105003.

[2] Ozma MA, Khodadadi E, Rezaee MA, Asgharzadeh M, Aghazadeh M, Zeinalzadeh E, Ganbarov K, Kafil HS. Bacterial Proteomics and its Application in Pathogenesis Studies. *Current Pharmaceutical Biotechnology.* 2022;23(10):1245-56.

[3] Abbasi A, Sabahi S, Bazzaz S, Tajani AG, Lahouty M, Aslani R, Hosseini H. An edible coating utilizing Malva sylvestris seed polysaccharide mucilage and postbiotic from Saccharomyces cerevisiae var. boulardii for the preservation of lamb meat. *International Journal of Biological Macromolecules.* 2023;246:125660.

[4] Kustatscher G, Collins T, Gingras A-C, Guo T, Hermjakob H, Ideker T, Lilley KS, Lundberg E, Marcotte EM, Ralser M. Understudied proteins: opportunities and challenges for functional proteomics. *Nature Methods.* 2022;19(7):774-9.

[5] Bian Y, Gao C, Kuster B. On the potential of micro-flow LC-MS/MS in proteomics. *Expert Review of Proteomics.* 2022;19(3):153-64.

[6] Green ER, Mecsas J. Bacterial secretion systems: an overview. *Virulence mechanisms of bacterial pathogens.* 2016:213-39.

[7] Abbasi A, Bazzaz S, Da Cruz AG, Khorshidian N, Saadat YR, Sabahi S, Ozma MA, Lahouty M, Aslani R, Mortazavian AM. A Critical Review on Akkermansia muciniphila: Functional Mechanisms, Technological Challenges, and Safety Issues. *Probiotics and Antimicrobial Proteins.* 2023:1-23.

[8] Weaver D, Amin D, King G. The conformations and basal conformational dynamics of translocation factor SecDF vary with translocon SecYEG interaction. *Journal of Biological Chemistry.* 2022;298(10).

[9] Hosseini H, Abbasi A, Sabahi S, Akrami S, Yousefi-Avarvand A. Assessing the Potential Biological Activities of Postbiotics Derived from Saccharomyces cerevisiae: An In Vitro Study. *Probiotics and Antimicrobial Proteins.* 2023:1-17.

[10] Qin S, Xiao W, Zhou C, Pu Q, Deng X, Lan L, Liang H, Song X, Wu M. Pseudomonas aeruginosa: Pathogenesis, virulence factors, antibiotic resistance, interaction with host, technology advances and emerging therapeutics. *Signal transduction and targeted therapy.* 2022;7(1):199.

[11] Abby SS, Denise R, Rocha EP. Identification of protein secretion systems in bacterial genomes using MacSyFinder version 2. *BioRxiv.* 2023:2023.01. 06.522999.

[12] Abbasi A, Bazzaz S, A. Ibrahim S, Hekmatdoost A, Hosseini H, Sabahi S, Sheykhsaran E, Rahbar Saadat Y, Asghari Ozma M, Lahouty M. A Critical Review on the Gluten-Induced Enteropathy/Celiac Disease: Gluten-Targeted Dietary and Non-Dietary Therapeutic Approaches. *Food Reviews International.* 2023:1-41.

[13] Gehrer CM, Mitterstiller A-M, Grubwieser P, Meyron-Holtz EG, Weiss G, Nairz M. Advances in ferritin physiology and possible implications in bacterial infection. *International Journal of Molecular Sciences.* 2023;24(5):4659.

[14] Naskar S, Hohl M, Tassinari M, Low HH. The structure and mechanism of the bacterial type II secretion system. *Molecular Microbiology.* 2021;115(3):412-24.

[15] Barret M, Egan F, O'Gara F. Distribution and diversity of bacterial secretion systems across metagenomic datasets. *Environmental microbiology reports.* 2013;5(1):117-26.

[16] Daveri A, Benigno V, van der Meer JR. Characterization of an atypical but widespread type IV secretion system for transfer of the integrative and conjugative element (ICE clc) in Pseudomonas putida. *Nucleic Acids Research.* 2023;51(5):2345-62.

[17] Fan E, Chauhan N, Udatha DG, Leo JC, Linke D. Type V secretion systems in bacteria. *Virulence Mechanisms of Bacterial Pathogens.* 2016:305-35.

[18] Abbasi A, Rad AH, Maleki LA, Kafil HS, Baghbanzadeh A. Antigenotoxicity and Cytotoxic Potentials of Cell-Free Supernatants Derived from Saccharomyces cerevisiae var. boulardii on HT-29 Human Colon Cancer Cell Lines. *Probiotics and Antimicrobial Proteins.* 2023:1-13.

[19] Trunk T. Characterization and comparative analyses of type Vd-secreted phospholipases expressed in pathogenic bacteria. 2020.

[20] Ho BT, Dong TG, Mekalanos JJ. A view to a kill: the bacterial type VI secretion system. *Cell host & microbe.* 2014;15(1):9-21.

[21] Sabahi S, Mortazavi SA, Nassiri M, Ghazvini K, Shahidi F, Abbasi A. Production of functional ice cream fortified by immunoglobulin Y against Escherichia coli O157: H7 and Helicobacter pylori. *Biointerface Research in Applied Chemistry.* 2022;13(2):188-98.

[22] Ozma MA, Lahouty M, Abbasi A, Rezaee MA, Kafil HS, Asgharzadeh M. Effective Bacterial Factors Involved in the Dissemination of Tuberculosis. 2022.

[23] Nicholson KR, Champion PA. Bacterial secretion systems: networks of pathogenic regulation and adaptation in mycobacteria and beyond. *PLoS Pathogens.* 2022;18(7):e1010610.

[24] Beckham KS, Ciccarelli L, Bunduc CM, Mertens HD, Ummels R, Lugmayr W, Mayr J, Rettel M, Savitski MM, Svergun DI. Structure of the mycobacterial ESX-5 type VII secretion system membrane complex by single-particle analysis. *Nature microbiology.* 2017;2(6):1-7.

[25] Hummels KR, Berry SP, Li Z, Taguchi A, Min JK, Walker S, Marks DS, Bernhardt TG. Coordination of bacterial cell wall and outer membrane biosynthesis. *Nature.* 2023;615(7951):300-4.

[26] Abbasi A, Aghebati-Maleki L, Homayouni-Rad A. The promising biological role of postbiotics derived from probiotic Lactobacillus species in reproductive health. *Critical Reviews in Food Science and Nutrition.* 2022;62(32):8829-41.

[27] Oldewurtel ER, Kitahara Y, Cordier B, Wheeler R, Özbaykal G, Brambilla E, Boneca IG, Renner, LD, van Teeffelen S. Cell envelope growth of Gram-negative bacteria proceeds independently of cell wall synthesis. *The EMBO Journal.* 2023:e112168.

[28] Abbasi A, Saadat TR, Saadat YR. Microbial exopolysaccharides–β-glucans–as promising postbiotic candidates in vaccine adjuvants. *International Journal of Biological Macromolecules.* 2022.

[29] Chandra H, Kovall RA, Yadav JS, Sun X. Host Immune Responses to Surface S-Layer Proteins (SLPs) of Clostridioides difficile. *Microorganisms.* 2023;11(2):380.

[30] Sheykhsaran E, Abbasi A, Baghi HB, Ghotaslou R, Sharifi Y, Sefidan FY, Laghousi D, Hosainzadegan H, Hasani A, Sadeghi J. Staphylococcus aureus: A bacterial candidate for multiple sclerosis incidence and progression. *Reviews and Research in Medical Microbiology.* 2022;33(4):212-20.

[31] Lynch MJ, Miller M, James M, Zhang S, Zhang K, Li C, Charon NW, Crane BR. Structure and chemistry of lysinoalanine crosslinking in the spirochaete flagella hook. *Nature chemical biology.* 2019;15(10):959-65.

[32] You Y, Ye F, Mao W, Yang H, Lai J, Deng S. An overview of the structure and function of the flagellar hook FlgE protein. *World Journal of Microbiology and Biotechnology.* 2023;39(5):126.

[33] Sinai L, Rosenberg A, Smith Y, Segev E, Ben-Yehuda S. The molecular timeline of a reviving bacterial spore. *Molecular cell.* 2015;57(4):695-707.

[34] Clair G, Esbelin J, Malléa S, Bornard I, Carlin F. The spore coat is essential for Bacillus subtilis spore resistance to pulsed light, and pulsed light treatment eliminates some spore coat proteins. *International journal of food microbiology.* 2020;323:108592.

[35] Combo S, Mendes S, Nielsen KM, da Silva GJ, Domingues S. The Discovery of the Role of Outer Membrane Vesicles against Bacteria. *Biomedicines.* 2022;10(10):2399.

[36] Sabahi S, Abbasi A, Mortazavi SA. Characterization of cinnamon essential oil and its application in Malva sylvestris seed mucilage edible coating to the enhancement of the microbiological, physicochemical and sensory properties of lamb meat during storage. *Journal of Applied Microbiology.* 2022;133(2):488-502.

[37] Abbasi A, Rad AH, Ghasempour Z, Sabahi S, Kafil HS, Hasannezhad P, Rahbar Saadat Y, Shahbazi N. The biological activities of postbiotics in gastrointestinal disorders. *Critical Reviews in Food Science and Nutrition.* 2022;62(22):5983-6004.

[38] Vestby LK, Grønseth T, Simm R, Nesse LL. Bacterial biofilm and its role in the pathogenesis of disease. *Antibiotics.* 2020;9(2):59.

[39] Hershey DM. Integrated control of surface adaptation by the bacterial flagellum. *Current opinion in microbiology.* 2021;61:1-7.

[40] Huang Z, Wang Y-H, Zhu H-Z, Andrianova EP, Jiang C-Y, Li D, Ma L, Feng J, Liu ZP, Xiang H. Cross talk between chemosensory pathways that modulate chemotaxis and biofilm formation. *MBio.* 2019;10(1):10.1128/mbio. 02876-18.

[41] Ozma MA, Abbasi A, Asgharzadeh M, Pagliano P, Guarino A, Köse Ş, Kafil HS. Antibiotic therapy for pan-drug-resistant infections. *Le infezioni in medicina.* 2022;30(4):525.

[42] Noval M, Banoub M, Claeys KC, Heil E. The battle is on: new beta-lactams for the treatment of multidrug-resistant Gram-negative organisms. *Current Infectious Disease Reports.* 2020;22:1-9.

[43] Abbasi A, Hajipour N, Hasannezhad P, Baghbanzadeh A, Aghebati-Maleki L. Potential in vivo delivery routes of postbiotics. *Critical Reviews in Food Science and Nutrition.* 2022;62(12):3345-69.

[44] Lozano C, Fernández-Fernández R, Ruiz-Ripa L, Gómez P, Zarazaga M, Torres C. Human mecC-carrying MRSA: Clinical implications and risk factors. *Microorganisms.* 2020;8(10):1615.

[45] Young JW, Zhao Z, Wason IS, Duong van Hoa F. A dual detergent strategy to capture a bacterial outer membrane proteome in peptidiscs for characterization by mass spectrometry and binding assays. *Journal of Proteome Research.* 2022;22(5):1537-45.

[46] Rodrigues IC, Rodrigues SC, Duarte FV, Costa PMd, Costa PMd. The role of outer membrane proteins in UPEC antimicrobial resistance: A systematic review. *Membranes.* 2022;12(10):981.

[47] Sabahi S, Homayouni Rad A, Aghebati-Maleki L, Sangtarash N, Ozma MA, Karimi A, Hosseini H, Abbasi A. Postbiotics as the new frontier in food and pharmaceutical research. *Critical Reviews in Food Science and Nutrition.* 2022:1-28.

[48] Jurėnas D, Fraikin N, Goormaghtigh F, Van Melderen L. Biology and evolution of bacterial toxin–antitoxin systems. *Nature Reviews Microbiology.* 2022;20(6):335-50.

[49] Popoff MR, Brüggemann H. Regulatory Networks Controlling Neurotoxin Synthesis in Clostridium botulinum and Clostridium tetani. *Toxins.* 2022;14(6):364.

[50] Hamad G, Hafez EE, Sobhy SE, Mehany T, Elfayoumy RA, Elghazaly EM, Eskander M, Tawfik, RG, Hussein SM, Pereira L. Detection of Clostridium botulinum in some Egyptian fish products, its control in vitro using Citrus leaves extracts, and applicability of Citrus limon leaf extract in Tuna. *Foods.* 2023;12(7):1466.

[51] Ozma MA, Abbasi A, Sabahi S. Characterization of postbiotics derived from Lactobacillus paracasei ATCC 55544 and its application in Malva sylvestris seed

mucilage edible coating to the improvement of the microbiological, and sensory properties of lamb meat during storage. *Biointerface Res Appl Chem.* 2022;13.

[52] Yang NJ, Isensee J, Neel DV, Quadros AU, Zhang H-XB, Lauzadis J, Liu SM, Shiers S, Belu A, Palan S. Anthrax toxins regulate pain signaling and can deliver molecular cargoes into ANTXR2+ DRG sensory neurons. *Nature neuroscience.* 2022;25(2):168-79.

[53] Abbasi A, Rad AH, Maleki LA, Kafil HS, Baghbanzadeh A. Cytotoxic Potentials of Cell-Free Supernatant Derived from Lactobacillus casei CRL431 on HCT-116 and HT-29 Human Colon Cancer Cell Lines. 2022.

[54] Ozma MA, Abbasi A, Akrami S, Lahouty M, Shahbazi N, Ganbarov K, Pagliano P, Sabahi S, Köse Ş, Yousefi M. Postbiotics as the key mediators of the gut microbiota-host interactions. *Le infezioni in medicina.* 2022;30(2):180.

[55] Ozma MA, Abbasi A, Ahangarzadeh Rezaee M, Hosseini H, Hosseinzadeh N, Sabahi S, Noori SMA, Sepordeh S, Khodadadi E, Lahouty M. A critical review on the nutritional and medicinal profiles of garlic's (Allium sativum L.) bioactive compounds. Food Reviews International. 2022:1-38.

[56] Abbasi A, Kafil HS, Ozma MA, Sangtarash N, Sabahi S. Can food matrices be considered as a potential carrier for COVID-19? *Le infezioni in medicina.* 2022;30(1):59.

[57] Homayouni-rad A, Aghebati-Maleki L, Samadi-Kafil H, Abbasi A, Khani N. Postbiotics as a safe alternative to live probiotic bacteria in the food and pharmaceutical industries. *HBI_Journals.* 2021;26:132-57.

[58] Ghotaslou R, Nabizadeh E, Memar MY, Law WMH, Ozma MA, Abdi M, Yekani M, Kadkhoda H, Bafadam S, Ghotaslou A. The metabolic, protective, and immune functions of Akkermansia muciniphila. *Microbiological Research.* 2022:127245.

[59] Rad AH, Aghebati-Maleki L, Kafil HS, Abbasi A. Molecular mechanisms of postbiotics in colorectal cancer prevention and treatment. *Critical reviews in food science and nutrition.* 2021;61(11):1787-803.

[60] Ozma MA, Moaddab SR, Hosseini H, Khodadadi E, Ghotaslou R, Asgharzadeh M, Abbasi, A, Kamounah FS, Aghebati Maleki L, Ganbarov K. A critical review of novel antibiotic resistance prevention approaches with a focus on postbiotics. *Critical Reviews in Food Science and Nutrition.* 2023:1-19.

[61] Mirzaei R, Kavyani B, Nabizadeh E, Kadkhoda H, Ozma MA, Abdi M. Microbiota metabolites in the female reproductive system: Focused on the short-chain fatty acids. *Heliyon.* 2023.

[62] Homayouni Rad A, Aghebati Maleki L, Samadi Kafil H, Abbasi A. Postbiotics: A novel strategy in food allergy treatment. *Critical reviews in food science and nutrition.* 2021;61(3):492-9.

[63] Abbasi A, Sheykhsaran E, Kafil HS. *Postbiotics: science, technology and applications:* Bentham Science Publishers; 2021.

[64] Kleniewska P, Hoffmann A, Pniewska E, Pawliczak R. The influence of probiotic Lactobacillus casei in combination with prebiotic inulin on the antioxidant capacity of human plasma. *Oxidative medicine and cellular longevity.* 2016;2016.

[65] Muñoz MdCC, Benomar N, Ennahar S, Horvatovich P, Lerma LL, Knapp CW, Gálvez A, Abriouel H. Comparative proteomic analysis of a potentially probiotic

Lactobacillus pentosus MP-10 for the identification of key proteins involved in antibiotic resistance and biocide tolerance. *International Journal of Food Microbiology.* 2016;222:8-15.
[66] Chikindas ML, Weeks R, Drider D, Chistyakov VA, Dicks LM. Functions and emerging applications of bacteriocins. *Current opinion in biotechnology.* 2018;49:23-8.
[67] Abbasi A, Sanej KD, Mohammadi A, Moradi S, Nayeri BD, Bazzaz S, Hosseini H. The Role of Postbiotics in Food Safety Promotion.
[68] Cotter PD, Ross RP, Hill C. Bacteriocins—a viable alternative to antibiotics? *Nature Reviews Microbiology.* 2013;11(2):95-105.
[69] Huang X, He Y, Zhong C, Zhao K, Shah NP, Tao X, Wei H. Screening of probiotic strains of Lactiplantibacillus plantarum from Hu sheep and its ability to inhibit Listeria monocytogenes in pasteurized milk. *LWT.* 2023;182:114883.
[70] Abbasi A, Aghebati-Maleki A, Yousefi M, Aghebati-Maleki L. Probiotic intervention as a potential therapeutic for managing gestational disorders and improving pregnancy outcomes. *Journal of reproductive immunology.* 2021;143:103244.
[71] Barouei J, Martinic A, Bendiks Z, Mishchuk D, Heeney D, Slupsky CM, Marco ML. Type 2–resistant starch and Lactiplantibacillus plantarum NCIMB 8826 result in additive and interactive effects in diet-induced obese mice. *Nutrition Research.* 2023;118:12-28.
[72] Turner S, Raisley B, Roach K, Bajaña S, Munroe ME, James JA, Coggeshall KM, Kovats S. Gram-Positive Bacteria Cell Wall Peptidoglycan Polymers Activate Human Dendritic Cells to Produce IL-23 and IL-1β and Promote TH17 Cell Differentiation. *Microorganisms.* 2023;11(1):173.
[73] Liu H, Komai-Koma M, Xu D, Liew FY. Toll-like receptor 2 signaling modulates the functions of CD4+ CD25+ regulatory T cells. *Proceedings of the National Academy of Sciences.* 2006;103(18):7048-53.
[74] Rad AH, Maleki LA, Kafil HS, Zavoshti HF, Abbasi A. Postbiotics as promising tools for cancer adjuvant therapy. *Advanced Pharmaceutical Bulletin.* 2021;11(1):1.
[75] Strahinic I, Kojic M, Tolinacki M, Fira D, Topisirovic L. The presence of prtP proteinase gene in natural isolate Lactobacillus plantarum BGSJ3–18. *Letters in applied microbiology.* 2010;50(1):43-9.
[76] Rad AH, Abbasi A, Kafil HS, Ganbarov K. Potential pharmaceutical and food applications of postbiotics: a review. *Current pharmaceutical biotechnology.* 2020;21(15):1576-87.
[77] Ji D, Ma J, Xu M, Agyei D. Cell-envelope proteinases from lactic acid bacteria: biochemical features and biotechnological applications. *Comprehensive Reviews in Food Science and Food Safety.* 2021;20(1):369-400.
[78] Rad AH, Maleki LA, Kafil HS, Zavoshti HF, Abbasi A. Postbiotics as novel health-promoting ingredients in functional foods. *Health promotion perspectives.* 2020;10(1):3-4.

Chapter 9

Postbiotics and Colorectal Cancer Treatment

Shirin Farsad[1,*], PhD,
and Alireza Rasouli[2], MSc
[1]Department of Microbiology, Faculty of Basic Sciences, Qom Branch, Islamic Azad University, Qom, Iran
[2]Microbial biotechnology, Developer of biological diagnostic systems, Qom, Iran

Abstract

Colorectal cancer is one of the most common and deadly cancers in the world. The microbiome of the digestive tract maintains the homeostasis of the body and in the case of dysbiosis, it leads to the development of colorectal cancer various factors cause this cancer and with the researchers then concluded that postbiotics Which are the metabolites from probiotics and are used indifferent mechanisms to treat many diseases, as well as improve the symptoms of colorectal cancer. Common methods of colorectal cancer treatment include surgery, radiotherapy and chemotherapy but due to side effects, it is better to use biological methods, based on this, the use of prebiotics, probiotics, postbiotics and fecal microbiome transplantation leads to the regulation of the hosts immune system, it becomes possible to change the type and amount of gut microbiota and change the activity of pathogens.

Introduction

Colorectal cancer is a fatal disease and accounted for about 9.4% death in 2020 (Sung et al., 2021). Despite the advancement of technology, the incidence rate

* Corresponding Author's Email: shfarsadi1i@gmail.com.

In: Exploring Microbiotics in Health and Disease
Editor: Edward L. Stillman
ISBN: 978-8-89113-410-2

of colorectal cancer is increasing in developed countries. The reason for the prevalence of colorectal cancer includes: a) modulation created in the APC gene (adenoma polyps), b) Wnt-B catenin pathway activation and cancer proliferation. c) lack of DNA repair. The development of colorectal cancer depends on environmental, genetic factor, immunity, metabolic function, epigenetic factor and type of gut microbiome of the host (Fong, Li, and Yu 2020). gut microbiota includes bacteria, fungi, viruses and protists (Richard and Sokol 2019). Gut microbiota under normal conditions have a beneficial commensal relationship with humans, but in the case of dysbiosis, the number and type of germs change and with the predominance of pathogenic bacteria it leads to infection, disruption of biological barrier function, severe inflammations, stimulation and activation of cancer pathways. Generation and production of their harmful metabolites destroy the normal functions of the host (Illiano, Brambilla, and Parolini 2020). But by restoring and rebuilding the gut microbiota, we can get closer to the path of recovery and treatment of colorectal cancer.

Gut Microbiota

Gut microbiota under normal conditions has several roles such as the development of the body's mucosal immune system, effective in the metabolic process, maintaining the integrity of the intestinal barriers, but in the case of eubiosis to dysbiosis and changing the type and number of alternative bacteria such as *fusobacterium nucleatum*, *Helicobacter pylori*, *Bacteroides fragilis*, *Enterococcus faecalis* (Gagnière et al., 2016). Is one of the main causes of colorectal cancer.

Intestinal microbiota uses certain mechanisms to cause colorectal cancer:

1. production of harmful metabolites
2. production of toxin -producing factor,
3. change in the regulation of immune system function (Sun and Kato 2016).

These factors cause chronic inflammation, gradually carcinogenesis is formed and finally cancer progress.

Probiotics

Probiotics are microorganisms including fungi, bacteria, and yeasts and if they are consumed enough, they improve human health. Probiotics stop and treat colorectal cancer through three processes: a) inhibiting the establishment and colonization of pathogenic bacteria, b) regulation and adjustment of the immune system, c) strengthening the biological barrier and protecting the intestinal epithelium.

Prebiotics

Prebiotics are nutrient that cannot be digested by the human digestive system, and after being consumed by probiotics, they will be useful compounds for human health. These compounds are fructo-oligosaccharide, galacto-oligosaccharide, inulin and fructan, the main functions of prebiotics include:

a) Fermentation of compounds by intestinal microbiota
b) Activation of beneficial bacteria in the digestive system
c) Inhibiting the establishment and colonization of pathogens
d) Complete absorption of prebiotics by the intestine with anti-inflammatory activity (Fong, Li, and Yu 2020).

Antibiotics

It seems that antibiotics reduce the diversity and number of intestinal bacteria (Maier et al., 2017, Azcarate-Peril et al., 2017). But some antibiotics play an important role in strengthening the biological barrier of intestine. high consumption of red meat due to percentage of colorectal cancer and leads to the proliferation of cancer cells. another role of antibiotics is to inhibit the production of microbial sulfides and maintain the integrity of the intestinal barrier and prevent excessive proliferation of cancer cells (Ijssennagger et al., 2015).

FMT

Infection of fecal bacteria from healthy people to sick people causes:

a) Balance of intestinal microbiome,
b) control of IBD,
c) inhibition of establishment and colonization of antibiotic- resistant bacteria,
d) the recovery of colorectal cancer in mice is according to Rosshart's theory (Rosshart et al., 2017).

Postbiotics

Using the supernatant of probiotics in research work is safer than live bacteria. The anticancer function of postbiotics is characterized by two mechanisms:

a) Selective anticancer activity of probiotics through inhibition of cancer cells
b) Epithelial protective role and increased secretion of IgA (Fong, Li, and Yu 2020).

Metabolic compounds obtained from *Lactobacillus plantarum* postbiotics are characterized by cytotoxicity and anti-proliferative effects (Chuah et al., 2019, Tukenmez et al., 2019). lee, by examining Lactobacillus fermentum cell free supernatant, proved its therapeutic effect on colorectal cell lines. CFS increases the expression of Bak, Bax, Caspase 3 and induces apoptosis (Chuah et al., 2019). konishi pointed out the effect of free chrome in the supernatant of Lactobacillus casei ATCC334 and the inhibition of colon cancer cells in the way that c- junc terminal kinase is activated and as a result apoptosis is induced. Another useful function of postbiotics is the ability to inhibit intestinal inflammation and maintain the integrity and coherence of the intestinal biological barrier. Izuddin showed that the consumption of Lactobacillus plantarum RG14 postbiotic supplements strengthens intestinal epithelial cells and for sheep after the lactation period and reduces the number of inflammatory cytokines (Konishi et al., 2016).

Like IL-10 and as a result. the integrity of intestinal barrier is improved through strong bonds (Izuddin et al., 2019). In another Gao studied Lactobacillus rhamnosus GG HM0539 has a role of protecting the integrity of the intestinal barrier and increases the amount of mucin (Gao et al., 2019).

In Vitro Postbiotic Biological Activities

1. Inhibiting the proliferation of cancer cells:
   a) Maintain replication signals
   b) Escape from growth suppression
   c) The possibility of repletion of acceptance
   d) Inflammatory tumor
   e) The invasion and metastasis
   f) Induction or vascular access
   g) Opposition of cell death
   h) Genome inconsistency and mutation (Holanda, Yiannikouris, and Kim 2020, Hanahan and Weinberg 2011).

2. Induction of apoptosis of cancer cells:
   i) shriveling and shrinkage of cells
   j) creating membrane bubbles
   k) chromatin thickening and nuclear shrinkage
   l) chromatid condensation
   m) Formation of cytoplasmic vesicle.

Postbiotics of Gut Bacterium

1. Heat -killed bacteria cell:

Different methods such as using chemicals, heat, sonication and UV rays can be used to kill bacteria (Deshpande, Athalye-Jape, and Patole 2018, Taverniti and Guglielmetti 2011, Zorzela et al., 2017). The killed from of two important strains of probiotics such as Bifidobacterium bifidum and lactobacillus have beneficial functions (Chen et al., 2020, Sugahara et al., 2017, Maeda et al., 2009, Donato et al., 2010, Lin et al., 2008, Li et al., 2009, Ueno et al., 2011). The action of Lactobacillus rhamnosus GG in the gastrointestinal tract leads to the reduction of intestinal inflammation and the maintenance of immune system responses, and probably plays an important.

Role in the treatment of irritable bowel syndrome (Pahumunto and Teanpaisan 2023, Donato et al., 2010, Lin et al., 2008). According to Li et al., 's research on Lactobacillus rhamnosus GG killed by heat, it reduces pro-inflammatory mediators caused by LPS and as a result increases anti-inflammatory mediator (Li et al., 2009). According to the studies conducted by Ueno, the use of heat-*killed Lactobacillus* brevis SBC8803 for the treatment of colorectal cancer controls inflammation and maintains homeostasis (Ueno et al., 2011). Wang showed that Akremensia muciniphila bacteria strongly prevents the development of colorectal cancer (Wang et al., 2020). Kim reported that heat-killed bacteria such as Lactobacillus ruteri MG5346, Lactobacillus casei MG4584, and Bifidobacterium MG 731 delay the growth of colorectal cancer (Kim et al., 2022).

2. Cell free supernatant:

supernatant without living cells consist of secretory metabolites from microorganisms. To prepare cell- free supernatant (CFS), culture medium containing microorganisms is first incubated, then centrifuged, and finally undesirable structures are removed (Rad et al., 2021). these are metabolites have antioxidant properties, antitumor and antimicrobial (Pahumunto and Teanpaisan 2023, Kim et al., 2020, Lee et al., 2020). supernatant free cell of *Bifidobacterium* and *Lactobacillus* stop cancer progression (Escamilla, Lane, and Maitin 2012).

Lactobacillus rhamnosus GG and Lactobacillus casei prevent cancer cells from attacking surrounding tissues (Escamilla, Lane, and Maitin 2012). After the studies done on Lactobacillus fermentum CSF, it was confirmed that it induces apoptosis (Lee et al., 2020). by studying the role of probiotics in inhibiting colorectal cancer, pahumunto found out that these bacteria inhibit the expression of pro-inflammatory cytokines in the caco-2 cancer cell line. This cell line and finally colorectal cancer is inhibited (Pahumunto and Teanpaisan 2023).

Cell Component

According to the research done by Far, it was found that the teichoic acid of bacterial cell wall is connected to the cytoplasmic membrane by covalent bond (Kleerebezem et al., 2010, Weidenmaier and Peschel 2008). Lipoteichoic acid of Lactobacillus plantarum promotes the phosphorylation of p38 kinase epk enzymes, which are the induction and activation factors of NF-Ϗβ and leads to the reduction of IL-8 production and as result inhibits inflammation in pig digestive epithelial cell (Noh et al., 2015).

1. Exopolysaccharides:

Exopolysaccharides, which are a subgroup of polysaccharides, are secreted from the cell walls of microbes with the property of binding to surfaces (Xiao and Zheng 2016).

Exopolysaccharides of bacterial origin are the most important industrial biopolymers and are very important from an economic point of view (Freitas, Alves, and Reis 2011). the beneficial effects of EPS on human health including colorectal cancer have been confirmed (Oerlemans et al., 2021). EPS from a wide group of bacteria, such as various Lactobacillus, bifidobacterial, which are effective in maintaining intestinal homeostasis (Salazar et al., 2016).

For example, Lactobacillus acidophilus inhibits the growth of colorectal cancer cell line caco-2 and in the same it induces apoptosis by simulating cell cycle arrest in the G0/G1 phase (Di et al., 2018).

2. Short chain fatty acids (SCFAs):

SCFAs are saturated fatty acids have a maximum of 6 carbons in their molecular structure are induce butyric acid, acetic acid, caproic acid, propionic acid and valeric acid. SCFAs are the result of the fermentation process from indigestible saccharide substrates by anaerobic bacteria living in the human intestine (Kannan and Quine 2012).

The advantage of sufficient production of SCFAs leads to limitation of human pathogenesis such asthma, cancers, metabolic disease (Tan et al., 2014). the effective immunological applications of SCFAs for treatment of colorectal cancer were confirmed in the 1980s. according to the theory of whitehead et al., butyric acid from the proliferation of LIM1215 cancer cell (Whitehead, Young, and Bhathal 1986). *In vivo* model, the functional role of SCFAs needs more research and investigations, but their anti-inflammatory role in reducing and inhibiting the risk factors of colon cancer such as inflammatory bowel syndrome and colitis seems essential (Tian et al., 2018, Parada Venegas et al., 2019).

The anti-inflammatory role of SCFAs is necessary to reduce colon inflammation by reducing the production of pro-inflammatory cytokines such as TNF-α, IL-16, IL-17

In colorectal cancer (Tian et al., 2018, Hu et al., 2016). in another study, researchers found that the growth of colorectal cancer cell line HT-29 inhibited by butyrate and propionate fatty acids (Gamet et al., 1992). Gibson concluded that the simultaneous use of appropriate concentrations of probiotics and prebiotics led to the production of butyric acid in target tissue (colon), which is an indicator of the protective function of this fermented substance in colorectal cancer. SCFAs such as valerate and propionate inhibit the differentiation of colorectal cancer cells and ultimately stop the growth of cancer cells (McIntyre, Gibson, and Young 1993).

3. ENZYMES:

Enzymes are biological catalysts and increase the speed of chemical reactions in living cells. Among other things the enzymatic reactions carried out in the microbial niches of the human digestive system have important effects on the relationship between the microbe and host (Jia et al., 2022). Early studies on colorectal cancer showed that there is no direct relationship between Lactic acid producing bifidobacterial living in digestive tract and colorectal cancer (Kosumi et al., 2018). The studies in mice show the role of active enzymes in Bifidobacterium longum and lactobacillus acidophilus in mice with colorectal cancer leads to an increase in nitro reductase and beta glucuronidase enzyme activity and also administration of Lactococcus lactis producing catalase enzyme inhibits colorectal cancers (Goldin and Gorbach 1980, Reddy and Rivenson 1993, Nalini, Manju, and Menon 2004, de Moreno de Leblanc et al., 2008).

Other Postbiotics

Colorectal cancer progression depends on the transfer of bile acids and the type of intestinal microbial metabolism.

1. Bile acid:

Excessive bile acids lead to the production of Reactive oxygen species (ROS), destruction of colon epithelial cells and tumorigenesis (Barrasa et al., 2011, Booth, Gilmore, and Bilton 1997, Bernstein et al., 2011).

2. Indole metabolite:

Indole metabolites are able to bind with the aryl hydrocarbon receptor and lead to the stimulation of regulatory T cells in the direction of the advancement of differentiation and reduction of anti-inflammatory reactions (Chen et al., 2008, Mezrich et al., 2010), also reducing colitis has a protective role against colorectal cancer (Busbee et al., 2020, Shimada Y. and et al., 2013).

3. Kynurenine:

Kynurenine reduces the permeability of CD8+ Tcell and escape from tumor cells (Campesato et al., 2020).

4. Serotonin:

Some scientists like to point out the effect of serotonin on the reduction of intestinal inflammation and some on the increase of intestinal inflammation (Kannen et al., 2020).

5. Tryptophan:

The role of tryptophan in the differentiation of regulatory T cells and the improvement of intestinal barrier function (Scott, Fu, and Chang 2020).

In Vivo Biological Activities of Postbiotics

1. Regulation gut microbiota composition and abundance by postbiotics:

Terada et al., investigated the role of enterococcus faecalis EC-12 killed in heat and observed that the number of Enterobacteriaceae and clostridium perfringens decreases with the increase of Lactobacilli and bifidobacterial (Terada et al., 2004). Bacteriocin obtained from lactic acid bacteria, as well as the use of lacidophyllin restores beneficial intestinal bacteria (De Vuyst and Leroy 2007). lacidophyllin quickly causes diversity in the intestinal microbiota after diarrhea caused by antibiotic use in mice (Li et al., 2017, Yang et al., 2022).

Following the use of lacidophyllin the diversity of lactobacilli increases and Bacteroides, Pasteurella and Para Bacteroides strains and decrease As pathogens (Yang et al., 2022). Kimoto-nira et al., investigated the long -term use of Lactococcus lactis strain G50 on the intestinal microflora of mice and showed that this bacterial strain inhibits the growth of H2S producing bacteria (Kimoto-Nira et al., 2009). This gas- producing bacteria such as salmonella, Citrobacter and shigella are involved in colorectal cancer (Huycke and Gaskins 2004).

2. Regulation of commensal microorganism population living in the gut by postbiotics:

The intestinal mucosal barrier, the first strong line of defense against gastrointestinal pathogens (epithelial cells), is protected by the host's mucosal layers (Turner 2009, Hansson 2020). intestinal mucosal layers contain mucin glycoprotein compounds that secreted by goblet cells (Martens, Neumann, and Desai 2018). It is the binding site of beneficial symbiotic intestinal bacteria and it is also able to isolate pathogens from the Caco2 cell line (Pelaseyed et al., 2014), on the other hand, pathogenic bacteria by releasing their harmful enzymes, first destroy the mucosal barrier and then attack the damaged mucosal surfaces, leading to the colonization and infection of pathogens (McGuckin et al., 2011). Short chain fatty acids synthesize mucus in germ-free mice (Wrzosek et al., 2013, Johansson et al., 2015). Butyric acids have been Used to treat the colorectal cell line type Ls174T and it has increased mucin protein expression and increased the binding rate of Bifidobacterium and lactobacilli and finally inhibited pathogens such as a *E. coli* (Jung et al., 2015, He et al., 2017). probiotics are attached to epithelial cells by having fimbriae and lectin, and block the binding site of pathogenic bacteria and remove pathogens by competitive inhibition (Tytgat et al., 2016, Petrova et al., 2016).

3. Improving the immune system with postbiotics:

By inhibiting the competition of binding to the target site and expression of regulatory genes, postbiotics change in the direction of improving the function of the biological barrier of an intestine and thus eliminate pathogens. after salmonella infection, the consumption of lactobacillus paracasei supernatant has an anti-inflammatory role (Tsilingiri et al., 2012). anti-inflammatory reactions occur due to the secretion of proinflammatory cytokines (Dinarello 2000). Acetic acids also reduce intestinal inflammation and ultimately inhibit colorectal cancer (Jia, Xie, and Jia 2018).

4. Regulation of host-microbiota relationship by postbiotics:

The relationship between the gut microbiota and the host's immune system is effective on the host 'health, the gut microbiota regulates the host's inflammatory reactions, the secretion of cytokines and the differentiation of inflammatory cells are effective on the host's immune system (Schirmer et al., 2016, Parolini 2019). In the case of digestive dysbiosis and the presence of pathogenic bacteria such as Fusobacterium, Wnt pathway is stimulated and by Fada binding to E-Cadherin, β-catenin is activated and carcinogenesis is activated (Rubinstein et al., 2013). Bacteroides fragilis toxins are also attached to the epithelial cells of the digestive tract and by Wnt stimulation NF-κβ signaling pathway is stimulated and by intensifying proinflammatory reactions, DNA damage and colorectal tumorigenesis are caused (Goodwin et al., 2011, Wu et al., 2009).

Conclusion

In recent years, the functional role of postbiotics for the treatment of various disease has been discussed. among the biological treatment methods, the use of probiotic supplements, the FMT and administration of postbiotics are of special importance due to their greater safety and efficiency, although all the different mechanisms are not known and require further investigations.

References

Azcarate-Peril, M. A., Andrew J. Ritter, Dennis Savaiano, Andrea Monteagudo-Mera, Carlton Anderson, Scott T. Magness, and Todd R. Klaenhammer. 2017. "Impact of short-chain galactooligosaccharides on the gut microbiome of lactose-intolerant individuals." *Proceedings of the National Academy of Sciences* 114 (3):E367-E375.

Barrasa, J. I., Nieves Olmo, Pablo Pérez-Ramos, Angélica Santiago-Gómez, Emilio Lecona, Javier Turnay, and M. Antonia Lizarbe. 2011. "Deoxycholic and chenodeoxycholic bile acids induce apoptosis via oxidative stress in human colon adenocarcinoma cells." *Apoptosis* 16:1054-1067.

Bernstein, C., Hana Holubec, Achyut K. Bhattacharyya, Huy Nguyen, Claire M. Payne, Beryl Zaitlin, and Harris Bernstein. 2011. "Carcinogenicity of deoxycholate, a secondary bile acid." *Archives of toxicology* 85:863-871.

Booth, L. A., I. T. Gilmore, and R. F. Bilton. 1997. "Secondary bile acid induced DNA damage in HT29 cells: are free radicals involved?" *Free radical research* 26 (2):135-144.

Busbee, P. B., Lorenzo Menzel, Haider Rasheed Alrafas, Nicholas Dopkins, William Becker, Kathryn Miranda, Chaunbing Tang, Saurabh Chatterjee, Udai P. Singh, and Mitzi Nagarkatti. 2020. "Indole-3-carbinol prevents colitis and associated microbial dysbiosis in an IL-22–dependent manner." *JCI insight* 5 (1).

Campesato, L. F., Sadna Budhu, Jeremy Tchaicha, Chien-Huan Weng, Mathieu Gigoux, Ivan Jose Cohen, David Redmond, Levi Mangarin, Stephane Pourpe, and Cailian Liu. 2020. "Blockade of the AHR restricts a Treg-macrophage suppressive axis induced by L-Kynurenine." *Nature communications* 11 (1):4011.

Chen, W., Xueqing Liang, Amanda J. Peterson, David H. Munn, and Bruce R. Blazar. 2008. "The indoleamine 2, 3-dioxygenase pathway is essential for human plasmacytoid dendritic cell-induced adaptive T regulatory cell generation." *The Journal of Immunology* 181 (8):5396-5404.

Chen, Y. T., P. S. Hsieh, H. H. Ho, S. H. Hsieh, Y. W. Kuo, S. F. Yang, and C. W. Lin. 2020. "Antibacterial activity of viable and heat-killed probiotic strains against oral pathogens." *Letters in applied microbiology* 70 (4):310-317.

Chuah, L. O., Hooi Ling Foo, Teck Chwen Loh, Noorjahan Banu Mohammed Alitheen, Swee Keong Yeap, Nur Elina Abdul Mutalib, Raha Abdul Rahim, and Khatijah Yusoff. 2019. "Postbiotic metabolites produced by Lactobacillus plantarum strains exert selective cytotoxicity effects on cancer cells." *BMC complementary and alternative medicine* 19:1-12.

de Moreno de Leblanc, A., Jean Guy LeBlanc, Gabriela Perdigon, Anderson Miyoshi, Philippe Langella, Vasco Azevedo, and Fernando Sesma. 2008. "Oral administration of a catalase-producing Lactococcus lactis can prevent a chemically induced colon cancer in mice." *Journal of Medical Microbiology* 57 (1):100-105.

De Vuyst, L., and Frédéric Leroy. 2007. "Bacteriocins from lactic acid bacteria: production, purification, and food applications." *Microbial Physiology* 13 (4):194-199.

Deshpande, G., Gayatri Athalye-Jape, and Sanjay Patole. 2018. "Para-probiotics for preterm neonates - The next frontier." *Nutrients* 10 (7):871.

Di, W., Lanwei Zhang, Huaxi Yi, Xue Han, Yingchun Zhang, and Liang Xin. 2018. "Exopolysaccharides produced by Lactobacillus strains suppress HT-29 cell growth via induction of G0/G1 cell cycle arrest and apoptosis." *Oncology letters* 16 (3):3577-3586.

Dinarello, C. A. 2000. "Proinflammatory cytokines." *Chest* 118 (2):503-508.

Donato, K. A., Mélanie G. Gareau, Yu Jing Jenny Wang, and Philip M Sherman. 2010. "Lactobacillus rhamnosus GG attenuates interferon-γ and tumour necrosis factor-α-induced barrier dysfunction and pro-inflammatory signalling." *Microbiology* 156 (11):3288-3297.

Escamilla, J., Michelle A. Lane, and Vatsala Maitin. 2012. "Cell-free supernatants from probiotic Lactobacillus casei and Lactobacillus rhamnosus GG decrease colon cancer cell invasion *in vitro*." *Nutrition and cancer* 64 (6):871-878.

Fong, W., Qing Li, and Jun Yu. 2020. "Gut microbiota modulation: a novel strategy for prevention and treatment of colorectal cancer." *Oncogene* 39 (26):4925-4943.

Freitas, F., Vitor D. Alves, and Maria A. M. Reis. 2011. "Advances in bacterial exopolysaccharides: from production to biotechnological applications." *Trends in biotechnology* 29 (8):388-398.

Gagnière, J., Jennifer Raisch, Julie Veziant, Nicolas Barnich, Richard Bonnet, Emmanuel Buc, Marie-Agnès Bringer, Denis Pezet, and Mathilde Bonnet. 2016. "Gut microbiota imbalance and colorectal cancer." *World journal of gastroenterology* 22 (2):501.

Gamet, L., Danièle Daviaud, Colette Denis-Pouxviel, Christian Remesy, and Jean-Claude Murat. 1992. "Effects of short-chain fatty acids on growth and differentiation of the human colon-cancer cell line HT29." *International journal of cancer* 52 (2):286-289.

Gao, J., Yubin Li, Yu Wan, Tongtong Hu, Liting Liu, Shaojie Yang, Zelong Gong, Qing Zeng, Yi Wei, and Weijun Yang. 2019. "A novel postbiotic from Lactobacillus rhamnosus GG with a beneficial effect on intestinal barrier function." *Frontiers in microbiology* 10:477.

Goldin, B. R., and Sherwood L. Gorbach. 1980. "Effect of Lactobacillus acidophilus dietary supplements on 1, 2-dimethylhydrazine dihydrochloride-induced intestinal cancer in rats." *Journal of the National Cancer Institute* 64 (2):263-265.

Goodwin, A. C., Christina E. Destefano Shields, Shaoguang Wu, David L. Huso, Xin Qun Wu, Tracy R. Murray-Stewart, Amy Hacker-Prietz, Shervin Rabizadeh, Patrick M. Woster, and Cynthia L. Sears. 2011. "Polyamine catabolism contributes to enterotoxigenic Bacteroides fragilis-induced colon tumorigenesis." *Proceedings of the National Academy of Sciences* 108 (37):15354-15359.

Hanahan, D., and Robert A Weinberg. 2011. "Hallmarks of cancer: the next generation." *cell* 144 (5):646-674.

Hansson, G. C. 2020. "Mucins and the microbiome." *Annual review of biochemistry* 89:769-793.

He, X., Qing Zeng, Santhosh Puthiyakunnon, Zhijie Zeng, Weijun Yang, Jiawen Qiu, Lei Du, Swapna Boddu, Tongwei Wu, and Danxian Cai. 2017. "Lactobacillus rhamnosus GG supernatant enhance neonatal resistance to systemic Escherichia coli K1 infection by accelerating development of intestinal defense." *Scientific reports* 7 (1):43305.

Holanda, D. M., Alexandros Yiannikouris, and Sung Woo Kim. 2020. "Investigation of the efficacy of a postbiotic yeast cell wall-based blend on newly-weaned pigs under a dietary challenge of multiple mycotoxins with emphasis on deoxynivalenol." *Toxins* 12 (8):504.

Hu, Y., Richard K. Le Leu, Claus T. Christophersen, Roshini Somashekar, Michael A. Conlon, Xing Q. Meng, Jean M. Winter, Richard J Woodman, Ross McKinnon, and Graeme P. Young. 2016. "Manipulation of the gut microbiota using resistant starch is associated with protection against colitis-associated colorectal cancer in rats." *Carcinogenesis* 37 (4):366-375.

Huycke, M. M., and H. Rex Gaskins. 2004. "Commensal bacteria, redox stress, and colorectal cancer: mechanisms and models." *Experimental biology and medicine* 229 (7):586-597.

Ijssennagger, N., Clara Belzer, Guido J. Hooiveld, Jan Dekker, Saskia W. C. van Mil, Michael Müller, Michiel Kleerebezem, and Roelof van der Meer. 2015. "Gut microbiota facilitates dietary heme-induced epithelial hyperproliferation by opening the mucus barrier in colon." *Proceedings of the National Academy of Sciences* 112 (32):10038-10043.

Illiano, P., Roberta Brambilla, and Cinzia Parolini. 2020. "The mutual interplay of gut microbiota, diet and human disease." *The FEBS journal* 287 (5):833-855.

Izuddin, W. I., Teck Chwen Loh, Hooi Ling Foo, Anjas Asmara Samsudin, and Ali Merzza Humam. 2019. "Postbiotic L. plantarum RG14 improves ruminal epithelium growth, immune status and upregulates the intestinal barrier function in post-weaning lambs." *Scientific reports* 9 (1):9938.

Jia, B., Xiao Han, Kyung Hyun Kim, and Che Ok Jeon. 2022. "Discovery and mining of enzymes from the human gut microbiome." *Trends in Biotechnology* 40 (2):240-254.

Jia, W., Guoxiang Xie, and Weiping Jia. 2018. "Bile acid–microbiota crosstalk in gastrointestinal inflammation and carcinogenesis." *Nature reviews Gastroenterology & hepatology* 15 (2):111-128.

Johansson, M. E. V., Hedvig E. Jakobsson, Jessica Holmén-Larsson, André Schütte, Anna Ermund, Ana M. Rodríguez-Piñeiro, Liisa Arike, Catharina Wising, Frida Svensson, and Fredrik Bäckhed. 2015. "Normalization of host intestinal mucus layers requires long-term microbial colonization." *Cell host & microbe* 18 (5):582-592.

Jung, T. H., Jeong Hyeon Park, Woo-Min Jeon, and Kyoung-Sik Han. 2015. "Butyrate modulates bacterial adherence on LS174T human colorectal cells by stimulating mucin secretion and MAPK signaling pathway." *Nutrition Research and Practice* 9 (4):343-349.

Kannan, M. M., and Sabarimuthu Darlin Quine. 2012. "Ellagic acid protects mitochondria from β-adrenergic agonist induced myocardial damage in rats; evidence from *in vivo*, *in vitro* and ultra structural study." *Food Research International* 45 (1):1-8.

Kannen, V., Michael Bader, Juliana Y. Sakita, Sergio A. Uyemura, and Jeremy A. Squire. 2020. "The dual role of serotonin in colorectal cancer." *Trends in Endocrinology & Metabolism* 31 (8):611-625.

Kim, S. J., Chang-Ho Kang, Gun-Hee Kim, and Hyosun Cho. 2022. "Anti-tumor effects of heat-killed L. reuteri MG5346 and L. casei MG4584 against human colorectal carcinoma through caspase-9-dependent apoptosis in xenograft model." *Microorganisms* 10 (3):533.

Kim, Y. J., Hwan Hee Yu, Yeong Jin Park, Na-Kyoung Lee, and Hyun-Dong Paik. 2020. "Anti-biofilm activity of cell-free supernatant of Saccharomyces cerevisiae against Staphylococcus aureus." *Journal of Microbiology and Biotechnology* 30 (12):1854.

Kimoto-Nira, H., Koko Mizumachi, Takashi Okamoto, Keisuke Sasaki, and Jun-ichi Kurisaki. 2009. "Influence of long-term consumption of a Lactococcus lactis strain on the intestinal immunity and intestinal flora of the senescence-accelerated mouse." *British journal of nutrition* 102 (2):181-185.

Kleerebezem, M., Pascal Hols, Elvis Bernard, Thomas Rolain, Miaomiao Zhou, Roland J. Siezen, and Peter A. Bron. 2010. "The extracellular biology of the lactobacilli." *FEMS microbiology reviews* 34 (2):199-230.

Konishi, H., Mikihiro Fujiya, Hiroki Tanaka, Nobuhiro Ueno, Kentaro Moriichi, Junpei Sasajima, Katsuya Ikuta, Hiroaki Akutsu, Hiroki Tanabe, and Yutaka Kohgo. 2016. "Probiotic-derived ferrichrome inhibits colon cancer progression via JNK-mediated apoptosis." *Nature communications* 7 (1):12365.

Kosumi, K., Tsuyoshi Hamada, Hideo Koh, Jennifer Borowsky, Susan Bullman, Tyler S. Twombly, Daniel Nevo, Yohei Masugi, Li Liu, and Annacarolina da Silva. 2018. "The amount of Bifidobacterium genus in colorectal carcinoma tissue in relation to tumor characteristics and clinical outcome." *The American journal of pathology* 188 (12):2839-2852.

Lee, J., Joo-Eun Lee, Seil Kim, Dukjin Kang, and Hee Min Yoo. 2020. "Evaluating cell death using cell-free supernatant of probiotics in three-dimensional spheroid cultures of colorectal cancer cells." *JoVE (Journal of Visualized Experiments)* (160):e61285.

Li, N., W. Michael Russell, Martha Douglas-Escobar, Nick Hauser, Mariela Lopez, and Josef Neu. 2009. "Live and heat-killed Lactobacillus rhamnosus GG: effects on proinflammatory and anti-inflammatory cytokines/chemokines in gastrostomy-fed infant rats." *Pediatric Research* 66 (2):203-207.

Li, Z., Weiwei Wang, Dan Liu, and Yuming Guo. 2017. "Effects of Lactobacillus acidophilus on gut microbiota composition in broilers challenged with Clostridium perfringens." *PloS one* 12 (11):e0188634.

Lin, P. W., Tala R. Nasr, Andrew J. Berardinelli, Amrita Kumar, and Andrew S. Neish. 2008. "The probiotic Lactobacillus GG may augment intestinal host defense by regulating apoptosis and promoting cytoprotective responses in the developing murine gut." *Pediatric research* 64 (5):511-516.

Maeda, N., Risa Nakamura, Yoshitaka Hirose, Shinji Murosaki, Yoshihiro Yamamoto, Tetsuo Kase, and Yasunobu Yoshikai. 2009. "Oral administration of heat-killed

Lactobacillus plantarum L-137 enhances protection against influenza virus infection by stimulation of type I interferon production in mice." *International immunopharmacology* 9 (9):1122-1125.

Maier, T. V., Marianna Lucio, Lang Ho Lee, Nathan C VerBerkmoes, Colin J. Brislawn, Jörg Bernhardt, Regina Lamendella, Jason E McDermott, Nathalie Bergeron, and Silke S. Heinzmann. 2017. "Impact of dietary resistant starch on the human gut microbiome, metaproteome, and metabolome." *MBio* 8 (5): https://doi.org/10.1128/mbio. 01343-17.

Martens, E. C., Mareike Neumann, and Mahesh S. Desai. 2018. "Interactions of commensal and pathogenic microorganisms with the intestinal mucosal barrier." *Nature Reviews Microbiology* 16 (8):457-470.

McGuckin, M. A., Sara K. Lindén, Philip Sutton, and Timothy H. Florin. 2011. "Mucin dynamics and enteric pathogens." *Nature Reviews Microbiology* 9 (4):265-278.

McIntyre, A., P. R. Gibson, and G. P. Young. 1993. "Butyrate production from dietary fibre and protection against large bowel cancer in a rat model." *Gut* 34 (3):386-391.

Mezrich, J. D., John H. Fechner, Xiaoji Zhang, Brian P. Johnson, William J. Burlingham, and Christopher A. Bradfield. 2010. "An interaction between kynurenine and the aryl hydrocarbon receptor can generate regulatory T cells." *The Journal of Immunology* 185 (6):3190-3198.

Nalini, N., Vaiyapuri Manju, and Venugopal P. Menon. 2004. "Effect of coconut cake on the bacterial enzyme activity in 1, 2-dimethyl hydrazine induced colon cancer." *Clinica Chimica Acta* 342 (1-2):203-210.

Noh, S. Young, Seok-Seong Kang, Cheol-Heui Yun, and Seung Hyun Han. 2015. "Lipoteichoic acid from Lactobacillus plantarum inhibits Pam2CSK4-induced IL-8 production in human intestinal epithelial cells." *Molecular Immunology* 64 (1):183-189.

Oerlemans, M. M. P., Renate Akkerman, Michela Ferrari, Marthe T. C. Walvoort, and Paul de Vos. 2021. "Benefits of bacteria-derived exopolysaccharides on gastrointestinal microbiota, immunity and health." *Journal of functional foods* 76:104289.

Pahumunto, N., and Rawee Teanpaisan. 2023. "Anti-cancer properties of potential probiotics and their cell-free supernatants for the prevention of colorectal cancer: An *in vitro* study." *Probiotics and Antimicrobial Proteins* 15 (5):1137-1150.

Parada Venegas, D., Marjorie K. De la Fuente, Glauben Landskron, María Julieta González, Rodrigo Quera, Gerard Dijkstra, Hermie J. M. Harmsen, Klaas Nico Faber, and Marcela A. Hermoso. 2019. "Short chain fatty acids (SCFAs)-mediated gut epithelial and immune regulation and its relevance for inflammatory bowel diseases." *Frontiers in immunology*:277.

Parolini, C. 2019. "Effects of fish n-3 PUFAs on intestinal microbiota and immune system." *Marine drugs* 17 (6):374.

Pelaseyed, T., Joakim H. Bergström, Jenny K. Gustafsson, Anna Ermund, George M. H. Birchenough, André Schütte, Sjoerd van der Post, Frida Svensson, Ana M. Rodríguez-Piñeiro, and Elisabeth E. L. Nyström. 2014. "The mucus and mucins of the goblet cells and enterocytes provide the first defense line of the gastrointestinal tract and interact with the immune system." *Immunological reviews* 260 (1):8-20.

Petrova, M. I., Nicole C. E. Imholz, Tine L. A. Verhoeven, Jan Balzarini, Els J. M. Van Damme, Dominique Schols, Jos Vanderleyden, and Sarah Lebeer. 2016. "Lectin-like molecules of Lactobacillus rhamnosus GG inhibit pathogenic Escherichia coli and Salmonella biofilm formation." *PloS one* 11 (8):e0161337.

Rad, A. H., Leili Aghebati-Maleki, Hossein Samadi Kafil, and Amin Abbasi. 2021. "Molecular mechanisms of postbiotics in colorectal cancer prevention and treatment." *Critical reviews in food science and nutrition* 61 (11):1787-1803.

Reddy, B. S., and Abraham Rivenson. 1993. "Inhibitory effect of Bifidobacterium longum on colon, mammary, and liver carcinogenesis induced by 2-amino-3-methylimidazo [4, 5-f] quinoline, a food mutagen." *Cancer Research* 53 (17):3914-3918.

Richard, M. L., and Harry Sokol. 2019. "The gut mycobiota: insights into analysis, environmental interactions and role in gastrointestinal diseases." *Nature Reviews Gastroenterology & Hepatology* 16 (6):331-345.

Rosshart, S. P., Brian G. Vassallo, Davide Angeletti, Diane S. Hutchinson, Andrew P. Morgan, Kazuyo Takeda, Heather D. Hickman, John A. McCulloch, Jonathan H. Badger, and Nadim J. Ajami. 2017. "Wild mouse gut microbiota promotes host fitness and improves disease resistance." *Cell* 171 (5):1015-1028. e13.

Rubinstein, M. R., Xiaowei Wang, Wendy Liu, Yujun Hao, Guifang Cai, and Yiping W. Han. 2013. "Fusobacterium nucleatum promotes colorectal carcinogenesis by modulating E-cadherin/β-catenin signaling via its FadA adhesin." *Cell host & microbe* 14 (2):195-206.

Salazar, N., Miguel Gueimonde, Clara G. De Los Reyes-Gavilán, and Patricia Ruas-Madiedo. 2016. "Exopolysaccharides produced by lactic acid bacteria and bifidobacteria as fermentable substrates by the intestinal microbiota." *Critical Reviews in Food Science and Nutrition* 56 (9):1440-1453.

Schirmer, M., Sanne P. Smeekens, Hera Vlamakis, Martin Jaeger, Marije Oosting, Eric A. Franzosa, Rob Ter Horst, Trees Jansen, Liesbeth Jacobs, and Marc Jan Bonder. 2016. "Linking the human gut microbiome to inflammatory cytokine production capacity." *Cell* 167 (4):1125-1136. e8.

Scott, S. A., Jingjing Fu, and Pamela V. Chang. 2020. "Microbial tryptophan metabolites regulate gut barrier function via the aryl hydrocarbon receptor." *Proceedings of the National Academy of Sciences* 117 (32):19376-19387.

Shimada Y., Kinoshita M., Harada K., Mizutani M., Masahata K., Kayama H., and Kiyoshi Takeda 2013. "Commensal Bacteria-dependent indole production enhances epithelial barrier function in the colon." *PLoS One*. doi: https://doi.org/10.1371/journal.pone.0080604.

Sugahara, H., R. Yao, T. Odamaki, and J. Z. Xiao. 2017. "Differences between live and heat-killed bifidobacteria in the regulation of immune function and the intestinal environment." *Beneficial microbes* 8 (3):463-472.

Sun, J., and Ikuko Kato. 2016. "Gut microbiota, inflammation and colorectal cancer." *Genes & diseases* 3 (2):130-143.

Sung, H., Jacques Ferlay, Rebecca L. Siegel, Mathieu Laversanne, Isabelle Soerjomataram, Ahmedin Jemal, and Freddie Bray. 2021. "Global cancer statistics 2020: GLOBOCAN estimates of incidence and mortality worldwide for 36 cancers in 185 countries." *CA: a cancer journal for clinicians* 71 (3):209-249.

Tan, J., Craig McKenzie, Maria Potamitis, Alison N. Thorburn, Charles R. Mackay, and Laurence Macia. 2014. "The role of short-chain fatty acids in health and disease." *Advances in immunology* 121:91-119.

Taverniti, V., and Simone Guglielmetti. 2011. "The immunomodulatory properties of probiotic microorganisms beyond their viability (ghost probiotics: proposal of paraprobiotic concept)." *Genes & nutrition* 6 (3):261-274.

Terada, A., Wakoto Bukawa, Tatsuhiko Kan, and Tomotari Mitsuoka. 2004. "Effects of the consumption of heat-killed Enterococcus faecalis EC-12 preparation on microbiota and metabolic activity of the faeces in healthy adults." *Microbial ecology in health and disease* 16 (4):188-194.

Tian, Y., Qing Xu, Liqun Sun, Ying Ye, and Guozhong Ji. 2018. "Short-chain fatty acids administration is protective in colitis-associated colorectal cancer development." *The Journal of Nutritional Biochemistry* 57:103-109.

Tsilingiri, K., Theolis Barbosa, Giuseppe Penna, Flavio Caprioli, Angelica Sonzogni, Giuseppe Viale, and Maria Rescigno. 2012. "Probiotic and postbiotic activity in health and disease: comparison on a novel polarised ex-vivo organ culture model." *Gut* 61 (7):1007-1015.

Tukenmez, U., Busra Aktas, Belma Aslim, and Serkan Yavuz. 2019. "The relationship between the structural characteristics of lactobacilli-EPS and its ability to induce apoptosis in colon cancer cells *in vitro*." *Scientific reports* 9 (1):8268.

Turner, J. R. 2009. "Intestinal mucosal barrier function in health and disease." *Nature reviews immunology* 9 (11):799-809.

Tytgat, H. L. P., François P. Douillard, Justus Reunanen, Pia Rasinkangas, Antoni P. A. Hendrickx, Pia K. Laine, Lars Paulin, Reetta Satokari, and Willem M. de Vos. 2016. "Lactobacillus rhamnosus GG outcompetes Enterococcus faecium via mucus-binding pili: evidence for a novel and heterospecific probiotic mechanism." *Applied and environmental microbiology* 82 (19):5756-5762.

Ueno, N., Mikihiro Fujiya, Shuichi Segawa, Toshie Nata, Kentaro Moriichi, Hiroki Tanabe, Yusuke Mizukami, Naoyuki Kobayashi, Kazutoshi Ito, and Yutaka Kohgo. 2011. "Heat-killed body of lactobacillus brevis SBC8803 ameliorates intestinal injury in a murine model of colitis by enhancing the intestinal barrier function." *Inflammatory bowel diseases* 17 (11):2235-2250.

Wang, L., Lei Tang, Yiming Feng, Suying Zhao, Mei Han, Chuan Zhang, Gehui Yuan, Jun Zhu, Shuyuan Cao, and Qian Wu. 2020. "A purified membrane protein from Akkermansia muciniphila or the pasteurised bacterium blunts colitis associated tumourigenesis by modulation of CD8+ T cells in mice." *Gut* 69 (11):1988-1997.

Weidenmaier, C., and Andreas Peschel. 2008. "Teichoic acids and related cell-wall glycopolymers in Gram-positive physiology and host interactions." *Nature Reviews Microbiology* 6 (4):276-287.

Whitehead, R. H., G. P. Young, and P. S. Bhathal. 1986. "Effects of short chain fatty acids on a new human colon carcinoma cell line (LIM1215)." *Gut* 27 (12):1457-1463.

Wrzosek, L., Sylvie Miquel, Marie-Louise Noordine, Stephan Bouet, Marie Joncquel Chevalier-Curt, Véronique Robert, Catherine Philippe, Chantal Bridonneau, Claire Cherbuy, and Catherine Robbe-Masselot. 2013. "Bacteroides thetaiotaomicron and Faecalibacterium prausnitzii influence the production of mucus glycans and the development of goblet cells in the colonic epithelium of a gnotobiotic model rodent." *BMC biology* 11:1-13.

Wu, S., Ki-Jong Rhee, Emilia Albesiano, Shervin Rabizadeh, Xinqun Wu, Hung-Rong Yen, David L. Huso, Frederick L. Brancati, Elizabeth Wick, and Florencia McAllister. 2009. "A human colonic commensal promotes colon tumorigenesis via activation of T helper type 17 T cell responses." *Nature medicine* 15 (9):1016-1022.

Xiao, R., and Yi Zheng. 2016. "Overview of microalgal extracellular polymeric substances (EPS) and their applications." *Biotechnology advances* 34 (7):1225-1244.

Yang, N., Yang Zhan, Jianhua Wan, Yingmeng Li, Xu Hu, and Wenjun Liu. 2022. "Effects of Lacidophilin tablets, yogurt, and bifid triple viable capsules on the gut microbiota of mice with antibiotic-associated diarrhea." *Canadian Journal of Infectious Diseases and Medical Microbiology* 2022.

Zorzela, L., S. K. Ardestani, L. V. McFarland, and S. Vohra. 2017. "Is there a role for modified probiotics as beneficial microbes: a systematic review of the literature." *Beneficial microbes* 8 (5):739-754.

Biographical Sketch

Shirin Farsad

Affiliation:

Department of Microbiology, Faculty of Basic Sciences, Islamic Azad University, Qom Branch, Qom, Iran.

Education: Microbiology PhD Student.

Business Address: Islamic Azad University, Qom Branch.

Research and Professional Experience:

Working on using probiotics for cancer treatment in the lab.

Professional Appointments: University research assistant.

Honors:

Publications from the Last 3 Years:

[1] *The effect of probiotics on the improvement of colorectal cancer* (2022).

[2] A review of the practical effects of ginseng and the treatment of disease. Bioremediation of polluted waters using microorganisms. A speech at the 5th international congress of Probiotics and Superbeneficial Foods entitled "*Probiotic Treatment of Skin Disease*" (2022).
[3] *A review article on the mechanisms of probiotics for the treatment of COVID-19 patients* (2022).

Alireza Rasouli

Affiliation:

Department of Microbiology, Faculty of Basic Sciences, Islamic Azad University, Qom Branch, Qom, Iran.

Education: MSc of Microbial Biotechnology.

Business Address: Islamic Azad University, Qom Branch.

Research and Professional Experience: Working on Optimization of bioethanol production.

Professional Appointments: University research assistant.

Honors:

Publications from the Last 3 Years:

[1] *Single-cell Oil Production Using Low-Cost Carbon Sources by Newly Isolated Kocuria Y205* (2021).
[2] *Bio-production of Single-cell Oil by Rhodococcus Erythropolis PTCC 1767 Bacterial using Low-cost Carbon Sources* (2020).

Chapter 10

Human Milk Oligosaccharides: Types, Physiological Effects and Production Processes

Zhenshang Xu
and Ting Wang*
State Key Laboratory of Biobased Material and Green Papermaking, Qilu University of Technology, Shandong Academy of Science, Jinan, Shandong Province, PR China

Abstract

Human milk is a complex biological liquid rich in nutrients and bioactive substances. Human milk oligosaccharides (HMOs) are a kind of complex carbohydrates that the human body cannot digest while the beneficial bacteria in the gut can utilize, and are the third largest nutrient in human milk. HMOs are complex mixtures of oligosaccharides, and more than 200 different types of HMOs have been identified. The types and contents of oligosaccharides in human milk were affected by various factors, but 2'-fucosyllactose (2'-FL) accounted for the highest proportion. HMOs are an important part of newborn protection and play an important role in infant growth and development. At present, many physiological functions of HMOs have been found, such as regulating intestinal flora, anti-adhesion of pathogenic bacteria, improving immunity and promoting brain development. In view of their important roles, many methods have been used to extract or synthesize HMOs, among which biosynthesis methods have been used to synthesize HMOs because they do not use toxic reagents and are convenient for large-scale production. In this study, the types, physiological functions and biosynthesis methods of HMOs are reviewed in order to make the future application of HMOs possible, such as additives for infant milk powder.

---

* Corresponding Author's Email: tingwang_97@hotmail.com.

In: Exploring Microbiotics in Health and Disease
Editor: Edward L. Stillman
ISBN: 978-8-89113-410-2

Keywords: human milk oligosaccharides, physiological functions, biosynthesis methods

1. Introduction

Human milk has always been regarded as the best food source for infants and young children. In addition to providing nutrients for normal growth of infants and young children, human milk also has many health promoting effects that cow milk does not have. The most important difference between human milk and cow milk is the type and structure of oligosaccharides. Human milk oligosaccharides (HMOs) are the third largest solid components after lactose and fat, and the content of oligosaccharides in human milk is 5-15 g/L, which is 100-300 times that of cow's milk (Bode, 2012). Human milk contains at least thousands of oligosaccharides, of which more than 200 have been identified (Ninonuevo et al., 2006). In the United States and Europe, chemically synthesized lacto-N-neotetraose (LNnT) and chemically or biologically synthesized 2' -fucosyllactose (2 '-FL) are under review as new additives in infant formula (Bode et al., 2016). Recent clinical trials have proved that these two oligosaccharides have an important impact on the establishment of intestinal flora in early infants (Alliet et al., 2016).

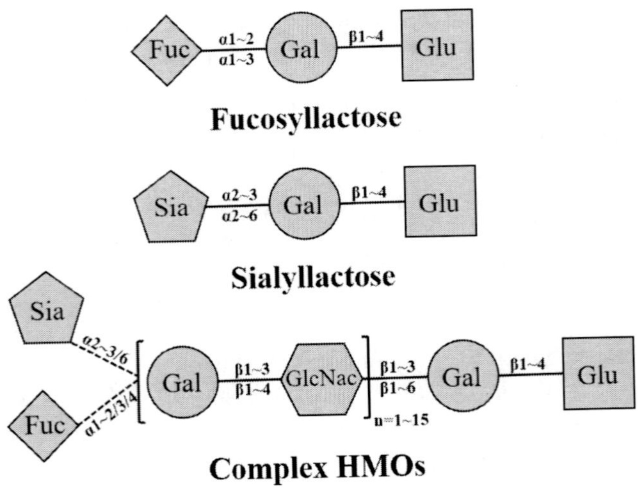

Figure 1. The structure of HMOs. Fuc, L-fucose; Sia, sialic acid; GlcNac, N-acetylglucosamine; Gal, D-galactose; Glu, D-glucose.

The special ingredients in human milk are suitable for babies with immature digestive and immune systems. It protects infants from infection and inflammation, promotes the development of their immune function and the maturation of their organs (Michaelsen et al., 2007). This is partly due to the presence of large amounts of HMOs. The infant's gut cannot digest HMOs, but it can provide multiple protective effects for newborns, such as helping regulate the gut microbiota, promoting intestinal development, preventing pathogenic infections, and stimulating immune system maturation (Kuntz et al., 2008). HMOs is an important magic weapon for the superiority of breastfeeding. For infants who cannot be breastfed, infant formula becomes an important source of nutrition. Especially in recent years, with the commercialization of HMOs abroad for the first time, HMOs research has become a hot spot in breast milk research.

So far, there are many methods to extract or synthesize HMOs, among which biosynthesis method is used to synthesize a variety of HMOs because it does not use toxic reagents and is convenient for large-scale production. The method of biosynthesis of HMOs can be divided into two steps, including carbon skeleton construction and fucosylation or sialylation (Lu et al., 2021). The production of HMOs can be achieved by constructing metabolic pathways in microorganisms. Using common carbon sources such as glucose, lactose, and glycerol, 2'-FL, 3'-fucosyllactose (3'-FL), 3'-sialyllactose (3'-SL), 6'-sialyllactose (6'-SL), lacto-N-tetraose (LNT), LNnT, and other oligosaccharides are relatively abundant in human milk can be obtained in microbial cell factories. At present, most of the metabolic pathways to synthesize HMOs are constructed in *Escherichia coli*. The research on the action mechanism and synthesis method of HMOs makes it possible to use them as a common additive in infant formula in the future.

2. Types of HMOs

2.1. Structural Characteristics of HMOs

So far, scientists have detected more than 200 HMOs molecules in human breast milk (Ninonuevo et al., 2006). Although HMOs is diverse and complex in structure, it is composed of five basic monosaccharide monomers, including D-glucose, D-galactose, N-acetylglucosamine, L-fucose, and sialic acid. The reduced terminus of HMOs usually contain a lactose structure with alternating

N-acetylglucosamine and D-galactose as the skeleton. N-acetylglucosamine is connected to D-galactose by the β-1, 6 bond and is modified with L-fucose or sialic acid at the end of its skeleton (Bode, 2012). As shown in Figure 1, the vast majority of HMOs had 3 to 9 degrees of polymerization, inwhich the 5 monomers were connected by different glucosidic bonds to form straight or branched chain structures. In addition, more complex structures could be formed after fucosylation or sialylation. According to the difference of modification groups, the types of HMOs can be mainly divided into three categories: neutral fucosylated, neutral non-fucosylated and acidic sialic sugars, which are distributed in content of 35%~50%, 42%~55% and 12%~14% (Totten et al., 2012).

2.2. Main Components and Content Differences of HMOs

The distribution of HMOs in individuals is very different. Therefore, the types and content of HMOs reported in different literatures are quite diverse. Samuel et al., (2019) studied 20 kinds of HMOs in the breast milk of mothers from 7 European countries, whose total content was between 6.7 and 13.1 g/L. Table 1 shows the content of common HMOs reported in literature, among which 2'-FL accounts for the highest proportion (Thurl et al., 2010). It should be noted that these changes, in addition to the analysis method, may be attributed to the maternal gestational age, genetic, lactating secretory state and lactation period.

Some of the most representative HMOs in breast milk, such as 2'-FL, Lacto-N-fucopentaose I (LNFP-I), and Lacto-N-fucopentaose II (LNFP-II), have significant genetic differences. For example, differences in α-1, 2 fucosylated HMOs depend on maternal fucosyltransferase gene expression (Bode et al., 2012). The structure and composition of HMOs vary during lactation, and a European study of breast milk reported that lactation, along with genetic blood type, is one of the biggest influences on HMOs variation (Samuel et al., 2019). The total HMOs concentration decreased with the prolongation of lactation time, while some HMOs may increase. The physiological status of the lactating mother (e.g., BMI) and the conditions of delivery (e.g., mode of delivery and number of births) may also influence the glycosylation of breast milk in the lactating mother and thus the composition of HMOs (Austin et al., 2019).

Table 1. Types and contents of common oligosaccharides in human milk

HMOs	abbreviation	Content (g/L)
2'-fucosyllactose	2'-FL	2.20~7.23
3'-fucosyllactose	3'-FL	0.31~1.62
3'-sialyllactose	3'-SL	0.17~0.30
6'-sialyllactose	6'-SL	0.039~0.87
Lacto-N-tetraose	LNT	0.25~1.74
Lacto-N-neotetraose	LNnT	1.61~1.97
Difucosyllactose	DFLac	0.2~0.41
Lacto-N-hexaose	LNH	0.05~0.13
Lacto-N-fucopentaose I	LNFP-I	0.16~1.99
Lacto-N-fucopentaose II	LNFP-II	0.22~0.47
Lacto-N-fucopentaose III	LNFP-III	0.35~0.49
Lacto-N-fucopentaose V	LNFP-V	0.02~0.49
Sialyllacto-N-tetraose b	LSTb	0.06~0.33
Sialyllacto-N-tetraose c	LSTc	0.13~1.31
Lacto-N-Difucohexaose I	LNDFH-I	1.22~1.28
Lacto-N-Difucohexaose II	LNDFH-II	0.02~0.41
Disialyl-Lacto-N-Tetraose	DSLNT	1.02~1.19

3. Physiological Functions of HMOs

The efficacy of HMOs has been one of the hot spots in HMOs research. Studies have reported that the beneficial effects of HMOs include the regulation of intestinal microbiota, anti-adhesion effect on pathogens, immune system regulation, and promotion of brain development.

3.1. Regulation of Intestinal Flora

HMOs is the most important prebiotic for babies. Since most HMOs are not destroyed by human stomach acid or decomposed by digestive enzymes, they can directly reach the large intestine. Subsequently, HMOs can be fermented and utilized by some bacteria to produce short-chain fatty acids and form an acidic environment, which is conducive to the growth of intestinal probiotics (*Bifidobacterium* and *Lactobacillus*) and effectively hinder the flora harmful to human health, thus maintaining human intestinal health (Jost et al., 2015). In the intestinal flora of breast-fed infants, *Bifidobacteria* are usually dominant, especially the enrichment of *Bifidobacterium longum* (Hoeflinger et al., 2015). According to genome sequencing, the uniqueness of *B. longum* lies in its possession of transporters and enzymes required to transport HMOs into cells and metabolize them in cells (Sela et al., 2008). Other *Bifidobacteria* possess enzymes that degrade HMOs in the outer membrane of the cell and transport the products into the cell for metabolism. There is evidence that breastfed babies have more *Bifidobacteria* than formula-fed babies. When infants were fed formula with addition of 2'-FL and LNnT, a unique fecal bacterial profile was developed that was more similar to that of breastfed infants compared to formula without addition of prebiotics (Garrido et al., 2012).

3.2. Anti-Adhesion Effect on Pathogens

Breast milk protects the intestines of infants from pathogens, in part because HMOs are abundant in breast milk. HMOs improves host defense mechanisms by enhancing intestinal barrier function. It can be used as an antimicrobial agent to directly reduce microbial infections and indirectly control pathogens by providing a competitive advantage to non-pathogenic microorganisms. Generally speaking, pathogenic microorganisms have the same pathogenic mechanism: they first recognize the cell, bind to its surface, and then enter the inside of the cell to release harmful substances and absorb internal nutrients, resulting in a variety of diseases (Ninonuevo et al., 2006). Many pathogens cause disease by adhering to cell surfaces, and the sugar chain structure of some HMOs and mucosal cell surfaces is similar, so HMOs may imitate the structure of viral receptors and indirectly inhibit the production of diseases by trapping pathogens (Newburg et al., 2005). In order to reduce the probability of diarrhea caused by *Campylobacter jejuni*, α-1, 2-fucosylated HMOs, which can be recognized by *C. jejuni*, was used as an anti-adhesion agent to prevent the combination of bacteria and human intestinal mucosal cells (Morrow et al., 2004).

3.3. Immune System Regulation

HMOs has the ability to regulate the infant immune system. They directly regulate the gene expression of intestinal cells, resulting in changes in the expression of glycans on the cell surface and other cellular reactions, and then indirectly affect the infant non-specific immune response (Hanson et al., 2007). The results of in vitro studies show that HMOs regulates the production of lymphocyte cytokines, stimulates the production of immune active substances in the body, improves cell vitality, and thus improves the immunity of the body to bacteria and various diseases (Kulinich et al., 2016). This physiological process plays an irreplaceable role in immune system information transmission and immune coordination. Plasma inflammatory cytokine concentrations were significantly lower in formula-fed infants supplemented with 2'-FL and were similar to those in the breastfed group (Goehring et al., 2016).

3.4. Promotion of Brain Development

Breast milk contains a certain amount of sialic acid, which is mainly derived from the sialic acid attached to the ends of HMOs. Studies have shown that sialyl gangliosides and polysialyl glycoproteins are important for brain development and cognition, so babies who are breastfed have better brain development, richer synapses, and more developed nervous systems (Wang, 2009).

4. Production of HMOs

At present, HMO synthesis methods include chemical method, enzymatic method, chemical-enzymatic method, and whole cell synthesis method. Chemical synthesis of HMOs has been developed earlier and the more mature method is fully automatic solid-phase synthesis. In solid phase synthesis, the synthesized oligosaccharides are connected to insoluble substances, which can achieve rapid separation of reaction products and excess reactants (Plante et al., 2001). In order to overcome the obstacle of electron and space in the glycosyl donor, which makes it difficult to form a sugar anhydride bond, it was determined to protect the glycosyl donor and acceptor with hydroxyl group and further activate it to synthesize oligosaccharides with stable structure (Nokami et al., 2013). In enzymatic methods, glycosyltransferase and glycosidase are two common enzymes that act on oligosaccharides and their precursors. Lactose was synthesized into fucosyllactose using α-1, 2-fucosyltransferase by improving the source of the enzyme and the limitations of the active substrate. Chen et al., (2015) cleverly used the high efficiency and selectivity of enzymatic method and flexibility of chemical method to synthesize tetrasaccharides with 81% yield by using a one-pot double-enzyme system. However, the use of toxic reagents and the low yield make chemical synthesis methods unsuitable for the production of food additives. Dumon et al., (2001) used lactose as a receptor to successfully prepare LNT and LNnT in recombinant *E. coli* cells. Since then, the whole cell biosynthesis of HMOs has received much attention and extensive research. Figure 2 showed the schematic representation of HMOs production in microbial cell factories.

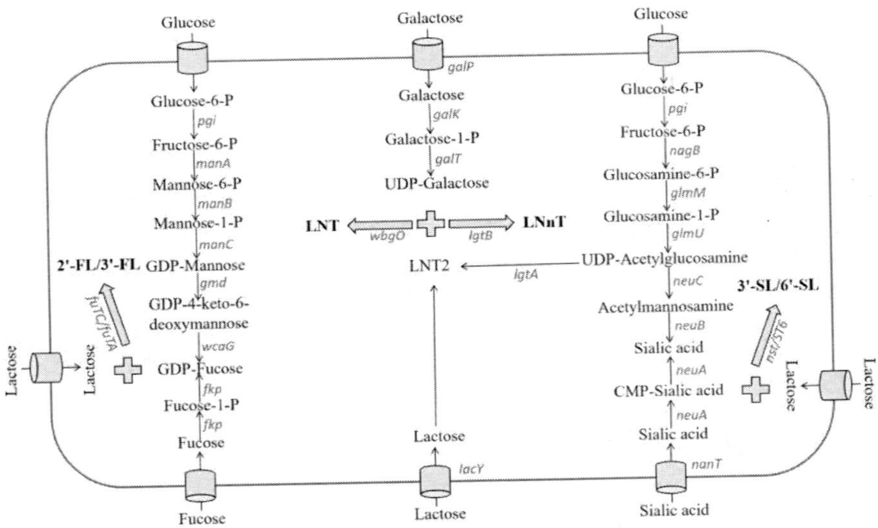

Figure 2. Schematic representation of HMOs production in microbial cell factories. manA, mannose-6-phosphate isomerase; manB, phosphomannomutase; manC, mannose-1-phosphate guanylyltransferase; gmd, GDP-mannose 4, 6-dehydratase; wcaG, GDP-4-keto-6-deoxymannose 3, 5-epimerase 4-reductase; fkp, L-fucokinase/GDP-L-fucose phosphorylase; fuTC, α-1, 2-fucosyltransferase; fuTA, α-1, 3-fucosyltransferase; lacY, lactose permease; nagB, glucosamine-6-phosphate deaminase; glmM, GDP-mannose mannosylhydrolase; glmU, bifunctional protein; neuA, CMP-Neu5Ac synthetase; neuB, sialic acid synthase; neuC, GlcNAc-6-phosphate 2 epimerase; nanT, sialic acid transporter; nst, α-2, 3-sialyltransferase; ST6, α-2, 6-sialyltransferase; galP, galactose permease; galK, galactokinase; galT, galctose-1-phosphate uridyltransferase, phosphoglycerate mutase; lgtA, β-1, 3-N-acetylglucosaminyltransferase; lgtB, β-1, 4-galactostltransferase; wbgO, β-1, 3-galactostltransferase.

4.1. Biosynthesis of Fucosyllactose

Fucosyllactose is a product of fucose linked to lactose via α-1, 2 or α-1, 3 glucoside bonds. Based on the different connection, fucosyllactose is divided into 2'-FL and 3'-FL (Huang et al., 2017). These two relatively simple oligosaccharides are the main components in HMOs, of which 2'-FL is the most abundant oligosaccharide in human milk. Under the action of fucosyltransferases, guanosine diphosphate-L-fucose (GDP-L-Fucose) and lactose undergo group substitution to form 2'-FL or 3'-FL and guanosine diphosphate (GDP) (Lee et al., 2012). GDP-L-fucose, which provides fucosylated donors for fucosylation, is a key substance in fucosyllactose synthesis. There are two synthesis pathways in bacteria, mammals and plants, namely *de novo* pathway and salvage pathway. *De novo* synthesis pathway can take glucose, glycerol, mannose, or lactose as the starting material (Chin et al., 2015). The biosynthesis process of FL is shown in Figure 2 (left).

4.2. Biosynthesis of Sialyllactose

The main sialyllactose in breast milk is 3'-SL and 6'-SL, which are the products of sialic acid linked to lactose via α-2,3 or α-2,6 glucoside bonds, respectively (Guo et al., 2014). Sialic acid plays an important role in infant brain development. Under the action of sialyltransferases, cytidylate monophosphate-sialic acid (CMP-Neu5Ac) and lactose undergo group translocation to form 3'-SL and 6'-SL in microbiota (Endo et al., 2000). The synthesis of CMP-Neu5Ac can be completed through the *de novo* pathway and the salvage pathway (Drouillard et al., 2010). The biosynthesis process of SL is shown in Figure 2 (right).

4.3. Biosynthesis of Complex HMOs

4.3.1. Synthesis of Lacto-N-tetraosaccharide Series HMOs

LNT and LNnT are oligosaccharides composed of four six-carbon sugar units, which can be further fucosylated to form a variety of oligosaccharides abundant in human milk. More and more biosynthesis methods have been used to obtain LNT and LNnT from *E. coli* using lactose, D-glucose and L-fucose as substrates. Overexpression of the *lgtA* gene encoding β-1, 3-N-acetylglucosamine transferase and the *wbgO* gene encoding β-1, 3-galactosyltransferase led to whole-cell biosynthesis of LNT (Baumgärtner et al., 2014). By expressing GDP-L-fucose via a salvage pathway and simultaneously expressing bacterial fucosyltransferase, LNT is further transformed into corresponding fucosylated HMOs. For example, *futC* encoding α-1, 2-fucosyltransferase catalyzed the LNT to further generate lacto-N-fucosylpentose I (LNFP-I), while *fuct14* encoding α-1, 4-fucosyltransferase catalyzed the formation of lacto-N-difucohexose (LNDFH-II) in *E. coli* (Baumgärtner et al., 2015). Overexpression of the *lgtA* gene and the *lgtB* gene encoding β-1, 4-galactostltransferase led to whole-cell biosynthesis of LNnT (Dong et al., 2019). The biosynthesis process of LNT and LNnT is shown in Figure 2 (middle).

4.3.2. Synthesis of Other Complex HMOs

Galactose and N-acetylglucosamine form N-disaccharide structure, and then multiple disaccharide structure repeat units form main chain or branch chain, the reducing end of which is linked to lactose to form lacto-N-biose (LNB) (Figure 1). After fucosylation or sialylation, complex fucosylated or sialated HMOs are formed. There are abundant complex oligosaccharides in HMOs, most of which are such structures (Bode, 2009). The expression of phospho-β-galactosidase encoded by gnbG of Lactobacillus casei BL23 in E. coli can catalyze the formation of LNB. The maximum yield of LNB is 10.7 g/L with the conversion rate of 69% (Bidart et al., 2017).

4.4. Host and Yield

E. coli is a well-studied model microorganism, and is widely used for fermentation products as microbial cell factories (Yang et al., 2020). Although it is currently an industrial strain used for some HMOs biosynthesis such as 2'-FL, *E. coli* itself has many problems. This species is not a traditional food industry strain, easy to infect phages, and will produce endotoxins (Rosano and Ceccarelli, 2014). Therefore, food grade hosts have greater advantages for HMOs production. Such potential hosts include yeast (*Saccharomyces cerevisiae*, *Pichia pastoris*), *Bacillus subtilis*, *Corynebacterium glutamicum* and *Lactobacillus*. At present, HMOs biosynthesis has been studied in the former four food-grade microbial hosts. As shown in Table 2, the HMO production in different hosts is presented (Lu et al., 2021).

Table 2. HMO production in different hosts

Engineering Strains	Characteristics	Product	Yield (g/L)	Reference
E. coli JM109(DE3)	Overexpressing *gmd* and *wcaG*. Introducing *fucT2*.	2'-FL	1.23	Lee et al., 2012
E. coli W3110	Introducing *futC*.	2'-FL	25	Merighi et al., 2012
E. coli JM109(DE3)	Overexpressing *manB*, *manC*, *gmd*, and *wcaG*. Introducing *fkp* and *futC*.	2'-FL	20.28	Baumgärtner et al., 2013
E. coli BL21(DE3)	Introducing *fucT2*. Deleting *lac* operon.	2'-FL	6.4	Chin et al., 2015
E. coli BL21(DE3)	Introducing *fkp* and *fucT2*. Deleting *lacZ*, *fucI*, and *fucK*.	2'-FL	23.1	Chin et al., 2016
E. coli BL21(DE3)	Overexpressing *glk*, *manB*, *manC*, *gmd*, and *wcaG*	2'-FL	10.75	Qin et al., 2016
E. coli BL21(DE3)	Overexpressing *fucT2*. Deleting *lacZ*.	2'-FL	15.4	Chin et al., 2017
E. coli BL21(DE3)	Overexpressing *wbgL*, *lacY*, *manB*, *manC*, *gmd*, *fcl*, and *gal*. Deleting *lacZ*.	2'-FL	42	Parkot et al., 2017
E. coli JM109	Introducing *fkp*. Deleting *fucI* and *fucK*	2'-FL	3.3	Guan et al., 2018
E. coli ΔLM15	Overexpressing *manB*, *manC*, *gmd*, and *wcaG*. Introducing *Te2FT*.	2'-FL	0.49	Seydametova et al., 2019
E. coli BL21(DE3)	Deleting *araA* and *rhaA*.	2'-FL	47	Jung et al., 2019
E. coli BL21(DE3)	Deleting *lacZ*, *gcd*, *glK*, *ptsG*, *pfKA*, and *wcaJ*.	2'-FL	60	Parschat et al., 2020
E. coli S17-3	Introducing *futC* and *wcfB*. Deleting *lacZ*, *wcaJ*, and *wcaI*.	2'-FL	0.62	Chen et al., 2020
E. coli C41(DE3)	Introducing *rcsA* and *rcsB*. Deleting *wcaJ*, *nudD*, and *nudK*.	2'-FL	66.8	Ni et al., 2020
E. coli BL21(DE3)	Introducing α-1,3-FTs coding gene.	3'-FL	0.58	Yu et al., 2018
E. coli BL21(DE3)	Overexpressing *futA*. Deleting *lacZ*.	3'-FL	4.6	Choi et al., 2019
E. coli ΔL-YA	Overexpressing *fucT*. Eliminating β-galactosidase. Deleting *wcaJ* and *ptsG*.	3'-FL	11.5	Jung et al., 2019
E. coli BL21(DE3)	Overexpressing *rcsA* and *lacY*. Introducing *fucT*. Deleting *lacZ*, *wcaJ*, and *Ion*.	2'-FL, 3'-FL	9.12, 12.43	Huang et al., 2017
E. coli JM107 (DE3)	Overexpressing *rcsA*. Introducing *lgtA*, *lgtB*, and *fucT*. Deleting *wcaJ* and *lacZ*.	LNnFP	3	Dumon et al., 2001
E. coli JM107 (DE3)	Introducing futA and rcsA. Deleting lacZ.	LNnDFH II, 3FL, LNnFPV, LNnT, LNnH	1.7, 0.5, 0.5, 1, 0.5	Dumon et al., 2004

Table 2. (Continued)

Engineering Strains	Characteristics	Product	Yield (g/L)	Reference
E. coli JM107	Overexpressing *lgtA* and *lgtB*. Introducing α1,2-FTs coding gene.	LNnFP I, 2′-FL, LNnT	1.7, 0.6, 0.7	Drouillard et al., 2006
E. coli LJ100	Introducing *lgtA*, *wbgO*, and *futC*.	LNFP I	0.27	Baumgärtner et al., 2015
E. coli LJ100	Introducing *lgtA*, *wbgO*, and *FucT14*.	LNDFH II	0.55	Baumgärtner et al., 2015
E. coli JM109	Overexpressing *lacY*. Introducing *lgtA* and *lgtB*. Deleting *lacZ*.	LNT2, LNnT	6, 5	Priem et al., 2002
E. coli LJ100	Introducing *lgtA* and *wbgO*.	LNT	0.22	Baumgärtner et al., 2014
E. coli LJ100	Overexpressing *lacY*. Introducing *lgtA* and *wbgO*. Deleting *lacZYA*.	LNT2, LNT	13.70, 12.72	Baumgärtner et al., 2015
E. coli NM522	Overexpressing the CMP-Neu5Ac synthetase, α2,3-sialyltransferase coding gene. Coupling CMP-Neu5Ac production system.	3'-SL	33	Endo et al., 2000
E. coli JM107	Introducing CMP-Neu5Ac synthase coding gene. Deleting *lacZ* and *nanA*.	3'-SL	2.6	Priem et al., 2002
E. coli DC	Decreasing expression of sialyltransferase gene. Increasing expression of *neuABC*. Deleting *nanA*, *nanK*, and *lacZ*.	6'-SL	34	Drouillard et al., 2010
E. coli BL21(DE3)	Introducing sialyltransferase coding gene.	3'-SL, 6'-SL	1.74, 2.11	Guo et al., 2014
S. cerevisiae D452-2	Introducing *fucT2*, *lac12*, and *fkp*.	2'-FL	0.503	Yu et al., 2018
S. cerevisiae D452-2	Overexpressing *gmd*, and *wcaG*. Introducing *fucT2* and *lac12*.	2'-FL	0.56	Liu et al., 2018
S. cerevisiae D452-2	Introducing *fucT2*, *gmd*, *wcaG*, and *wbgL*.	2'-FL	25.5	Lee et al., 2020
P. pastoris	Introducing β-N-acetylhexosaminidase coding gene.	LNT2, LNnT	8.6, 2	Liu et al., 2020
B. subtilis 168	Increasing expression of *fkp* and *futC*. Decreasing expression of *purR*.	2'-FL	0.674	Deng et al., 2019
B. subtilis 168	Introducing *fkP*, *futC*, and *lac12*. Deleting *yesZ*.	2'-FL	5.01	Deng et al., 2019
B. subtilis 168	Introducing *lacY*, *lgtA*, and *lgtB*.	LNnT	4.52	Dong et al., 2019
B. subtilis BY24	Introducing *lgtB*. Decreaing expression of *pfkA*, *pyk*, *zwf*, and *mnaA* . Deleting *tuaD*.	LNnT	5.41	Dong et al., 2020
C. glutamicum	Overexpressing *manB* and *manC*. Introducing *fucT2*, *gmd*, *wcaG*, and *lacY*.	2'-FL	8.1	Seo et al., 2018

Conclusion and Perspective

In recent years, more and more studies have been reported on different aspects of HMOs. There are many kinds of HMOs. To date, more than 200 types have been identified. Nevertheless, the discovery and identification of novel oligosaccharides is still a problem. The content of different types of HMOs varies greatly. Among which, the oligosaccharides with higher content such as 2'-FL has been clearly understood. Therefore, the future needs to clarify whether those oligosaccharides with lower content will play an unexpected role. This is also a common problem in the field of separation, purification and functional research of HMOs. Of course, the new functional investigation of well-studied HMOs are equally important.

Biosynthesis of HMOs has the advantages of green, safe and economical, which provides a great possibility for the wide application of HMOs in the future. At present, the problems that need to be studied or solved in biosynthesis of HMOs include the following aspects. (1) Mining and modification of enzymes to improve the production efficiency of HMOs in microorganisms or in vitro. (2) Try to take advantage of novel host with higher safety to produce HMOs, such as lactic acid bacteria. (3) Optimization of metabolic pathways in microorganisms, including the expression intensity of different genes in the product metabolic flow, and metabolic blocking of by-products. (4) Co-culture with other strains to overcome the problem of insufficient nucleotide substrate. (5) Simultaneous synthesis of multiple HMOs products to improve the conversion rate of substrates and the production efficiency of cell factories.

References

Austin, S., De Castro, C. A., Sprenger, N., Binia, A., Affolter, M., Garcia-Rodenas, C. L., Beauport, L., Tolsa, J. F., Fischer Fumeaux, C. J. (2019) Human Milk Oligosaccharides in the Milk of Mothers Delivering Term versus Preterm Infants. *Nutrients*. 11(6):1282.

Baumgärtner, F., Conrad, J., Sprenger, G. A., Albermann, C. (2014) Synthesis of the human milk oligosaccharide lacto-Ntetraose in metabolically engineered, plasmid-free E. coli. *ChemBioChem* 15 (13), 1896-1900.

Baumgärtner, F., Jurzitza, L., Conrad, J., Beifuss, U., Sprenger, G. A., Albermann, C. (2015) Synthesis of fucosylated lacto-Ntetraose using whole-cell biotransformation. *Bioorg. Med. Chem.* 23 (21), 6799-6806

Baumgärtner, F., Seitz, L., Sprenger, G. A., Albermann, C. (2013) Construction of Escherichia coli strains with chromosomally integrated expression cassettes for the synthesis of 2′-fucosyllactose. *Microb. Cell Fact.* 12, 40.

Baumgärtner, F., Sprenger, G. A., Albermann, C. (2015) Galactose-limited fed-batch cultivation of Escherichia coli for the production of lacto-N-tetraose. *Enzyme Microb. Technol.* 75-76, 37-43.

Bode, L. (2009) Human milk oligosaccharides: prebiotics and beyond. *Nutr. Rev.* 67 Suppl 2: S183-191.

Bode, L. (2012) Human milk oligosaccharides: Every baby needs a sugar mama. *Glycobiology.* 22: 1147-1162.

Bode, L., Contractor, N., Barile, D., Pohl, N., Prudden, A. R., Boons, G. J., Jin, Y. S., Jennewein, S. (2016) Overcoming the limited availability of human milk oligosaccharrides: challenges and opportunities for research and application. *Nutr. Rev.* 74: 635-644.

Bode, L., Jantscher-krenn, E. (2012) Structure-function relationships of human milk oligosaccharides. *Adv. Nutr.* 3(3): 383S-391S.

Bidart, G.N., Rodríguez-Díaz, J., Palomino-Schätzlein, M., Monedero, V., Yebra, M.J. (2017) Human milk and mucosal lacto-and galacto-N-biose synthesis by transgalactosylation and their prebiotic potential in Lactobacillus species. *Appl. Microbiol. Biotechnol.* 101: 205-215.

Chen, C., Zhang, Y., Xue, M., Liu, X., Li, Y., Chen, X., Wang, P., Wang, F., Cao, H. (2015) Sequential one-pot multienzyme （OPME） synthesis of lacto-N-neotetraose and its sialyl and fucosyl derivatives. *Chem. Commun.* 51: 7689-7692.

Chen, Q., Wu, H., Ji, M., Xie, Y., Li, S., Li, Y., Shi, J., Sun, J. (2020) Engineering a colanic acid biosynthesis pathway in E. coli for manufacturing 2′-fucosyllactose. *Process Biochem.* 94, 79-85.

Chin, Y. W., Kim, J. Y., Kim, J. H., Jung, S. M., Seo, J. H. (2017) Improved production of 2′-fucosyllactose in engineered Escherichia coli by expressing putative α-1,2-fucosyltransferase, WcfB from Bacteroides f ragilis. *J. Biotechnol.* 257, 192-198.

Chin, Y. W., Kim, J. Y., Lee, W. H., Seo, J. H. (2015) Enhanced production of 2′-fucosyllactose in engineered Escherichia coli BL21star(DE3) by modulation of lactose metabolism and fucosyltransferase. *J. Biotechnol.* 210, 107-115.

Chin, Y. W., Seo, N., Kim, J. H., Seo, J. H. (2016) *Metabolic engineering of Escherichia coli to produce 2′-fucosyllactose via salvage pathway of guanosine 5′-diphosphate (GDP)-l-fucose.*

Choi, Y. H., Park, B. S., Seo, J. H., and Kim, B. G. (2019) Biosynthesis of the human milk oligosaccharide 3-fucosyllactose in metabolically engineered Escherichia coli via the salvage pathway through increasing GTP synthesis and β-galactosidase modification. *Biotechnol. Bioeng.* 116 (12), 3324-3332.

Deng, J., Chen, C., Gu, Y., Lv, X., Liu, Y., Li, J., LedesmaAmaro, R., Du, G., Liu, L. (2019) Creating an in vivo bifunctional gene expression circuit through an aptamer-based regulatory mechanism for dynamic metabolic engineering in Bacillus subtilis. *Metab. Eng.* 55, 179-190.

Deng, J., Gu, L., Chen, T., Huang, H., Yin, X., Lv, X., Liu, Y., Li, N., Liu, Z., Li, J., Du, G., Liu, L. (2019) Engineering the Substrate Transport and Cofactor Regeneration

Systems for Enhancing 2′-Fucosyllactose Synthesis in Bacillus subtilis. *ACS Synth. Biol.* 8 (10), 2418-2427.

Dong, X., Li, N., Liu, Z., Lv, X., Li, J., Du, G., Wang, M., Liu, L. (2019) Modular pathway engineering of key precursor supply pathways for lacto-N-neotetraose production in Bacillus subtilis. *Biotechnol. Biofuels* 12 (1), 212.

Dong, X., Li, N., Liu, Z., Lv, X., Shen, Y., Li, J., Du, G., Wang, M., Liu, L. (2020) CRISPRi-Guided Multiplexed Fine-Tuning of Metabolic Flux for Enhanced Lacto-N-neotetraose Production in Bacillus subtilis. *J. Agric. Food Chem.* 68 (8), 2477-2484.

Drouillard, S., Driguez, H., Samain, E. (2006) Large-Scale Synthesis of H-Antigen Oligosaccharides by Expressing Helicobacter pylori α1,2-Fucosyltransferase in Metabolically Engineered Escherichia coli Cells. Angew. *Chem., Int. Ed.* 45 (11), 1778-1780.

Drouillard, S., Mine, T., Kajiwara, H., Yamamoto, T., Samain, E. (2010) Efficient synthesis of 6′-sialyllactose, 6,6′-disialyllactose, and 6′-KDO-lactose by metabolically engineered E. coli expressing a multifunctional sialyltransferase from the Photobacterium sp. JT-ISH-224. *Carbohydr. Res.* 345 (10), 1394-1399.

Dumon, C., Priem, B., Martin, S. L., Heyraud, A., Bosso, C., Samain, E. (2001) In vivo fucosylation of lacto-N-neotetraose and lacto-N-neohexaose by heterologous expression of Helicobacter pylori α-1,3 fucosyltransferase in engineered Escherichia coli. *Glycoconjugate* 18 (6), 465-474.

Dumon, C., Priem, B., Martin, S. L., Heyraud, A., Bosso, C., Samain E. (2001) In vivo fucosylation of lacto-N-neotetraose and lacto-N-neohexaose by heterologous expression of Helicobacter pylori alpha-1,3 fucosyltransferase in engineered Escherichia coli. *Glycoconj. J.* 18(6):465-74.

Dumon, C., Samain, E., Priem, B. (2004) Assessment of the Two Helicobacter pylori α-1,3-Fucosyltransferase Ortholog Genes for the Large-Scale Synthesis of LewisX Human Milk Oligosaccharides by Metabolically Engineered Escherichia coli. *Biotechnol. Prog.* 20, 412-419.

Endo, T., Koizumi, S., Tabata, K., Ozaki, A. (2000) Largescale production of CMP-NeuAc and sialylated oligosaccharides through bacterial coupling. *Appl. Microbiol. Biotechnol.* 53, 257-261.

Garrido, D., Barile, D., Mills, D. A. (2012) A molecular basis for bifidobacterial enrichment in the infant gastrointestinal tract. *Adv. Nutr.* 3(3): 415S-421S.

Goehring, K. C., Marriage, B. J., Oliver, J. S., Wilder, J. A., Barrett, E. G., Buck, R. H. (2016) Similar to those who are breastfed, infants fed a formula containing 2'-fucosyllactose have lower inflammatory cytokines in a randomized controlled trial. *J. Nutr.* 146(12): 2559-2566.

Guan, N., Shin, H. D., Long, L., Azadi, P., Chen, R. (2018) TCA cycle-powered synthesis of fucosylated oligosaccharides. *Glycobiology* 28 (7), 468-473.

Guo, Y., Jers, C., Meyer, A. S., Arnous, A., Li, H., Kirpekar, F., Mikkelsen, J. D. (2014) A Pasteurella multocida sialyltransferase displaying dual trans-sialidase activities for production of 3′-sialyl and 6′-sialyl glycans. *J. Biotechnol.* 170, 60-67.

Hoeflinger, J. L., Davis, S. R., Chow, J., Miller, M. J. (2015) In vitro impact of human milk oligosaccharides on Enterobacteriaceae growth. *J. Agric. Food Chem.* 63: 3295-3302.

Huang, D., Yang, K., Liu, J., Xu, Y., Wang, Y., Wang, R., Liu, B., Feng, L. (2017) Metabolic engineering of Escherichia coli for the production of 2′-fucosyllactose and 3-fucosyllactose through modular pathway enhancement. *Metab. Eng*. 41, 23-38.

Jost, T., Lacroix, C., Braegger, C., Chassard, C. (2015) Impact of human milk bacteria and oligosaccharides on neonatal gut microbiota establishment and gut health. *Nutr. Rev.* 73(7): 426-437.

Jung, S. M., Chin, Y. W., Lee, Y. G., Seo, J. H. (2019) Enhanced production of 2′-fucosyllactose from fucose by elimination of rhamnose isomerase and arabinose isomerase in engineered Escherichia coli. *Biotechnol. Bioeng*. 116 (9), 2412-2417.

Jung, S. M., Park, Y. C., and Seo, J. H. (2019) Production of 3-Fucosyllactose in Engineered Escherichia coli with α-1,3-Fucosyltransferase from Helicobacter pylori. *Biotechnol. J.* 14 (6), e1800498.

Kulinich, A., Liu, L. (2016) Human milk oligosaccharides: The role in the fine-tuning of innate immune responses. *Carbohydr. Res.* 432: 62-70.

Kuntz, S., Rudloff, S., Kunz, C. (2008) Oligosaccharides from human milk influence growth-related characteristics of intestinally transformed and non-transformed intestinal cells. *J. Nutr.* 99"462-471.

Lee, J. W., Kwak, S., Liu, J. J., Yu, S., Yun, E. J., Kim, D. H., Liu, C., Kim, K. H., Jin, Y. S. (2020) Enhanced 2′-Fucosyllactose production by engineered Saccharomyces cerevisiae using xylose as a co-substrate. *Metab. Eng*. 62, 322-329.

Lee, W. H., Pathanibul, P., Quarterman, J., Jo, J. H., Han, N. S., Miller, M. J., Jin, Y. S., Seo, J. H. (2012) Whole cell biosynthesis of a functional oligosaccharide, 2′-fucosyllactose, using engineered Escherichia coli. *Microb. Cell Fact.* 11, 48.

Liu, J. J., Kwak, S., Pathanibul, P., Lee, J. W., Yu, S., Yun, E. J., Lim, H., Kim, K. H., Jin, Y. S. (2018) Biosynthesis of a Functional Human Milk Oligosaccharide, 2′-Fucosyllactose, and l-Fucose Using Engineered Saccharomyces cerevisiae. *ACS Synth. Biol.* 7 (11), 2529-2536.

Liu, Y., Yan, Q., Ma, J., Yang, S., Li, T., Jiang, Z. (2020) Production of Lacto-N-triose II and Lacto-N-neotetraose from Chitin by a Novel β-N-Acetylhexosaminidase Expressed in Pichia pastoris. *ACS Sustainable Chem. Eng.* 8 (41), 15466-15474.

Lu, M., Mosleh, I., Abbaspourrad, A. (2021) Engineered Microbial Routes for Human Milk Oligosaccharides Synthesis. *ACS Synth. Biol.* 10(5):923-938.

Merighi, M., Mccoy, J. M., Heidtman, M. I. (2012) Biosynthesis of human milk oligosaccharides in engineered bacteria. *US Patent App.* US20120208181A1.

Michaelsen, K. (2007) Advance in our understanding of the biology of human milk and its effects on the offsprong. *J. Nutr.* 137:503-510.

Morrow, A. L., Ruiz-Palacios, G. M., Altaye, M., Jiang, X., Guerrero, M. L., Meinzen-Derr, J. K., Farkas, T., Chaturvedi, P., Pickering, L. K., Newburg, D. S. (2004) Human milk oligosaccharides are associated with protection against diarrhea in breast-fed infants. *J. Pediatr.* 145(3):297-303.

Newburg, D. S., Ruiz-Palacios, G. M., Morrow, A. L. (2005) Human milk glycans protect infants against enteric pathogens. *Annu. Rev. Nutr*. 25:37-58.

Ni, Z., Li, Z., Wu, J., Ge, Y., Liao, Y., Yuan, L., Chen, X., Yao, J. (2020) Multi-Path Optimization for Efficient Production of 2′-Fucosyllactose in an Engineered Escherichia coli C41 (DE3) Derivative. *Front. Bioeng. Biotechnol.* 8, 611900.

Ninonuevo, M. R., Park, Y., Yin, H., Zhang, J., Ward, R. E., Clowers, B. H., German, J. B., Freeman, S. L., Killeen, K., Grimm, R., Lebrilla, C. B. (2006) A strategy for annotating the human milk glycome. *J. Agric. Food Chem.* 54(20):7471-80.

Nokami, T., Hayashi, R., Saigusa, Y., Shimizu, A., Liu, C., Tony Mong, K., Yoshida, J. (2013) Automated solution-phase synthesis of oligosaccharides via iterative electrochemical assembly of thioglycosides. *Org. Lett.* 15:4520-4523.

Parkot, J., Huefner, E., Jennewein, S., Elling, L., Engels, L. (2017) Fucosyltransferases and their applications. *Patent* US9611285B2.

Parschat, K., Schreiber, S., Wartenberg, D., Engels, B., Jennewein, S. (2020) High-Titer De Novo Biosynthesis of the Predominant Human Milk Oligosaccharide 2′-Fucosyllactose from Sucrose in Escherichia coli. *ACS Synth. Biol.* 9 (10), 2784-2796.

Plante, O. J., Palmacci, E. R., Seeberger, P. H. (2001) Automated solid-phase synthesis of oligosaccharides. *Science.* 291:1523-1527.

Priem, B., Gilbert, M., Wakarchuk, W. W., Heyraud, A., Samain, E. (2002) A new fermentation process allows large-scale production of human milk oligosaccharides by metabolically engineered bacteria. *Glycobiology* 12 (4), 235-240.

Qin, H. M., Li, S., Zhang, Y. F., Wang, J. W., Li, J., Song, S., Lu, F., Li, Y. (2016) Multienzymatic cascade synthesis of fucosyloligosaccharide via a two-step fermentation strategy in Escherichia coli. *Biotechnol. Lett.* 38 (10), 1747-1752.

Rosano, G. L., Ceccarelli, E. A. (2014) Recombinant protein expression in Escherichia coli: advances and challenges. *Front. Microbiol.* 5:172.

Samuel, T. M., Binia, A., de Castro, C. A., Thakkar, S. K., Billeaud, C., Agosti, M., Al-Jashi, I., Costeira, M. J., Marchini, G., Martínez-Costa, C., Picaud, J. C., Stiris, T., Stoicescu, S. M., Vanpeé, M., Domellöf, M., Austin, S., Sprenger, N. (2019) Impact of maternal characteristics on human milk oligosaccharide composition over the first 4 months of lactation in a cohort of healthy European mothers. *Sci. Rep.* 9(1):11767.

Sela, D. A., Chapman, J., Adeuya, A., Kim, J. H., Chen, F., Whitehead, T. R., Lapidus, A., Rokhsar, D. S., Lebrilla, C. B., German, J. B., Price, N. P., Richardson, P. M., Mills, D. A. (2008) The genome sequence of Bifidobacterium longum subsp. infantis reveals adaptations for milk utilization within the infant microbiome. *Proc. Natl. Acad. Sci. U S A.* 105(48): 18964-18969.

Seo, J. H., Chin, Y. W., Jo, H. Y. (2018) Method of producing 2′-fucosyllactose using Corynebacterium glutamicum. *US Patent App.* US20180298389A1.

Seydametova, E., Yu, J., Shin, J., Park, Y., Kim, C., Kim, H., Yu, S. H., Park, Y., Kweon, D. H. (2019) Search for bacterial α1,2- fucosyltransferases for whole-cell biosynthesis of 2′-fucosyllactose in recombinant Escherichia coli. *Microbiol. Res.* 222, 35-42.

Thurl, S., Munzert, M., Henker, J., Boehm, G., Müller-Werner, B., Jelinek, J., Stahl, B. (2010) Variation of human milk oligosaccharides in relation to milk groups and lactational periods. *Br. J. Nutr.* 104(9):1261-71.

Totten, S. M., Zivkovic, A. M., Wu, S., Ngyuen, U., Freeman, S. L., Ruhaak, L. R., Darboe, M. K., German, J. B., Prentice, A. M., Lebrilla, C. B. (2012) Comprehensive profiles of human milk oligosaccharides yield highly sensitive and specific markers for determining secretor status in lactating mothers. *J. Proteome Res.* 11(12): 6124-6133.

Wang, B. (2009) Sialic acid is an essential nutrient for brain development and cognition. *Annu. Rev. Nutr.* 29:177-222.

Yang, D., Park, S. Y., Park, Y. S., Eun, H., Lee, S. Y. (2020) Metabolic Engineering of Escherichia coli for Natural Product Biosynthesis. *Trends Biotechnol.* 38(7):745-765.

Yu, J., Shin, J., Park, M., Seydametova, E., Jung, S. M., Seo, J. H., Kweon, D. H. (2018) Engineering of α-1,3-fucosyltransferases for production of 3-fucosyllactose in Escherichia coli. *Metab. Eng.* 48, 269-278.

Yu, S., Liu, J. J., Yun, E. J., Kwak, S., Kim, K. H., Jin, Y. S. (2018) Production of a human milk oligosaccharide 2′-fucosyllactose by metabolically engineered Saccharomyces cerevisiae. *Microb. Cell Fact.* 17, 101.

Chapter 11

Potential Applications of Postbiotics in Functional Foods and Their Effects on Human Health

Seyedeh Zahra Nasirifar
Amin Abbasi
Leila Mirmoghtadaie*
and Hedayat Hosseini
Department of Food Science and Technology,
National Nutrition and Food Technology Research Institute,
Faculty of Nutrition Science and Food Technology,
Shahid Beheshti University of Medical Sciences, Tehran, Iran

Abstract

According to the clinical research, there is a relationship among style of life, particularly food, diseases, and health status of humans. On this point, functional foods can be effective on humans' health and quality of life. Probiotics were consumed as functional compounds to improve health status of life. But probiotic bacterial cells must be survived in improper situation of food processes and digestive system to exert their effects on health. In addition of viable probiotic cells, the byproducts of non-viable microorganisms which is called postbiotics, have been reported to show biological activity in host. So, probiotics can successfully replace with postbiotics. They show immunomodulatory, antihypertensive, anti-inflammatory, antioxidative effects and growth prohibiting activity against abnormal cell duplication. The postbiotics,

* Corresponding Author's Email: mirmoghtadaie@sbmu.ac.ir.

In: Exploring Microbiotics in Health and Disease
Editor: Edward L. Stillman
ISBN: 978-8-89113-410-2

can be used in a wide range of functional food products such as the matrix of fermented and non-fermented foods. Therefore, the aim of this chapter was to approach the advantages of application of postbiotics as functional components in foods.

Keywords: functional foods, postbiotics, probiotics, shelf life, health status

Introduction

Recently, functional foods have attracted a lot of attention from consumers and businesses interested in foods with positive health effects. Probiotics and prebiotics also are classified as a type of functional componenets due to their confirmed positive impact on human health [1]. The most often employed bacterial genera in numerous functional foods include *Bifidobacterium*, *Lactobacillus*, *Pediococcus*, *Enterococcus*, *Streptococcus*, *Bacillus*, and *Escherichia* [2]. Probiotic bacteria that enter the body through food must be able to endure stomach and intestinal circumstances, as well as stick to the intestinal epithelium and colonize and achieve a suitable quantity there. In addition, bacteria's metabolites can be able to have a positive impact on human health. All these conditions are not always present in every individual. As a result, the definitions of "paraprobiotic" and "postbiotic" have changed the understanding of probiotics today. The use of live probiotic bacteria is limited by drawbacks including the inability of living microorganisms to maintain cell viability at the desired level due to numerous factors affecting their viability in the gastrointestinal tract, their potential to transfer antibiotic resistance genes to pathogenic bacteria, the risks of increasing acute inflammation, and mortality rates. Postbiotics, however, draw attention to their benefits, including being more readily generated on an industrial scale and being simple to store (Aydın 2022). Additionally, probiotics are live bacteria with concerns with dose uniformity and unpredictability. However, postbiotics are not connected to these issues. In addition to having a longer shelf life, postbiotics are also simple to transport, store, and maintain (probiotics require a lower storage temperature). In comparison to probiotics (excluding bacterial lysates), postbiotics' production method and quantitative control are faster and more accurate. Postbiotics are more secure than probiotics in terms of safety.

However, postbiotics are not related to these issues. Furthermore, to having a longer shelf life, postbiotics also have simple transportion, store, and maintenance (probiotics require a lower storage temperature). In comparison to probiotics (excluding bacterial lysates), postbiotics' production method and quantitative control are faster and more accurate. Postbiotics are more secure than probiotics in terms of safety. Furthermore, unlike probiotics, postbiotics avoid the issues of absorbing virulence factors as well as antibiotic resistance genes. Postbiotics protect against live bacteria in a child's early development since they have an underdeveloped and weak immune system, as well as a permeable intestinal barrier. Postbiotics are thought to be a viable alternative for therapeutic interventions for a variety of allergy illnesses due to their ability to improve immune system maturation by restoring the balance between Th1/Th2 mediated immunity (Kaur, Thukral et al. 2021). Therefore, researchers have focused on postbiotics, the metabolites of non-viable microorganisms that demonstrate biological activity in the host, in an effort to overcome these difficulties. In addition to their potential to prevent aberrant cell replication, postbiotics have demonstrated immunomodulatory, antihypertensive, anti-inflammatory, and antioxidative properties [3]. As a result, postbiotics have become a potentially effective replacement for probiotics in the creation of functional foods.

Functional Foods

The demand for functional foods has grown as people become more aware of the unique relationship between human health and food. As a result, developments in the food industry over the past few years have mostly concentrated on new scientific and technical methods for processing food and creating unique cuisines [4]. Foods nowadays are made not only to satisfy hunger and provide humans with the nutrients they require, but also to prevent diseases caused by inadequate nutrition and to improve both physical and mental health. According to the WHO and the FAO, a variety of dietary patterns and lifestyle choices are significant modifiable risk factors for the emergence of coronary heart disease, cancer, type 2 diabetes, obesity, osteoporosis, and periodontal disease. Functional foods are quite essential in this regard. The rising cost of healthcare, the continuous increase in life expectancy, and the desire of older people for better quality of life in their later years can all explain the rising demand for such foods [5]. Abedin, Chourasia [4] classified them as functional foods contain one or more bioactive components and have health-enhancing effects when added to a typical diet.

According to Ballini, Charitos [6] a unique feature of these foods is the fact that they have of several definition. An "official" definition of functional foods is, that it has a positive impact on one or more physiological functions in addition to its basic nutritional activity, such as enhancing general health and/or lowering the chance of developing disease. As a result, they are foods that provide health benefits in addition to nutritional value. Henry [7] mention that Any of the five methods described below can be used to functionally enhance a food product: (1) Removing a substance known to or suspected of having a negative impact upon consumption (such as an allergic protein). Boosting the concentration of a naturally occurring food ingredient to a level where it would produce the desired benefits (for instance, fortifying meals with a micronutrient to achieve a daily consumption greater than the advised daily intake). (3) Including a substance that isn't often included in most foods and isn't necessary a macronutrient or a micronutrient but has been demonstrated to have positive benefits (like a non-vitamin antioxidant or prebiotic fructans, for example). (4) Substituting a component, typically a macronutrient (fats), whose consumption is typically excessive with a component for which advantageous effects have been demonstrated (modified starch); (5) Increasing the bioavailability or stability of a component known to produce a functional effect or to lower the disease-risk potential of the food.

Table 1. The important probiotic strains [6]

Probiotic Bacteria		
Lactobacillaceae	***Bifidobacteriaceae***	**Others**
Lactobacillus acidophilus *Lactobacillus casei* *Lactobacillus crispatus* *Lactobacillus gasseri* *Lactobacillus helveticus* *Lactobacillus johnsonii* *Lactobacillus reuteri* *Lactobacillus rhamnosus* *Lactobacillus salivarius* *Lactobacillus plantarum subsp plantarum* *Lactobacillus faecium* *Lactobacillus mesenteroides*	*Bifidobacterium longum* *Bifidobacterium animalis* *Bifidobacterium breve* *Bifidobacterium infantis* *Bifidobacterium adolescentis* *Bifidobacterium lactis* *Bifidobacterium bifidum*	*Saccharomyces cerevisiae* *Saccharomyces boulardii* *Aspergillus niger* *Aspergillus oryzae* *Clostridium butyricum* *Escherichia coli*

Functional foods can be supplemented with vitamins, minerals, probiotics, prebiotics, and fibers. Probiotics are microorganisms that, when consumed in appropriate amounts, improve the health of the host. They are the subject of both academic research and business endeavors. Probiotic products are progressively increasing their market share, mostly in industrialized countries such as Europe, Japan, Australia, and the United States. Probiotic strains are incorporated or encapsulated in a variety of food products, including juices, yoghurts, cheeses, jams, biscuits, and food supplements [6].

Probiotics

FAO and WHO describe probiotics as viable microorganisms that, when consumed in adequate amounts, may benefit the host's health [6, 8]. *Lactobacillaceae* family, *Bifidobacteria* spp., and yeasts like *Saccharomyces boulardii* are the most probiotic species used in functional foods (dairy and nondairy).

The other lactic acid bacteria (LAB) that have positive effects on the gastrointestinal system include Lactobacillus, Lactococcus, Enterococcus, Carnobacterium, Propionibacterium, Streptococcus, Leuconostoc, Pediococcus, and Weissella. Most of our fundamental nutritional and therapeutic supplement needs could be met by probiotics, due to their essential functional qualities. Since most of them are regarded as having a qualified presumption of safety (QPS) or generally recognized as safe (GRAS) status, LAB are important industrial microorganisms that are used all over the world in a variety of industrial food fermentation, such as in the dairy, bakery, meat, legume, and beverage industries [4] because LABs can survive and produce metabolites in harsh environments.

Additionally, probiotics' anti-diabetic, anti-pathogenicity, anti-inflammatory, anti-obesity, anti-allergic, angiogenic, and anti-cancer characteristics have been documented. Further, probiotics could activate particular genes in localized host cells, activating, modifying, and controlling the host's immune response. They even influence the release of gastrointestinal hormones as part of the gut-brain axis and control brain activity through bidirectional neuronal communication [9]. They can create several physiologically active metabolites in addition to probiotic action, including reuterin, reutericyclin, gama aminobutyric acid (GABA), exopolysaccharides (EPSs), conjugated linoleic acid (CLA), and bacteriocins [10]. Polyphenols, bioactive peptides, beta-glucans, and the inulin type of fructans, fatty acids, and polyols are examples of the bioactive substances obtained from the substrate that are created during lactic acid fermentation. According to Abedin, Chourasia [4], these chemicals have a variety of potential health and nutritional advantages, such as increased food nutritional value and the ability to reduce intestinal infections, serum cholesterol levels, and even certain cancer. Furthermore, IBS patients typically have dysbiosis, which indicates that their gut balance is disrupted, and their microorganisms are fewer and less diverse. Probiotics, according to research, have the potential to be used as a treatment for IBS patients [11].

Postbiotics

The most common usage of the word "biotic" is in reference to a nutritional approach that benefits the gut flora. To maintain the host's health in the best possible condition, it also entails monitoring the effects of nutrition. The term "biotic," which is derived from the Greek word "biotikós," means "pertaining to life," and is used to describe the study of the bio-ecological community, which is primarily made up of living things and the physiological environments in which they live [12]. The term "postbiotic" refers to substances made by living bacteria or released after the lysis of bacteria. It is sometimes referred to as "metabiotic," "biogenic," or "metabolite/cell-free supernatant". Short-chain fatty acids (SCFA), peptides, organic acids, enzymes, teichoic acid, exopolysaccharides, muropeptides, cell surface proteins, and vitamins are some of these products [13-15]. Fermentation is the most prevalent source of postbiotics in both food and medicinal technologies. Another outstanding example of postbiotic fermentation is the rise in B vitamin concentration in wheat grains. The B group of vitamins are present in grains in significant amounts. These vitamins are frequently lost during milling or degraded during heat processing. Cereal fermentation and LAB pretreatment boost bacterial production, increasing the amount of vitamins B1, B2, B3, B9, B11, and B12 in the food. It may be a tactic to raise the amount of B vitamins in cereal products. *In vitro* levels of total lysine, protein fractions, sugars, soluble dietary fiber, and Ca, Fe, and Zn bioavailability were all significantly increased by LAB fermentation of cereals. Furthermore, antihypertensive angiotensin I converting enzyme (ACE)-inhibitory peptides, gama aminobutyric acid (GABA), and antioxidant peptides may be produced from wheat through LAB fermentation [16].

Postbiotics Health Beneficial

Postbiotics have systemic effects such as antioxidant, anticancer, antihypertensive, and hypocholesterolemic effects in addition to local effects on health such as antimicrobial, anti-inflammatory, and immune regulation [17-19]. A number of mechanisms, including enhanced epithelial barrier function, beneficial microbiota regulation, immune response modulation, systemic metabolism modulation, and nervous system signaling, are used by postbiotics to produce therapeutic effects [13, 20, 21]. By increasing the creation of tight junction proteins, which aid in preserving the integrity of the intestinal lining, postbiotics can enhance gut barrier performance. To stop dangerous compounds from entering the bloodstream, a strong intestinal barrier is necessary [22, 23]. Postbiotics are also used to keep food fresh longer. Also, they are a prospective substitute for antibiotics due to their strong antibacterial action. According to certain research, probiotics can move from the gut lumen, which may be premature, inflammatory, or leaky, to the bloodstream and then onto important organs, where they can cause systemic infections [24]. Postbiotics, on the other hand, have a considerable signaling potential with different tissues and organs, high stability, and are adequately absorbed and digested. Postbiotics can be utilized as a valuable antibacterial ingredient to stop food spoiling in the food industry due to their special qualities (shelf life up to 5 years, non-toxicity, easy transportation, and low-cost maintenance) [25, 26].

Postbiotics have potential for treating several medical diseases. Folate, for instance, is a vitamin that is known to be an antioxidant and plays a crucial role in the synthesis, methylation, and repair of DNA. Folate made in the intestines might therefore have an impact on the entire body. Higher levels of vitamin B12 and folate serum levels and a lower prevalence of anemia have been linked to the probiotic addition of Lactobacillus acidophilus to yogurt [12].

Streptococcus mutans, *Porphyromonas gingivalis*, *Fusobacterium nucleatum*, and *Aggregatibacter actinomycetemcomitans* were the oral pathogens against which Chen, Hsieh [28] tested the antibacterial activity of viable and heat-killed probiotic strains. Strong antipathogenic activity were shown by the probiotic strains *L. salivarius* subsp. *salicinius* AP-32, *L. rhamnosus* CT-53, *L. paracasei* ET-66, and *B. animalis* subsp. *lactis* CP-9, whereas heat-killed AP-32, CT-53, and ET-66 showed significant pathogen inhibition. The production of H_2O_2 was not linked to the antibacterial properties of 50 of these probiotics; *L. acidophilus* TYCA02 produced significant quantities of H_2O_2 but only had moderate antibacterial properties.

Probiotic oral pills, especially those with live probiotics, shown favorable inhibitory effects against oral infections. Insights into the antipathogenic efficacy of various probiotic species and their potential significance in functional foods that improve oral health are provided by their results, which show that probiotics inhibit the growth of oral pathogens and enhance oral health.

P. aculeata juice was employed as a carbon source in another work by Lara-Cervantes, Carrillo-Inungaray [29] to encourage the growth of two probiotic *Lactobacillus* strains during submerged fermentation. The Taguchi method using the orthogonal array L9 was used to improve the culture conditions. A kinetic culture monitoring some postbiotic features was used to validate the optimal treatment after evaluating the three-level variables of pH, agitation, and inoculum concentration. The amount of *L. plantarum* 14917 in the cells increased 1.76 times, and the main postbiotics produced were short-chain fatty acids such succinic, formic, acetic, propionic, and lactic acids, which are linked to probiotic metabolism and are crucial for human health. To the best of our knowledge, this study is the first to describe the valorization of *P. aculeata* juice as a substrate for probiotic strain growth, and additional research is needed to acquire additional uses in the manufacturing of functional foods.

Postbiotics Functional Foods

The application of postbiotics in functional foods is highly versatile. They can be incorporated into a wide range of food products, including dairy products, fermented vegetables, cereals, and beverages [30-32]. The incorporation of postbiotics not only enhances the nutritional value of these foods but also provides consumers with additional health benefits [33, 34].

The potential of postbiotics in the creation of functional foods has been investigated in a number of research [35, 36]. One study focused on the collagen-peptide microencapsulation of five probiotic strains to enhance bacterial protection under different conditions [37]. The researchers found that low-molecular-weight collagen-peptide improved the viability of probiotics after freeze-drying, simulated gastrointestinal conditions, and heat treatment. This finding suggests that postbiotics can enhance the stability and survival of probiotic bacteria in various food processing and digestion environments.

Another study looked at how *E. coli* Nissle 1917-produced postbiotics affected functional labneh that had been added galactooligosaccharides [38]. The cell surface and adhesive qualities of some probiotic strains were found to benefit from postbiotics, according to the researchers. This finding suggests that postbiotics can enhance the adhesion abilities of probiotics, potentially inhibiting the adhesion of foodborne pathogens to intestinal cells.

Furthermore, the production of postbiotics from yogurt cape gooseberry was found to significantly increase antimicrobial, anti-tumor, and antioxidant activities [39]. This study highlights the potential of postbiotics to enhance the functional properties of fermented foods, offering additional health benefits beyond the probiotic content. Similarly, the supplementation of red ginseng extract in a fermented medium led to immune-enhancing effects, including the production of immune-related cytokines and the enhancement of NK cell activity [40]. These findings demonstrate the potential of postbiotics to enhance the immune response in functional foods.

Numerous foods are naturally high in prebiotics or postbiotics or their precursors, such as acids, vitamins, and polyphenols [41, 42]. Classic postbiotic-rich diets include fermented foods like yogurt, sauerkraut, pickled vegetables, and kombucha. In nature, there are more than 4000 different flavonoids that can be obtained through diet. The majority of these phenolic substances are not absorbed in the gut. These polyphenols' intricate interactions with the intestinal flora produce microbial transformation products. It has been demonstrated that these compounds inhibit the growth of pathogenic strains of *Clostridium* spp., whereas the effects on commensal bacteria were either less severe or beneficial. In obese people, long-term tea polyphenol consumption was associated with a decrease in body weight. Bacteriodetes have a selective advantage over Firmicutes because they produce more of the glycosidases needed to break down polyphenols. Therefore, it has been proposed that the Firmicutes' restoration may lead to weight loss:Compared to their healthy peers, bacteria ratio [43].

Biopolymers, which are naturally occurring polymers made from plants, animals, or microorganisms, are one of the classes of postbiotics. Microorganisms make biopolymers as they expand, and these polymers can be discharged beyond the bacterial cell wall to form a heterogeneous collection of compounds known as EPS. Kefiran and dextran are two polymers from the kefir microflora that are part of this category. Kefir is made up of acid-lactic bacteria, yeasts, and 6 the primary exopolysaccharide of kefir grains. On the chemical level, this polysaccharide is a repetitive branched unit of hexa or hepta-saccharide, which is composed of a regular unit of pentasaccharides, in which one or two residues are randomly attached. It is composed equally of galactose and glucose, and it is responsible for binding the microorganisms in the kefir grains and keeping the microbiota attached to the matrix that will be multiplied. Kefiran cannot be absorbed since the digestive enzymes from the human gastrointestinal tract cannot hydrolyze it due to its chemical structure. However, microorganisms from the colon can ferment it. The presence of *Lactobacillus kefiranofaciens* and *Lactobacillus kefiri* in the grains, particularly the first one, which activates after 48 hours of cultivation, is associated to its production [44]. Traditional Mexican foods, such as those made from maize, agave varieties, nopal, and beans, have been identified as potential sources of synbiotics [45]. These fermented foods contain beneficial microorganisms, antioxidants, and short-chain fatty acids (SCFAs), all of which contribute to their functional properties. The utilization of these traditional foods as a source of postbiotics offers a unique opportunity to develop novel functional foods that combine the benefits of probiotics and prebiotics [46].

The Strategy of Adding Postbiotic to Functional Foods

To fully harness the potential of postbiotics in functional foods, researchers have explored various technological advancements [47]. The use of near-infrared spectroscopy (NIRS) as a trustworthy and quick substitute to conventional microbiology techniques for assessing probiotic viability is one such development [48, 49]. This non-destructive technique offers a promising approach to quickly and accurately assess the viability of probiotic supplements, ensuring their effectiveness in functional food products.

Encapsulation techniques have also been developed to protect postbiotics and enhance their delivery to the specific site within the gastrointestinal tract [50, 51]. Smart hydrogels and nanostructured platforms have shown potential in improving the viability and stability of postbiotics, ensuring their successful delivery to the target site [52, 53].

Aspect of Sensory Characteristics

One significant concern pertaining to the application of postbiotics in functional food processing revolves around their implementation for the aim of ensuring food safety and their impact on the sensory attributes of the end product. To mitigate fungal spoilage, Garnier et al. (2019) [54] included postbiotics derived from lactic acid bacteria into sour semi-hard cheese and cream during their taste study. Based on the findings of the research, it was seen that the use of postbiotics resulted in a reduction of the fungal population in cheese, while not affecting its sensory acceptability. However, it was noted that the use of postbiotics at levels of 2% and 5% (w/w) had an adverse effect on the sensory attributes of sour cream.

The sensory evaluation revealed that there was a notable increase in consumer acceptance of functional yoghurt that was enriched with cape gooseberry (*Physalis peruviana* L.) and contained postbiotics produced by *E. coli*. This increase in acceptance was observed across various sensory aspects, including appearance, sourness, mouthfeel, smoothness, and overall acceptance. The only characteristic of the product that exhibited a subpar contrast in comparison to the control sample was its colour [39].

In contrast, Ramos et al. (2022) [55] conducted the first investigation on *Leuconostoc* strains found in sheep's milk, focusing on their ability to produce postbiotic chemicals, including GABA, ornithine, tryptophan, and lactic acid. According to the authors' findings, several selected bacterial strains show potential as viable candidates for incorporation into functional dairy products.

Future Trends

It has been shown that non-viable bacterial compounds called postbiotics contain bioactivities such antibacterial, antioxidant, anti-inflammatory, and anti-proliferative [56]. They are created by microbes used in food or are released in complicated microbial cultures, food, or the intestine after cell lysis. Postbiotics have recently piqued the interest of scientists due to their potential application in pharmaceutical formulations and commercial food-based goods [57]. Postbiotics can be used as promising instruments in the food and pharmaceuticals industries to develop health benefits and therapeutic purposes since they are safer than their parent living cells, according to a review article that was published in 2022 [3]. Additionally, according to the same article, postbiotics might possess special qualities in terms of medical, technological, and financial aspects. The postbiotic market's present and future prospects with drugs that are now on the market are highlighted in another article that was released in 2023. The writers of this paper make various examples to illustrate the knowledge gaps and potential clinical uses.

They also examine the postbiotics market's recent and projected trends. In conclusion, because of their bioactivities, postbiotics have demonstrated significant promise for application in functional foods. The use of postbiotics in pharmaceutical formulations and commercial food-based products for health promotion, illness prevention, and complementary medicine is predicted to continue in the future. To completely comprehend the mechanisms of action of postbiotics and their potential uses in a variety of disciplines, more research is necessary.

Conclusion

In conclusion, postbiotics offer a promising avenue for the development of functional foods with enhanced health benefits. Their immunomodulatory, antihypertensive, anti-inflammatory, antioxidative, and anti-cancer properties make them valuable components in the matrix of fermented and non-fermented foods. The application of postbiotics in functional foods has the potential to improve human health and contribute to a better quality of life. It is becoming clearer and clearer how useful postbiotics can be in functional diets. Postbiotics present a possible alternative to probiotics in the creation of functional food items due to their capacity to increase the stability and survival of probiotic bacteria as well as their own biological activity [58]. The possibilities for incorporating these advantageous substances into functional foods are further expanded by improvements in encapsulation methods and the investigation of traditional foods as a source of postbiotics. The subject of functional foods is set for additional innovation and development as research into the advantages of postbiotics continues.

References

[1] Lemos Junior, W. J. F., Guerra, A. F., Tarrah, A., da Silva Duarte, V., Giacomini, A., Luchese, R. H., and Corich, V. (2020). Safety and stability of two potentially probiotic lactobacillus strains after *in vitro* gastrointestinal transit. *Probiotics and antimicrobial proteins*, 12, 657-66.

[2] Tarrah, A. (2022). Probiotics, prebiotics, and their application in the production of functional foods. *MDPI*, p. 154.

[3] Sabahi, S., Rad., H. A., Aghebati-Maleki, L., Sangtarash, N., Ozma, M. A., Karimi, A, Hosseini, H., and Abbasi, A. (2022). Postbiotics as the new frontier in food and pharmaceutical research. *Critical Reviews in Food Science and Nutrition*, 1-28.

[4] Abedin, M. M., Chourasia, R., Phukon, L. C., Sarkar, P., Ray, R. C., Singh, S. P., and Rai, A. K. (2023). Lactic acid bacteria in the functional food industry: Biotechnological properties and potential applications. *Critical Reviews in Food Science and Nutrition*, 1-19.

[5] Betoret, E., Betoret, N., Vidal, D., and Fito, P. (2011). Functional foods development: Trends and technologies. *Trends in Food Science & Technology*, 22(9), 498-508.

[6] Ballini, A., Charitos, I. A., Cantore, S., Topi, S., Bottalico, L., and Santacroce, L. (2023). About Functional Foods: The Probiotics and Prebiotics State of Art. *Antibiotics*, 12(4), 635.

[7] Henry, C. (2010). Functional foods. *European Journal of Clinical Nutrition*, 64(7), 657-9.

[8] Harald, B. (2019). Probiotics and prebiotics in clinical tests: an update. *F1000Research*, 8.

[9] Leeuwendaal, N. K., Stanton, C., O'Toole, P. W., and Beresford, T. P. (2022). Fermented foods, health and the gut microbiome. *Nutrients*, 14(7), 1527.

[10] Chourasia, R., Abedin, M. M., Chiring Phukon, L., Sahoo, D., Singh, S. P., and Rai, A. K. (2021). Biotechnological approaches for the production of designer cheese with improved functionality. *Comprehensive Reviews in Food Science and Food Safety*, 20(1), 960-79.

[11] Song, M. W., Kim, K. T., and Paik, H. D. (2023). Probiotics as a functional health supplement in infant formulas for the improvement of intestinal microflora and immunity. *Food Reviews International*, 39(2), 858-74.

[12] Kaur, S., Thukral, S. K., Kaur, P., and Samota, M. K. (2021). Perturbations associated with hungry gut microbiome and postbiotic perspectives to strengthen the microbiome health. *Future Foods*, 4, 100043.

[13] Aydın, B. (2022). Postbiotics And Paraprobiotics: A New Trend For Functional Foods.

[14] Rad, A. H., Abbasi, A., Kafil, H. S., and Ganbarov, K. (2020). Potential pharmaceutical and food applications of postbiotics: a review. *Current pharmaceutical biotechnology*, 21(15), 1576-87.

[15] Rad, A. H., Maleki, L. A., Kafil, H. S., Zavoshti, H. F., and Abbasi, A. (2020). Postbiotics as novel health-promoting ingredients in functional foods. *Health promotion perspectives*, 10(1), 3-4.

[16] Tomasik, P., and Tomasik, P. (2020). Probiotics, non-dairy prebiotics and postbiotics in nutrition. *Applied Sciences*, 10(4), 1470.

[17] Abbasi, A., Sabahi, S., Bazzaz, S., Tajani, A. G., Lahouty, M., Aslani, R., and Hosseini, H. (2023). An edible coating utilizing Malva sylvestris seed polysaccharide mucilage and postbiotic from Saccharomyces cerevisiae var. boulardii for the preservation of lamb meat. *International Journal of Biological Macromolecules*, 246, 125660.

[18] Abbasi, A., Sanej, K. D., Moradi, S., Bazzaz, S., Esmaeili, A., Ghafourian, K., Sabahi., S., Lahouty., M., Akrami., S., Aslani., R., and Hosseini., H. (2023). Bioactive Compounds and Biological Activities of *Allium sativum L. Bioactive Compounds in the Storage Organs of Plants*: Springer, p. 1-40.

[19] Abbasi, A., Bazzaz, S., Da Cruz, A. G., Khorshidian, N., Saadat, Y. R., Sabahi, S., Ozma, M. A., Lahouty, M., Aslani, R., and Mortazavian, A. M. (2023). A Critical Review on Akkermansia muciniphila: Functional Mechanisms, Technological Challenges, and Safety Issues. *Probiotics and Antimicrobial Proteins*, 1-23.

[20] Hosseini, H., Abbasi, A., Sabahi, S., Akrami, S., and Yousefi-Avarvand, A. (2023). Assessing the Potential Biological Activities of Postbiotics Derived from Saccharomyces cerevisiae: An *In Vitro* Study. *Probiotics and Antimicrobial Proteins*, 1-17.

[21] Abbasi, A., Aghebati-Maleki, A., Yousefi, M., and Aghebati-Maleki, L. (2021). Probiotic intervention as a potential therapeutic for managing gestational disorders and improving pregnancy outcomes. *Journal of reproductive immunology*, 143, 103244.

[22] KIVANÇ, M. (2023). Postbiotics and Their Application in Food and Nutrition: A Perspective. *Food Science & Applied Microbiology Reports*, 2(2), 55-7.

[23] Ozma, M. A., Moaddab, S. R., Hosseini, H., Khodadadi, E., Ghotaslou, R., Asgharzadeh, M., Abbasi, A., Kamounah, F. S., Maleki, L. A., Ganbarov, K., and Kafil, H. S. (2023). A critical review of novel antibiotic resistance prevention approaches with a focus on postbiotics. *Critical Reviews in Food Science and Nutrition*, 1-19.

[24] Rad, A. H., Maleki, L. A., Kafil, H. S., Zavoshti, H. F., and Abbasi, A. (2021). Postbiotics as promising tools for cancer adjuvant therapy. *Advanced Pharmaceutical Bulletin*, 11(1), 1.

[25] Rad, A., Aghebati-Maleki, L., Kafil, H., Gilani, N., Abbasi, A., and Khani, N. (2021). Postbiotics, as dynamic biomolecules, and their promising role in promoting food safety. *Biointerface Res Appl Chem*, 11, 14529–14544.

[26] Sheykhsaran, E., Abbasi, A., Ebrahimzadeh Leylabadlo, H., Sadeghi, J., Mehri, S., Naeimi Mazraeh, F., Feizi, H., and Bannazadeh Baghi, H. (2023). Gut microbiota and obesity: an overview of microbiota to microbial-based therapies. *Postgraduate medical journal*, 99(1171), 384-402.

[27] Yeşilyurt, N., Yılmaz, B., Ağagündüz, D., and Capasso, R. (2021). Involvement of probiotics and postbiotics in the immune system modulation. *Biologics*, 1(2), 89-110.

[28] Chen, Y. T., Hsieh, P. S., Ho, H. H., Hsieh, S. H., Kuo, Y. W., Yang, S. F., and Lin, C. W. (2020). Antibacterial activity of viable and heat-killed probiotic strains against oral pathogens. *Letters in applied microbiology*, 70(4), 310-7.

[29] Lara-Cervantes, T. d. J., Carrillo-Inungaray, M. L., Balderas-Hernández, V. E., Aguilar-Zárate, P., and Veana, F. (2022). Valorization of Parmentiera aculeata juice in growth of probiotics in submerged culture and their postbiotic production: A first approach to healthy foods. *Archives of Microbiology*, 204(11), 679.

[30] Ozma, M. A., Abbasi, A., Akrami, S., Lahouty, M., Shahbazi, N., Ganbarov, K., et al. (2022). Postbiotics as the key mediators of the gut microbiota-host interactions. *Le infezioni in medicina*, 30(2), 180.

[31] Homayouni-rad, A., Aghebati-Maleki, L., Samadi-Kafil, H., Abbasi, A., and Khani, N. (2021). Postbiotics as a safe alternative to live probiotic bacteria in the food and pharmaceutical industries. *HBI_Journals*, 26, 132-57.

[32] Homayouni Rad, A., Aghebati Maleki, L., Samadi Kafil, H., and Abbasi, A. (2021). Postbiotics: A novel strategy in food allergy treatment. *Critical reviews in food science and nutrition*, 61(3), 492-9.

[33] Salmerón, I. (2017). Fermented cereal beverages: From probiotic, prebiotic and synbiotic towards Nanoscience designed healthy drinks. Letters in applied microbiology, 65(2), 114-24.

[34] Abbasi, A., Bazzaz, S., Ibrahim, S, A., Hekmatdoost, A., Hosseini, H., Sabahi, S., Sheykhsaran, E., Saadat, Y. R., Ozma, M. A., and Lahouty, M. (2023). A Critical Review on the Gluten-Induced Enteropathy/Celiac Disease: Gluten-Targeted Dietary and Non-Dietary Therapeutic Approaches. *Food Reviews International*, 1-41.

[35] Rad, A. H., Aghebati-Maleki, L., Kafil, H. S., and Abbasi, A. (2021). Molecular mechanisms of postbiotics in colorectal cancer prevention and treatment. *Critical reviews in food science and nutrition*, 61(11), 1787-803.

[36] Abbasi, A., Sheykhsaran, E., and Kafil, H. S. (2021). Postbiotics: science, technology and applications: Bentham Science Publishers.

[37] Kim, S. I., Kim, J. W., Kim, K. T., and Kang, C. H. (2021). Survivability of Collagen-Peptide Microencapsulated Lactic Acid Bacteria during Storage and Simulated Gastrointestinal Conditions. *Fermentation*, 7(3), 177.

[38] Khojah, E., Gomaa, M. S., Elsherbiny, E. G., Elawady, A., and Darwish, M. S. (2022). The *In Vitro* Analysis of Postbiotics in Functional Labneh to Be Used as Powerful Tool to Improve Cell Surfaces Properties and Adherence Potential of Probiotic Strains. *Fermentation*, 8(3), 122.

[39] Darwish, M. S., Qiu, L., Taher, M. A., Zaki, A. A., Abou-Zeid, N. A., Dawood, D. H., Shalabi, O. M. A. K., Khojah, E., and Elawady, A. A. (2022). Health benefits of postbiotics produced by E. coli Nissle 1917 in functional yogurt enriched with cape gooseberry (Physalis peruviana L.). *Fermentation*, 8(3), 128.

[40] Mo, S. J., Nam, B., Bae, C. H., Park, S. D., Shim, J. J., and Lee, J. L. (2021). Characterization of novel Lactobacillus paracasei HY7017 capable of improving physiological properties and immune enhancing effects using red ginseng extract. *Fermentation*, 7(4), 238.

[41] Abbasi, A., Rad, A. H., Maleki, L. A., Kafil, H. S., and Baghbanzadeh, A. (2023). Antigenotoxicity and Cytotoxic Potentials of Cell-Free Supernatants Derived from Saccharomyces cerevisiae var. boulardii on HT-29 Human Colon Cancer Cell Lines. *Probiotics and Antimicrobial Proteins*, 1-13.

[42] Sabahi, S., Mortazavi, S. A., Nassiri, M., Ghazvini, K., Shahidi, F., and Abbasi, A. (2022). Production of functional ice cream fortified by immunoglobulin Y against Escherichia coli O157: H7 and Helicobacter pylori. *Biointerface Research in Applied Chemistry*, 13(2), 188-98.

[43] Chaluvadi, S., Hotchkiss, A. T., and Yam, K. L. (2015). Gut microbiota: Impact of probiotics, prebiotics, synbiotics, pharmabiotics, and postbiotics on human health. *Probiotics, prebiotics, and synbiotics: Bioactive foods in health promotion*: Elsevier Inc., 515-23.

[44] de Lima Barros, S. É., dos Santos Rocha, C., de Moura, M. S. B., Barcelos, M. P., and da Silva Hage-Melim, L. I. (2021). Potential beneficial effects of kefir and its postbiotic, kefiran, on child food allergy. *Food & Function*, 12(9), 3770-86.

[45] Torres-Maravilla, E., Méndez-Trujillo, V., Hernández-Delgado, N. C., Bermúdez-Humarán, L. G., and Reyes-Pavón, D. (2022). Looking inside mexican traditional food as sources of synbiotics for developing novel functional products. *Fermentation*, 8(3), 123.

[46] Hernández-Granados, M. J., and Franco-Robles, E. (2020). Postbiotics in human health: Possible new functional ingredients? *Food Research International*, 137, 109660.

[47] Abbasi, A., Rad, A. H., Ghasempour, Z., Sabahi, S., Kafil, H. S., Hasannezhad, P., Saadat, Y. R., and, Shahbazi, N. (2022). The biological activities of postbiotics in gastrointestinal disorders. *Critical Reviews in Food Science and Nutrition*, 62(22), 5983-6004.

[48] Aguinaga, Bósquez, J. P., Oğuz, E., Cebeci, A., Majadi, M., Kiskó, G., Gillay, Z., and Kovacs, Z. (2022). Characterization and viability prediction of commercial probiotic supplements under temperature and concentration conditioning factors by NIR spectroscopy. *Fermentation*, 8(2), 66.

[49] Abbasi, A., Aghebati-Maleki, L., and Homayouni-Rad, A. (2022). The promising biological role of postbiotics derived from probiotic Lactobacillus species in reproductive health. *Critical Reviews in Food Science and Nutrition*, 62(32), 8829-41.

[50] Garcia-Brand, A. J., Quezada, V., Gonzalez-Melo, C., Bolaños-Barbosa, A. D., Cruz, J. C., and Reyes, L. H. (2022). Novel developments on stimuli-responsive probiotic encapsulates: from smart hydrogels to nanostructured platforms. *Fermentation*, 8(3), 117.

[51] Abbasi, A., Saadat, T. R., and Saadat, Y. R. (2022). Microbial exopolysaccharides–β-glucans–as promising postbiotic candidates in vaccine adjuvants. *International Journal of Biological Macromolecules*.

[52] Sabahi, S., Abbasi, A., and Mortazavi, S. A. (2022). Characterization of cinnamon essential oil and its application in Malva sylvestris seed mucilage edible coating to the enhancement of the microbiological, physicochemical and sensory properties of lamb meat during storage. *Journal of Applied Microbiology*, 133(2), 488-502.

[53] Abbasi, A., Hajipour, N., Hasannezhad, P., Baghbanzadeh, A., and Aghebati-Maleki, L. (2022). Potential *in vivo* delivery routes of postbiotics. *Critical Reviews in Food Science and Nutrition*, 62(12), 3345-69.

[54] Garnier, L., Mounier, J., Lê, S., Pawtowski, A., Pinon, N., Camier, B., et al. (2019). Development of antifungal ingredients for dairy products: From *in vitro* screening to pilot scale application. *Food microbiology*, 81, 97-107.

[55] Ramos, I. M., Rodríguez-Sánchez, S., Seseña, S., Palop, M. L., and Poveda, J. M. (2022). Assessment of safety characteristics, postbiotic potential, and technological stress response of Leuconostoc strains from different origins for their use in the production of functional dairy foods. *LWT*, 165, 113722.

[56] Ozma, M. A., Abbasi, A., and Sabahi, S. (2022). Characterization of postbiotics derived from Lactobacillus paracasei ATCC 55544 and its application in Malva

sylvestris seed mucilage edible coating to the improvement of the microbiological, and sensory properties of lamb meat during storage. *Biointerface Res Appl Chem*, 13.

[57] Abbasi, A., Rad, A. H., Maleki, L. A., Kafil, H. S., and Baghbanzadeh, A. (2022). Cytotoxic Potentials of Cell-Free Supernatant Derived from Lactobacillus casei CRL431 on HCT-116 and HT-29 Human Colon Cancer Cell Lines.

[58] Abbasi, A., Sanej, K. D., Mohammadi, A., Moradi, S., Nayeri, B. D., Bazzaz, S., and Hosseini, H. The Role of Postbiotics in Food Safety Promotion.

Chapter 12

Functional Action Mechanisms of Postbiotics in Food Allergies

Mohammad Rastegarpour
Amin Abbasi
Fahimeh Ebrahimi
Mohammad Sina*
and Hedayat Hosseini
Department of Food Science and Technology,
National Nutrition and Food Technology Research Institute,
Faculty of Nutrition Science and Food Technology,
Shahid Beheshti University of Medical Sciences, Tehran, Iran

Abstract

The prevalence and severity of food allergy clinical manifestations have increased over the last two decades. In most cases, food allergies can be associated with a breakdown in the immune system's tolerance responses. Scientists have discovered that a significant increase in the incidence of food allergies is associated with changes in gut microbes' composition and function. Specific metabolic byproducts of the probiotics called postbiotics have been identified during investigations on appropriate probiotic strains. Postbiotics, due to their unique characteristics (safe profile, longer shelf life, resistance to mammalian enzymes, and stability in digestive system conditions), may have safety superiority against their parent live cells, and as a novel strategy, they can be applied for improved immune tolerance and the treatment of food

* Corresponding Author's Email: mohamadsina1996@gmail.com.

In: Exploring Microbiotics in Health and Disease
Editor: Edward L. Stillman
ISBN: 978-8-89113-410-2

allergies without any undesirable side-effects or human opportunistic infections, particularly in infants and pediatrics. In this chapter, we discuss the therapeutic benefits of different postbiotic compounds for the therapy of food allergies in light of the numerous publications demonstrating the high biological function and safety of postbiotics.

Keywords: food allergy, immune system, postbiotics, gut microbes

Introduction

Food allergy is a frequent immunological disorder originating from a breakdown of immune tolerance, defined by an unfavorable immune reaction to ingested food proteins [1, 2]. More than 170 foods have been identified as causing food allergies, and the majority of the more severe reactions may be linked to consumption of fish, shellfish, peanuts, milk, tree nuts, soy, wheat, seeds, and eggs, which may vary depending on the individual, national, and geographical context [3]. The main risk factors for the emergence of food allergies are linked to genetics, the environment, and how those variables combine to impair immunological tolerance. However, there is mounting evidence that the population and make-up of the gut microbiota play a significant role in the maturation of the immune system and are crucial in controlling reactions to food allergies. Therefore, early-life gut microbiota eubiosis may have an impact on the emergence of food allergies [2]. Additionally, studies have shown a substantial correlation between the gut microbiota's variety and composition and a person's lifestyle, including their choice of delivery method (vaginal vs. cesarean section), method of baby feeding (formula vs. nursing), birth order, usage of antibiotics, and diet (low fiber/high fat) [1]. In the community of gut microbes that are linked to disease, dysbiosis is often defined as an imbalance. Intestinal barrier degradation and increased intestinal permeability are frequently associated with gut microbiota dysbiosis, which increases the likelihood that allergens will enter the bloodstream and cause allergic sensitization. As a result, microbiome therapy may help to prevent or lessen food allergies [1]. Preclinical and clinical research from recent years has demonstrated that probiotics significantly affect food allergies by fostering immunological tolerance [2]. The innate immune system is primarily responsible for these probiotics' positive effects. Several mechanisms contribute to the probiotics' functionality, including: 1) encouraging immune cells to secrete regulatory cytokines; 2) improving gut

IgA responses; 3) interacting with intestinal cells and controlling gut permeability and mucus thickness; 4) stimulating the production of sIgA and beta-defensins; and 5) regulating gut microbiota population and function [2]. The volume of probiotic cells, the kind of probiotic carrier, and the microbial species or strains from which they generate postbiotics all have a significant impact on the effectiveness of probiotics. In this sense, both their viable (probiotic) and particularly their non-viable metabolites and/or byproducts (postbiotic) might be associated with the health-promoting effects of gut-beneficial bacteria [2, 4]. This chapter discussed new findings about the involvement of the gut microbiota in food allergies and the use of postbiotics as a preventative measure.

Main Mechanism of Food Allergy

Atopic diseases, which include food allergies, can be roughly categorized as IgE-mediated, mixed, and non-IgE-mediated. And the most well-studied form is IgE-mediated food allergy [5], which is mostly covered in this chapter. For general health, the immune system has to be able to differentiate between harmful environmental antigens and pathogenic ones. Food antigens reach the subepithelium after digestion in the digestive system to cause immunological tolerance or an allergic reaction with the help of the appropriate immune cells. Immune-tolerant or healthy people typically do not react to dietary protein antigens that are typically harmless [1]. When exposed to several common food allergens, patients with a history of food allergies are more likely to experience an inappropriate inflammatory immune response and a breakdown of oral tolerance to food antigens. Potential food antigens can be captured from the gut lumen through two main pathways, the paracellular pathway and the transcellular pathway, when they are transferred to the intestinal barrier. Gut-associated lymphoid tissue (GALT) plays a key role in immune tolerance, with a series of immune cells involved in this process. For instance, goblet cells (GCs) produce goblet cell-associated antigen passages (GAPs) to convey luminal antigens to CD103+ dendritic cells (DCs). Furthermore, M cell-mediated transcytosis enables CD103+ DCs to capture antigens. Sometimes, CD103+ DCs can extend a process through an M cell's transcellular pore or do periscope activity to get antigens directly from the lumen. Additionally, soluble antigens can pass through IECs through both the paracellular channel and the transcellular pathway, and food antigens are taken up by macrophages and given to CD103+ DCs [6–8]. Major Histocompatibility Complex (MHC) class II molecules on CD103+ DCs surfaces convey antigens to naïve T lymphocytes after CD103+ DCs pick up antigens and move to mesenteric lymph nodes (MLNs) [1].

A type of DC called CD103+ made transforming growth factor (TGF) and retinoic acid (RA), which turned naive T cells into regulatory cells (Tregs) that were specific to the antigen and expressed the FOXP3 protein. Additionally, retinoic acid can increase the expression of integrin in Tregs, which causes them to migrate to the gut and support immune system activity. The enzyme indoleamine 2, 3-dioxygenase (IDO), which is made by CD103+ DCs, changes tryptophan into kynurenines. This causes Treg differentiation. Additionally, macrophages can activate type 3 innate lymphocytes (ILC3) to produce granulocyte-macrophage colony stimulating factor (GM-CSF), which can start the oral tolerance established by CD103+ DCs, in order to directly convey food antigens to CD103+ DCs. Additionally, it appears that macrophages release interleukin-10 (IL-10), which encourages the growth of Tregs that have moved from the MLN to the intestinal lamina propria and generates significant levels of IL-10 and TGF, therefore establishing or sustaining oral tolerance [1].

Modulation of Food Allergy by the Gut Microbiome

Given the interaction between the immune system and the gut microbiome, it is conceivable that variables impacting the microbiome's composition and function might be used to indirectly lower the risk of developing food allergies. The consensus opinion, supported by the available research, is that probiotics can alter the makeup of the gut microbiota and its metabolites, enhancing intestinal barrier performance and modulating immune responses to avoid the development of food allergies. Surprisingly, prebiotics, synbiotics, and postbiotics could also be the catalyst for the onset of remission from food allergies. Probiotics, prebiotics, synbiotics, and postbiotics all have distinct effects and workings in the prevention and treatment of food allergies. Understanding their possible impact and underlying processes will help create a new food allergy management strategy [1].

Mechanisms of Gut Microbiota in Food Allergy Regulation

The Role of Microorganisms in the Development of Food Allergies

There is mounting evidence that changes in the makeup of the gut microbiota have a role in the etiology of food allergies [1]. Low-diversity microbiota or opportunistic pathogens can disrupt the IEC barrier, which can cause uncontrolled translocation of food antigens, particular pathogens, and pathogen-associated molecular patterns into the intestinal mucosa [9]. Additionally, dysbiosis and certain opportunistic infections may cause dietary antigens to partially breakdown, resulting in immunogenic peptides that cross the mucosal barrier more effectively than non-partially digested antigens [10, 11].

Gut Microbiota's Impact on Food Allergies

Food allergies were controlled by the gut microbiota in three different ways, including: 1) the impact of the gut microbiota on the performance of the mucosal barrier; 2) the gut microbiota's impact on immunity; and 3) the impact of metabolites from the gut microbiome on food allergies [12].

The Impact of Gut Microbiota on the Performance of the Mucosal

There are several things that can make the gut mucosal barrier less strong: the epithelium not being able to repair the barrier well, coming into contact with substances that weaken the barrier, epithelial inflammation, opportunistic pathogen colonization, microbial dysbiosis, and less biodiversity [13, 14]. Multiple studies have shown that barrier disruption plays a role in the development of food allergies. For instance, it has been shown that individuals with allergic proctitis had thinner mucus gel layers in their rectal mucosa, but mucus recovered after avoiding dietary allergens, indicating that allergens are what cause mucus depletion [1, 15].

Gut Microbiota's Impact on Immunity

By controlling type 2 immunity, fostering immunological maturation and tolerance, and influencing basophil population regulation, the gut microbiota affects a person's vulnerability to food allergies.. Basophils upregulate blood IgE levels, which causes an exaggerated reaction to food allergens [1, 16, 17].

The Impact of Metabolites from the Gut Microbiome on Food Allergies

Microbial metabolites acted as a second layer of communication between the commensal microbes and the host in the meanwhile. Numerous studies have shown that microbial metabolism, including SCFAs and tryptophan derivatives, can directly modify mucosal immune function and improve intestinal barrier integrity, which in turn affects an individual's propensity for food sensitivity [18, 19]. The central gut microbiota produces compounds called SCFAs that have immunomodulatory characteristics [20, 21]. Numerous investigations revealed that compared to healthy non-allergic controls, food allergy sufferers had considerably lower SCFAs concentrations [22, 23]. Benefits of SCFAs and hypothesized pathways for preventing food allergies have recently been postulated. SCFAs may stimulate the production of Reg3 and beta-defensin via activating the mTOR/STAT3 pathway through G protein-coupled receptors, such as GPR41, GPR43, and GPR109a [24]. One of the necessary amino acids is tryptophan. Numerous bacterial species, such as *Escherichia coli*, *Clostridium*, *Bacteroides*, *Peptostreptococcus*, *Eubacterium*, and *Lactobacillus* species, as well as *Ruminococcus gnavus*, may catabolize around 4–6% of tryptophan into indole and its metabolites [1]. Numerous studies have shown how tryptophan metabolites from the microbiota support the development of the immune system and preservation of barrier function, primarily through activating the aryl hydrocarbon receptor (AhR) [25, 26]. These bioactive metabolites are comprehensively discussed in the next section.

Postbiotics: Novel and Promising Tool in Biomedical

Postbiotics are soluble substances that come from probiotic cells and include cell corpses, cell components, cell-wall fractions, cellular secretions, and metabolites [27]. If consumed in large enough quantities, postbiotics can have beneficial effects on the host's health [28]. Additionally, postbiotics demonstrate how probiotic bacteria exert therapeutic benefits after passing through gastrointestinal defense barriers and supporting the health effects of their metabolites [29]. The word "postbiotic," on the other hand, refers to soluble metabolites produced by live bacteria or liberated from their structure upon lysis [30]. These byproducts give the host increased biological activity and certain physiological consequences. The two primary mechanisms by which intestinal microbiomes affect health are as follows: the probiotics-dependent crucial pathway, which depends on the microbiome's vitality, and the postbiotics-dependent novel pathway, which depends on non-living microbiome products [31, 32]. Examples of soluble postbiotics generated by probiotic species include short-chain fatty acids (SCFAs), teichoic acids, enzymes, peptidoglycans formed from muropeptides, peptides, exo-polysaccharides, vitamins, plasmalogens, cell surface proteins, and organic acids [33].

Classification of Postbiotics

The essential compositions of the postbiotic components may be used to categorize them, including lipids (butyrate, propionate, acetate, lactate, and dimethyl acetyl-derived plasmalogen), organic acids (propionic and 3-phenyllactic acid), proteins (lactocepin, p40, and p75 molecules (soluble proteins), carbohydrates (galactose-rich polysaccharides and teichoic acids), complex molecules (lipoteichoic acids and peptidoglycan-derived muropeptides), and vitamins (B-group vitamins) or through their biological activities such as antioxidant, antihypertensive, immunomodulatory, anti-inflammatory, hypocholesterolemic, and antiproliferative effects [33, 34].

Safety of Postbiotics

The findings of the studies showed that probiotics have health-promoting effects on postbiotics, but that eating items with live probiotics isn't always safe. In this context, an *ex vivo* investigation found that some probiotic bacteria trigger localized inflammatory responses that are comparable to those brought on by *Salmonella spp*. Live probiotic bacteria found in food and medicine have also been linked to some side effects, such as gastrointestinal problems (bloating, dysbiosis of the gut microbiome, and transmission of the gene for antibiotic resistance between gut microbiomes) and a weakened immune system[35]. After intestinal absorption, these substances' distinctive chemical structures allow them to communicate with many tissues and cells in the host, which is one of their possible mechanisms for establishing and sustaining homeostasis. Postbiotics' beneficial effects on food allergies are one of their therapeutic uses in food and nutrition [33]. A food allergy is an immune system condition that significantly lowers a patient's quality of life. Evidence suggests that a number of postbiotic metabolites, including short-chain fatty acids, have a significant effect on easing the symptoms of food allergies. These postbiotics increase immune cell responses in the host, lowering the host's vulnerability to benign antigens [33].

Functional Action Mechanisms of Postbiotics in Food Allergies

The results of studies show that allergic illnesses like food allergies are solely related to the host's gut microbiota because inflammatory reactions take place on the epidermal barrier. The gut microbiota plays important roles in the digestive process and defense against the invasion of harmful microbes [36]. Additionally, it is the primary complex of biomolecules originating from microorganisms that has significant potential to support epithelial barrier function and trigger a suitable immune response. The makeup of the gut microbiota can be altered by a number of factors, including genetics, environment, nutrition, psychological stress, using medications, infections, well-being, and lifestyle. However, when a person has dysbiosis in their digestive system, the predominant microbial population in the intestine shifts in favor of pathogenic microorganisms. As a result, the host's health is negatively impacted by the growth of this microbial population, its occupation of epithelial cell surfaces, and the production of secondary metabolites like toxins. In this regard, the presence of substances like SCFAs (butyrate, acetate, and lactate) and bacteriocins is credited with being the most significant antibacterial mechanism of postbiotics [37]. The capacity of postbiotics to limit the bioavailability of oxygen in the intestinal lumen is another key mechanism in this regard. Following frequent usage, these substances interact with host eukaryotic cells, modify immune system activity, and activate the pertinent signaling pathways to promote gastrointestinal homeostasis [38]. Additionally, they have the capacity to prevent allergic sensitization, reduce food allergen accessibility to the systemic circulation, support the integrity of epithelial cells, and communicate with immune cells (dendritic cells and macrophages) via both direct and indirect mechanisms of action.

The unique functions of gut-associated lymphoid tissues (GALT), mucosal immune cells such as Th1, Th2, and Th17 cells, antimicrobial peptides such as defensins, secretory IgA, and gut commensal microbes and their byproducts (postbiotics) are what primarily create and maintain gastrointestinal homeostasis.. The use of postbiotic components is regarded as a unique strategy to preserve the integrity of the epithelial barrier and enhance its activities [39]. In this context, the primary postbiotic processes identified in *in vitro* and *in vivo* research comprise: 1) activation of genes encoding components of tight junctions; 2) activating transcription factors like STAT3 and SP1 to assemble proteins; 3) increase in transepithelial electrical resistance in Caco-2 and T84 human colonic cells; 4) using intestinal epithelial cells (IECs) to produce antimicrobial peptides (AMPs); and 5) restoring the function of the epithelial barrier in inflammatory diseases such as inflammatory bowel disease (IBD). In addition, the colonic Lamina Propria (LP) was stimulated by the colonization of allergy-protective commensal bacteria (Clostridia) and their metabolites (SCFAs) to produce the barrier-protective cytokine IL-22. By modifying the mucus release from goblet cells and the formation of AMPs by paneth cells, IL-22 production increased epithelial barrier effectiveness. These IL-22-related functional responses significantly diminish allergy sensitization and the accessibility of food antigens to the host's systemic circulation. The activation of the host immune cells to induce non-responsiveness to non-offensive antigens by SCFAs, notably butyrate, contributes to protection against the development of FA, according to preclinical and clinical studies.

In order to stimulate intestinal dendritic cells and macrophages to produce IL-10 and regulate the development of Tregs (source of tolerogenic cytokines) in the mesenteric lymph nodes, postbiotic SCFAs have been shown to give colonocytes energy and attach to G protein-coupled receptors (GPRs) (expressed in the apical membrane of colonocytes, enterocytes, and immune cells) [40]. This suppresses allergic and inflammatory reactions. In order to protect gut homeostasis from excessive inflammation, a lipoteichoic acid (LTA) postbiotic may be a useful strategy. LTA affects cytokine-mediated immune responses. Through a TLR-2-affiliated mechanism, the LTA postbiotics generated from Lactobacillus plantarum block the NF-jB and Mitogen-Activated Protein Kinase (MAPK) signaling pathways in *in vitro* settings (HT-29 cells) by downregulating TNF-a-driven inflammatory cytokine production. Functionality of postbiotics in FA therapy is mediated by many key pathways, including: 1) inhibiting Histone Deacetylase (HDAC) to control Treg activity; 2) capacity of GPRs, primarily GPR43 and GPR109A, to signal 3) as the primary energy source for intestinal epithelial cells; 4) the DNA methylation rate is decreased while the production of the cytokines IL-10 and IFN-c is stimulated. Notably, the effectiveness of postbiotics is largely influenced by the parent microbial strains, the choice of various preparation techniques, the presence of a wide range of bioactive molecules, dosage, and the choice of suitable delivery mechanisms (pharmaceutical orfunctional food) [41].

As a result, the scientific literature now available supports the use of postbiotic components as a novel technique to enhance immunological tolerance and treat food allergies without causing any unfavorable side effects or human opportunistic infections, especially in babies and pediatrics [2, 42]. EVs of *Bifidobacterium longum* KACC 91563 were found to specifically bind and induce mast cell apoptosis without affecting the T-cell-mediated immune response, according to some studies of the effectiveness of postbiotics in animal models of food allergies.. For instance, injection of family 5 extracellular solute-binding protein, the main component of EVs, has the ability to reduce the number of mast cells and the occurrence of diarrhea in a food allergy mouse model [43]. Food allergies may be treated with *Bifidobacterium longum* KACC 91563. In a related investigation, oral treatment of bacterial lysates decreased allergen-specific IgE and IgG levels while increasing IL-10 levels and improving intestinal permeability in rats with OVA sensitization. Additionally, in infants with a family history of atopic reactions disease, non-hydrolyzed fermented infant formula with heat-killed *Bifidobacterium breve* C50 and *Streptococcus thermophilus* 065 reduced the risk of developing anaphylaxis during the first few months of life and after this formula was discontinued. Additionally, it has been demonstrated that SCFA, a byproduct of microbial fermentation, favorably influences food allergies.. Mice with a lack of the SCFA receptors GPR43 or GPR109A experienced worse allergy responses and had fewer CD103+ DCs [1].

Interestingly, OIT+ butyrate may limit cow's milk protein-induced basophil activation, impair acute allergic skin, and cause reactivity and mast cell degranulation, with increasing Treg-mediated BMMC inhibition [44]. Although there is no concrete proof that postbiotics other than those mentioned above can be engaged in the efficient relief of food allergies, mechanically speaking, they have a great deal of potential to influence the emergence of food allergies through their numerous physiological roles. For instance, the health advantages of SLPs include improving probiotic life and adherence to IECs, maintaining intestinal barrier integrity, and controlling immune cell activities [45, 46]. Postbiotics are currently being used extensively in a variety of sectors, including cancer, obesity, colitis, intestine repair, immunological modulation, and many more. Future research on postbiotic therapies may prove to be interesting. Despite encouraging results from human and animal studies, there is presently insufficient data to support the prophylactic or therapeutic use of postbiotics in the treatment of food allergies. Therefore, more research is required to describe novel postbiotics, investigate their roles in the prevention and treatment of food allergies, and determinethe right dosage and frequency of administration [1, 47] (Figure 1).

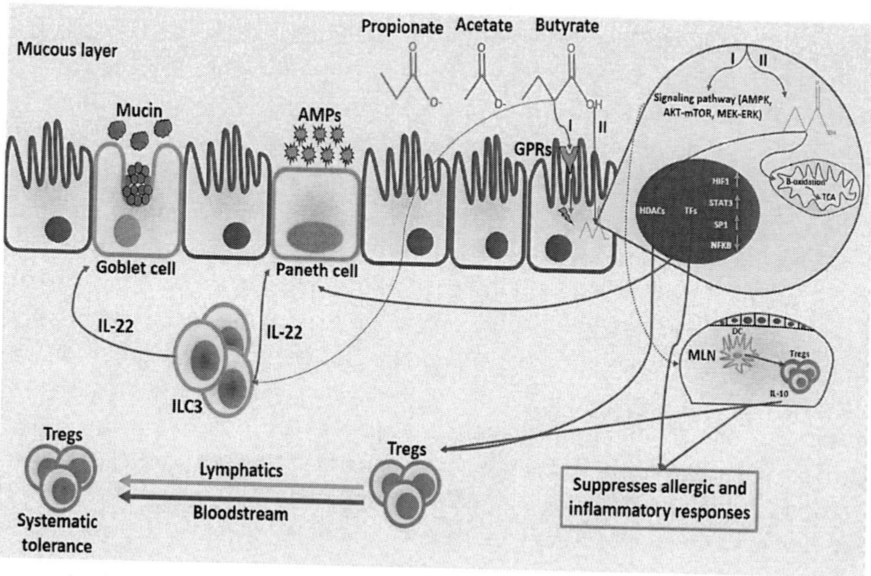

Figure 1. A function gut epithelial barrier in association with postbiotics is necessary for protection versus allergic sensitization. In healthy people, allergy-protective commensal microbes and their metabolites (SCFAs) preserve gut epithelial barrier integrity via driving ILC3s to generate IL-22. This response (IL-22) stimulates the generation of AMPs from Paneth cells and mucus from goblet cells and also diminishes the capability of diet allergens to obtain access to the systemic circulation. Postbiotics, particularly SCFAs, straightly stimulate Treg development and circulating Tregs develop systemic tolerance. On the other hand, in colonocytes, butyrate (one of the best known SCFAs) is β-oxidized to Acetyl-CoA and establishes the significant source of energy by log-in the TCA cycle. Besides, butyrate initiates triggering/suppression signaling pathway via GPRs and/or straightly suppresses HDACs, therefore up-regulating (HIF-1, STAT3 and SP1) or down-regulating (NF-κB) transcription factors (TFs), which lead to the improvement of gut epithelial barrier efficacy, AMPs generation, and reduce inflammation. GPRs, G-protein coupled receptors; AMP, antimicrobial peptide; ILC3, type 3 innate lymphoid cell; Treg, regulatory T cell; DC, dendritic cell; MLN, mesenteric lymph node; HDACs, histone deacetylase; TFs, transcription factors; TCA, tricarboxylic acid.

Conclusion

The occurrence and severity of food allergy clinical signs have significantly increased, according to the results of these studies. Currently, no definitive cure or disease-modifying treatment for food allergies has been confirmed by national or international food drug regulatory authorities. There is now clear evidence of the fundamental protective role of the intestinal microbiota and its metabolites (postbiotics) in food allergies. A key role in immunological development is played by the population and composition of the gut microbiota, which also affects food allergy responses. Gut bacteria, which are associated with a significant increase in food allergies across the United States, will be affected by changes in living conditions and dietary structure, as well as the abuse of antibiotics. To date, postbiotic therapy has been extensively implemented in a variety of areas, including inflammation control, intestine reconstruction, obesity, colitis, asthma, pregnancy neurodevelopment, and cancer. Postbiotics, due to their unique properties (chemical structures, safe profile, longer shelf life, resistance to mammalian enzymes, and stability to digestive system conditions), may be safer than their living parent cells and may be used as a novel strategy to improve immune tolerance and treat food allergies. They can represent a promising target for the prevention and treatment of food allergies. Although promising clinical and animal studies have been conducted, there is still a lack of solid evidence to support the preventive or therapeutic role of postbiotics in food allergies. Therefore, further studies of novel postbiotic substances are needed to assess their effect on the prevention and treatment of food allergies. To determine the correct dose and optimum frequency of administration of postbiotic supplements, it is also necessary to conduct clinical studies.

References

[1] Shi, J., Wang, Y., Cheng, L., Wang, J., and Raghavan, V. (2022). Gut microbiome modulation by probiotics, prebiotics, synbiotics and postbiotics: A novel strategy in food allergy prevention and treatment. *Critical Reviews in Food Science and Nutrition*, 1-17.

[2] Homayouni Rad, A., Aghebati, Maleki, L., Samadi, Kafil, H., and Abbasi, A. (2021). Postbiotics: A novel strategy in food allergy treatment. *Critical reviews in food science and nutrition*, 61(3), 492-9.

[3] Abbasi, A., Bazzaz, S., Ibrahim, S. A., Hekmatdoost, A., Hosseini, H., Sabahi, S., Sheykhsaran, E., Saadat, Y. R., Ozma, M. A., and Lahouty, M. (2023). A Critical

Review on the Gluten-Induced Enteropathy/Celiac Disease: Gluten-Targeted Dietary and Non-Dietary Therapeutic Approaches. *Food Reviews International*, 1-41.

[4] Abbasi, A., Rad, A. H., Maleki, L. A., Kafil, H. S., and Baghbanzadeh, A. (2023). Antigenotoxicity and Cytotoxic Potentials of Cell-Free Supernatants Derived from Saccharomyces cerevisiae var. boulardii on HT-29 Human Colon Cancer Cell Lines. *Probiotics and Antimicrobial Proteins*, 1-13.

[5] Yu, W., Freeland, D. M. H., and Nadeau, K. C. (2016). Food allergy: immune mechanisms, diagnosis and immunotherapy. *Nature Reviews Immunology*, 16(12), 751-65.

[6] Kobayashi, A., Donaldson, D. S., Erridge, C., Kanaya, T., Williams, I. R., Ohno, H., Mahajan, A., and Mabbott, N. A. (2013). The functional maturation of M cells is dramatically reduced in the Peyer's patches of aged mice. *Mucosal immunology.*, 6(5), 1027-37.

[7] Perrier, C., and Corthesy, B. (2011). Gut permeability and food allergies. *Clinical & Experimental Allergy.*, 41(1), 20-8.

[8] Satitsuksanoa, P., Jansen, K., Głobińska, A., Van de Veen, W., and Akdis, M. (2018). Regulatory immune mechanisms in tolerance to food allergy. *Frontiers in immunology.*, 9, 2939.

[9] Tan, J., McKenzie, C., Vuillermin, P. J., Goverse, G., Vinuesa, C. G., Mebius, R. E., Macia, L., and Mackay, C. R. (2016). Dietary fiber and bacterial SCFA enhance oral tolerance and protect against food allergy through diverse cellular pathways. *Cell reports.*, 15(12), 2809-24.

[10] Caminero, A., Galipeau, H. J., McCarville, J. L., Johnston, C. W., Bernier, S. P., Russell, A. K., et al. (2016). Duodenal bacteria from patients with celiac disease and healthy subjects distinctly affect gluten breakdown and immunogenicity. *Gastroenterology.*, 151(4), 670-83.

[11] Abbasi, A., Aghebati-Maleki, L., and Homayouni-Rad, A. (2022). The promising biological role of postbiotics derived from probiotic Lactobacillus species in reproductive health. *Critical Reviews in Food Science and Nutrition.*, 62(32), 8829-41.

[12] Lee, K. H., Song, Y., Wu, W., Yu, K., and Zhang, G. (2020). The gut microbiota, environmental factors, and links to the development of food allergy. *Clinical and Molecular Allergy.*, 18(1), 1-11.

[13] Akdis, C. A. (2021). Does the epithelial barrier hypothesis explain the increase in allergy, autoimmunity and other chronic conditions? *Nature Reviews Immunology.*, 21(11), 739-51.

[14] Di Tommaso, N., Gasbarrini, A., and Ponziani, F. R. (2021). Intestinal barrier in human health and disease. *International journal of environmental research and public health.*, 18(23), 12836.

[15] Abbasi, A., Saadat, T. R., and Saadat, Y. R. (2022). Microbial exopolysaccharides–β-glucans–as promising postbiotic candidates in vaccine adjuvants. *International Journal of Biological Macromolecules.*

[16] Sabahi, S., Abbasi, A., and Mortazavi, S. A. (2022). Characterization of cinnamon essential oil and its application in Malva sylvestris seed mucilage edible coating to

the enhancement of the microbiological, physicochemical and sensory properties of lamb meat during storage. *Journal of Applied Microbiology*., 133(2), 488-502.

[17] Abbasi, A., Rad, A. H., Ghasempour, Z., Sabahi, S., Kafil, H. S., Hasannezhad, P., Saadat, Y. R., and Shahbazi, N. (2022). The biological activities of postbiotics in gastrointestinal disorders. *Critical Reviews in Food Science and Nutrition*., 62(22), 5983-6004.

[18] Caminero, A., Meisel, M., Jabri, B., and Verdu, E. F. (2019). Mechanisms by which gut microorganisms influence food sensitivities. *Nature Reviews Gastroenterology & Hepatology*., 16(1), 7-18.

[19] Hamer, H. M., Jonkers, D., Venema, K., Vanhoutvin, S., Troost, F., and Brummer, R. J. (2008). The role of butyrate on colonic function. *Alimentary pharmacology & therapeutics*., 27(2), 104-19.

[20] Luu, M., Monning, H., and Visekruna, A. (2020). Exploring the molecular mechanisms underlying the protective effects of microbial SCFAs on intestinal tolerance and food allergy. *Frontiers in immunology*., 11, 1225.

[21] Ozma, M. A., Abbasi, A., Ahangarzadeh, Rezaee, M., Hosseini, H., Hosseinzadeh, N., Sabahi, S, et al. (2022). A critical review on the nutritional and medicinal profiles of garlic's (*Allium sativum* L.) bioactive compounds. *Food Reviews International*., 1-38.

[22] Gio-Batta, M., Spetz, K., Barman, M., Bråbäck, L., Norin, E., Björkstén, B., Wold, A. E., and Sandin, A. (2022). Low concentration of fecal valeric acid at 1 year of age is linked with eczema and food allergy at 13 years of age: findings from a Swedish birth cohort. *International Archives of Allergy and Immunology*., 183(4), 398-408.

[23] Goldberg, M. R., Mor, H., Magid, Neriya, D., Magzal, F., Muller, E., Appel, M. Y., et al. (2020). Microbial signature in IgE-mediated food allergies. *Genome Medicine*., 12, 1-18.

[24] Seo, K., Seo, J., Yeun, J., Choi, H., Kim, Y. I., and Chang, S. Y. (2021). The role of mucosal barriers in human gut health. *Archives of Pharmacal Research*., 44(4), 325-41.

[25] Muku, G. E., Murray, I. A., and Perdew, G. H. (2019). Activation of the Ah receptor modulates gastrointestinal homeostasis and the intestinal microbiome. *Current Pharmacology Reports*., 5, 319-31.

[26] Yu, M., Wang, Q., Ma, Y., Li, L., Yu, K., Zhang, Z., et al. (2018). Aryl hydrocarbon receptor activation modulates intestinal epithelial barrier function by maintaining tight junction integrity. *International journal of biological sciences*., 14(1), 69.

[27] Ozma, M. A., Abbasi, A., and Sabahi, S. (2022). Characterization of postbiotics derived from Lactobacillus paracasei ATCC 55544 and its application in Malva sylvestris seed mucilage edible coating to the improvement of the microbiological, and sensory properties of lamb meat during storage. *Biointerface Res Appl Chem*., 13.

[28] Abbasi, A., Sanej, K. D., Moradi, S., Bazzaz, S., Esmaeili, A., Ghafourian, K., et al. (2023). Bioactive Compounds and Biological Activities of *Allium sativum* L. *Bioactive Compounds in the Storage Organs of Plants*: Springer. p. 1-40.

[29] Abbasi, A., Sabahi, S., Bazzaz, S., Tajani, A. G., Lahouty, M., Aslani, R., et al. (2023). An edible coating utilizing Malva sylvestris seed polysaccharide mucilage and postbiotic from Saccharomyces cerevisiae var. boulardii for the preservation of lamb meat. *International Journal of Biological Macromolecules*., 246, 125660.

[30] Abbasi, A., Bazzaz, S., Da Cruz, A. G., Khorshidian, N., Saadat, Y. R., Sabahi, S., Ozma, M. A., Lahouty, M., Aslani, R., and Mortazavian, A. M. (2023). A Critical Review on Akkermansia muciniphila: Functional Mechanisms, Technological Challenges, and Safety Issues. *Probiotics and Antimicrobial Proteins*., 1-23.

[31] Hosseini, H., Abbasi, A., Sabahi, S., Akrami, S., and Yousefi-Avarvand, A. (2023). Assessing the Potential Biological Activities of Postbiotics Derived from Saccharomyces cerevisiae: An *In Vitro* Study. *Probiotics and Antimicrobial Proteins*., 1-17.

[32] Abbasi, A., Rad, A. H., Maleki, L. A., Kafil, H. S., and Baghbanzadeh, A. (2022). Cytotoxic Potentials of Cell-Free Supernatant Derived from Lactobacillus casei CRL431 on HCT-116 and HT-29 Human Colon Cancer Cell Lines.

[33] Sabahi, S., Homayouni Rad, A., Aghebati-Maleki, L., Sangtarash, N., Ozma, M. A., Karimi, A., Hosseini, H., and Abbasi, A. (2022). Postbiotics as the new frontier in food and pharmaceutical research. *Critical Reviews in Food Science and Nutrition*., 1-28.

[34] Ozma, M. A., Moaddab, S. R., Hosseini, H., Khodadadi, E., Ghotaslou, R., Asgharzadeh, M., et al. (2023). A critical review of novel antibiotic resistance prevention approaches with a focus on postbiotics. *Critical Reviews in Food Science and Nutrition*., 1-19.

[35] Abbasi, A., Hajipour, N., Hasannezhad, P., Baghbanzadeh, A., and Aghebati-Maleki, L. (2022). Potential *in vivo* delivery routes of postbiotics. *Critical Reviews in Food Science and Nutrition*., 62(12), 3345-69.

[36] Ozma, MA., Abbasi, A., Akrami, S., Lahouty, M., Shahbazi, N., Ganbarov, K., et al. (2022). Postbiotics as the key mediators of the gut microbiota-host interactions. *Le infezioni in medicina*., 30(2), 180.

[37] Homayouni-rad, A., Aghebati-Maleki, L., Samadi-Kafil, H., Abbasi, A., and Khani, N. (2021). Postbiotics as a safe alternative to live probiotic bacteria in the food and pharmaceutical industries. *HBI_Journals*., 26, 132-57.

[38] Rad, A. H., Aghebati-Maleki, L., Kafil, H. S., and Abbasi, A. (2021). Molecular mechanisms of postbiotics in colorectal cancer prevention and treatment. *Critical reviews in food science and nutrition*., 61(11), 1787-803.

[39] Abbasi, A., Sheykhsaran, E., and Kafil, H. S. (2021). Postbiotics: science, technology and applications: Bentham Science Publishers.

[40] Abbasi, A., Aghebati-Maleki, A., Yousefi, M., and Aghebati-Maleki, L. (2021). Probiotic intervention as a potential therapeutic for managing gestational disorders and improving pregnancy outcomes. *Journal of reproductive immunology*., 143, 103244.

[41] Rad, A. H., Maleki, L. A., Kafil, H. S., Zavoshti, H. F., and Abbasi, A. (2021). Postbiotics as promising tools for cancer adjuvant therapy. *Advanced Pharmaceutical Bulletin*., 11(1), 1.

[42] Rad, A. H., Abbasi, A., Kafil, H. S., and Ganbarov, K. (2020). Potential pharmaceutical and food applications of postbiotics: a review. *Current pharmaceutical biotechnology*., 21(15), 1576-87.

[43] Kim, J. H., Jeun, E. J., Hong, C. P., Kim, S. H., Jang, M. S., Lee, E. J., et al. (2016). Extracellular vesicle–derived protein from Bifidobacterium longum alleviates food allergy through mast cell suppression. *Journal of Allergy and Clinical Immunology*., 137(2), 507-16. e8.

[44] Vonk, M. M., Blokhuis, B. R., Diks, M. A., Wagenaar, L., Smit, J. J., Pieters, R. H., et al. (2019). Butyrate enhances desensitization induced by oral immunotherapy in cow's milk allergic mice. *Mediators of Inflammation*., 2019.

[45] Shao, H., Min, F., Huang, M., Wang, Z., Bai, T., Lin, M., Li, X., and Chen, H. (2022). Novel perspective on the regulation of food allergy by probiotic: The potential of its structural components. *Critical Reviews in Food Science and Nutrition*., 1-15.

[46] Abbasi, A., Sanej, K. D., Mohammadi, A., Moradi, S., Nayeri, B. D., Bazzaz, S., and Hosseini, H. The Role of Postbiotics in Food Safety Promotion.

[47] Rad, A. H., Maleki, L. A., Kafil, H. S., Zavoshti, H. F., and Abbasi, A. (2020). Postbiotics as novel health-promoting ingredients in functional foods. *Health promotion perspectives*., 10(1), 3-4.

Chapter 13

Postbiotics as Novel Bio-Preservation Strategies in the Food Industry

Mohammad Sina[1], MSc
Amin Abbasi[1], PhD
Anahita Ghorbani Tajani[2], PhD
Mohammad Rastegarpour[1,*], MSc
and Hedayat Hosseini[1,†], PhD
[1]Department of Food Science and Technology,
National Nutrition and Food Technology Research Institute,
Faculty of Nutrition Science and Food Technology,
Shahid Beheshti University of Medical Sciences, Tehran, Iran
[2]Department of Animal Science, University of Wyoming, Laramie, Wyoming, USA

Abstract

The utilization of probiotics and prebiotics for modifying gut microbiota has grown significantly over the past years. The identification and determination of new biologically active molecules called postbiotics have been made possible by advances in laboratory techniques. Postbiotics refer to substances that are secreted by microorganisms via their metabolic activity and affect the host directly or indirectly. The advantages and disadvantages of postbiotics have been discussed over the last few years, as well as their potential to be a replacement for other biologic agents. Their employment as bio-preservatives is one of their novel biocompatible applications. To inhibit the growth of spoilage and

---

* Corresponding Author's Email: hedayat@sbmu.ac.ir.
† Corresponding Author's Email: mohamad.rastegarpour@gmail.com.

In: Exploring Microbiotics in Health and Disease
Editor: Edward L. Stillman
ISBN: 978-8-89113-410-2

pathogenic organisms in food matrices, a postbiotic-based bio-preservation approach can be considered. It is a biological approach that aims at minimizing the use of chemical additives in foods. A review of the most recent applications of postbiotics for food bio-preservation and maintenance their microbial safety status, current challenges, and future perspectives is provided in this chapter.

Keywords: bio-preservatives, food safety, food packaging, postbiotics

Introduction

Food plays an essential role in life, providing vital nutrients that support growth and health. People are increasingly linking healthy foods with lower levels of additives or chemical substances called "clean label" products [1], and this awareness highlights the significance of studying natural substances in order to ensure food safety and satisfy consumer demand for a healthier diet. Antimicrobial agents are chemical or natural substances that can enhance safety and prolong the shelf life of food commodities by eliminating foodborne pathogens and spoilage organisms and/or inhibiting their growth [2, 3]. These agents comprise substances prepared from different sources. In particular, because of its natural and renewable nature, antimicrobial agents of microbial origin have gained more credibility over the years. For the production of antimicrobial agents, various microorganisms have been used as a source. Among them, probiotics are particularly important due to their ability to alter human and food microbiota in addition to their known health benefits and lower infection risk [4]. Incompatibility with the variety of matrices and environmental conditions that are hindering their growth and survival in foods is an essential challenge to use Live starter/probiotic cultures directly on food. Probiotics are capable of producing a number of metabolites called "Postbiotics" that can inhibit the growth of other organisms. As an alternative, the negative interactions between primary and secondary starters and food can be avoided by using postbiotics [5, 6]. For example, in terms of food safety and quality, antimicrobial agents of lactic acid bacteria, such as nisin, which is considered a bacteriocin, are of significant importance to the industry [7, 8]. Thus, the broad-spectrum antimicrobial activity of postbiotics, synergistic activities between organic acids and other metabolites as well as their high heat stability are fully exploited by using them instead of living microorganisms [9]. Due to its specific chemical composition, safety, ease of use and storage and stability in the broad range of pH and temperature, along with a wide spectrum of antibiotic activity, postbiotics have been recognized as superior to probiotics for industry applications [10]. This chapter provides an overview on how postbiotics can be used to bio-preserve and package a variety of foods as an accessible and effective strategy.

Bio-Preservatives

In ancient times people used salt, drying and smoking in order to preserve their food. New methods of preservation including packaging, freezing and the addition of chemicals have been developed over time. Nevertheless, these methods can cause a loss of nutrients and natural taste as well as health risks. To overcome these constraints, advanced techniques are being explored for the preservation of food quality and texture. Bio-preservation is one of these methods, which has been shown to be very effective in maintaining safety and preservation of the quality of food with low loss of nutrients and flavor [11]. Bio-preservatives improve the quality and safety of foodstuffs by adding antimicrobial substances derived from natural sources or produced through fermentation. These additives originate from natural microorganism, plants, animals and their metabolites are environmentally friendly and their antimicrobial properties make them useful to a broad range of foodborne microbes [12-14].

The process of preserving and extending the shelf life of perishable foods using biological agents, such as microbes and their metabolites, phages, enzymes, or natural antimicrobials, is known as "bio-preservation" [15]. The public and the food industry are very much benefiting from technological advances in this method of preservation. To limit microbial growth and to ensure the safety of food, biological preservation can be successfully achieved by combining a variety of natural additives. Furthermore, it provides supplementary nutrition and protection of food quality as well as dietary properties [12]. Due to their historical roles in the production of fermented foods, ability to produce antimicrobial metabolites, and safety for consumption, certain strains of lactic acid bacteria (LAB), *Bacillus* spp., *Bifidobacterium* spp., and *Saccharomyces cerevisiae* are common probiotics or food cultures for this purpose [12].

Probiotics may have advantages for humans, but they may also have disadvantages, such as the potential for adverse reactions in some individuals, uncertainty about their effects on the microbiome, worries about the quality and viability of supplements during pre- to post-processing, and the possibility of antibiotic resistance developing with excessive use [16]. Therefore, using compounds that outperform probiotics in terms of benefits while lacking their drawbacks can be beneficial.

Postbiotics, also known as metabiotics, biogenics, or cell-free supernatants, are becoming more popular as the focus of food bio-preservation research. In culture media or fermentation process, food, or the gastrointestinal system, helpful bacteria, in particular probiotics (i.e., LAB, *Bifidobacterium* spp., *S. cerevisiae*, and *Bacillus* spp.), create postbiotics [17].

Postbiotics may be of great interest because they differ from probiotics in a number of ways, including increased safety and better processability. Postbiotics can be added to foods with the highest levels of acidity before thermal processing because they are naturally stable throughout a wide range of temperatures and pH levels [18]. Additionally, postbiotics can be added to nondairy drinks where probiotics cannot thrive due to the low pH and water activity. Notably, the majority of postbiotics interact with other food ingredients infrequently or not at all. furthermore, it is not necessary to think about preserving postbiotic activity while storing and transporting postbiotic products. Additionally, because postbiotics lost their ability to reproduce and migrate, avoiding bacteremia or fungemia, they are anticipated to be safer than probiotics [19].

Postbiotics

The two primary pathways by which intestinal microbiomes affect health are as follows; the probiotics-dependent crucial pathway, which depends on the microbiome's viability, and the postbiotics-dependent novel pathway, which depends on non-living microbiome products [20, 21]. Cell structures or physiological functions of bacteria may change with the inactivation of bacterial cells through physical chemical methods. Therefore, the microbial cells are not able to grow after the use of these methods, but they will continue to have a positive effect [22, 23]. Postbiotics are soluble substances that come from probiotic cells and include cell corpses, cell components, cell-wall fractions, cellular secretions, and metabolites. If consumed in large enough quantities, postbiotics can have beneficial effects on the host's health. Postbiotics, in addition, provide evidence for the health benefits of probiotics metabolites and show how those probiotics can be used to treat GI problems after they have passed over intestinal defenses. The word "postbiotic," on the other hand, refers to soluble metabolites secreted by living bacteria or liberated from their structure upon lysis. These byproducts give the host increased biological activity and certain physiological consequences [23, 24].

The stability of postbiotics is among their most important advantages [25]. Postbiotics are far more robust and resistant to heat, light, and stomach acids than many probiotics, which can be inactivated by these elements [26, 27]. Safety is another benefit of postbiotics over probiotics. Probiotics are generally thought to be safe for healthy people, but those with weakened immune systems run the risk of infection or overgrowth. Postbiotics, in contrast, do not carry the same danger of infection or overgrowth because they are not living bacteria. Additionally, postbiotics are practical and simple to include in diets. Postbiotics, as opposed to probiotics, can be added to food and beverages without specific precautions, although probiotics frequently need refrigeration and cautious storage to retain their efficacy [28]. They can be included into a variety of foods and beverages because they are also more resistant to pH changes [26]. Postbiotics also contain conjugated linoleic acid, organic acids, short-chain fatty acids (SCFA), proteins, bioactive peptides, bacteriocins, biosurfactants, enzymes, and vitamins. Postbiotics also contain several substances that are safe for eukaryotic cells and frequently have antioxidant and antibacterial properties [29, 30].

Postbiotics have potential uses in the food industry, such as the development of functional foods, the use of postbiotics as biofilm inhibitors and removers [31], and the incorporation of postbiotics into food formulations and packaging materials to guarantee the safety and quality of food [32, 33]. For instance, recent research has revealed that postbiotics made from the bacteria Pediococcus acidilactici and *L. sakei* include flavonoids, phenolics, and their metabolites that can drastically lower the amount of foodborne pathogens in food [34, 35]. Postbiotics can be incorporated into active antimicrobial food packaging systems in a variety of ways, including coating or adsorbing a thin layer of postbiotics onto the polymer surface, attaching specific postbiotics, such as bacteriocins and enzymes to polymers via ion or covalent linkages, incorporating postbiotics directly into the packaging polymer matrix, and laminating the postbiotic-loaded active film between two external layers to enhance postbiotic adhesion [4, 36]. Postbiotics' stability is also unaffected because they can be integrated into the polymer matrix. Bio-preservation and packaging are the main topics of the majority of studies on the use of postbiotics in food.

Classification of Postbiotics

The host's intestine is a suitable environment for the microbiome community, with numerous metabolites that are very low molecular weight during this life cycle which play an important role in regulating growth and development of good bacteria, cellular communication and protection from certain stress factors [23, 37]. Some of these soluble metabolites secrete by live bacteria or release into the host's intestinal environment where they create a specified physiological effect from altering cellular processes or metabolic pathways [38]. The postbiotic components can be divided into different categories based on their basic chemical structures, such as lipids (butyrate, propionate, acetate, lactate, dimethylacetyl-derived plasmalogen), organic acids (propionic and 3-phenyl lactic acid), proteins (lactocepin, p40, and p75 molecules (soluble proteins)), carbohydrates (galactose-rich polysaccharides, and teichoic acids), complex molecules (lipoteichoic acids and peptidoglycan-derived muropeptides), and vitamins (B-group vitamins) or by their biological processes, such as their anti-oxidant, anti-hypertensive, immunomodulatory, anti-inflammatory, low-cholesterol, and anti-proliferative actions [39]. It's also vital to remember that postbiotics, like prebiotic substances, promote the development of probiotics in each person's digestive system as opposed to introducing new strains of bacteria to the gut microbiota [23]. In order to use postbiotics in pharmaceutical or food formulations, it is necessary to optimize various extraction and identification methods of their chemical composition, evaluate their safety, and research their function in biological systems [40]. Some postbiotics such as bacteriocins and organic acids also offer significant possibilities in food biological preservatives, food packaging, and biofilm management due to their bacteriostatic capacity [41].

Methods of Applying Postbiotics in Food

Depending on the type of food and postbiotic form, postbiotics have been generated from and used in liquid or lyophilized form in numerous research. Postbiotics in dry form were used in formulations of foods such as fish, ground meat, cheese, bakery, and liquid food in either free or encapsulated forms. On the other hand, postbiotic solutions were sprayed on or mixed into coatings or films for fish and meat fillets, poultry, fruits, and vegetables [42]. Although postbiotics are frequently given directly to foods, their integration into coating and film matrices has been carefully studied by researchers. Other techniques, like spraying and washing, have also been used. The qualities of the food, the type of postbiotics, and the physical characteristics of the film and coatings solutions are only a few of the variables that affect each method's benefits and drawbacks [43, 44].

Postbiotics as Novel Bio-Preservation Strategy in Food Industry

Bacteriostatic postbiotics have been used extensively in recent years to enhance food quality, according to reports. For instance, the only bacteriocin that has been licensed for use as a food preservative is nisin (a postbiotic of lantibiotic generated by particular *L. lactis* subsp. *lactis* strains), which is frequently used in dairy products, bakery, baby food, and canned soup [19]. Additionally, *P. pentosaceus* produces bacteriocins, which include both hydrophilic and hydrophobic areas, and which are widely used in food packaging due to their ability to suppress the growth of Gram-positive bacteria like *L. monocytogenes* [45].

In dairy products, the genera Lactobacillus and Pediococcus have frequently been used. Pediocin, a heat- and acid-resistant chemical produced by the Pediococcus genus, has been recognized for its usage in dairy products because most dairy products experience heat treatment during processing. Among these, *L. plantarum* stands out for its capacity to prevent the growth of fungi by destroying cell structure utilizing a variety of metabolites, such as lactic acid, fatty acids, peptides, and bacteriocin (plantaricin), which are phenolic compounds. Additionally, *L. plantarum* produces metabolites that bind to mycotoxins, including organic acids, amino acids, and enzymes [46]. Furthermore, Cell-free supernatant from *L. plantarum* YML007 can be used as potential biological preservation to prevent soybean grains from a variety of food spoilage molds and bacteria and to extend their shelf life to two months [19]. Additionally, the bacteriostatic properties of the organic acids produced by microbes such as phenyllactic acid, lactic, acetic, propionic, butyric acids, and epsilon-polylysine could enhance the quality and shelf life of some foods. For example, phenyllactic acid generated by lactic acid bacteria is a key broad-spectrum antibacterial chemical that inhibits the growth of unwanted germs through numerous ways and has been widely employed in dairy and bakery products [47].

There is an increasing emphasis on ingesting nondairy probiotic foods, such as fruits and vegetables, as some people are unable to take probiotic dairy products due to lactose intolerance, milk protein allergy, cholesterol concerns, or vegetarianism. Probiotics can, however, be challenging to add to fruits and vegetables [48, 49]. Typically, probiotics can adversely alter the physical features (for example, fruit color), sensory aspects, and acceptability of food when they directly create organic acids in the food matrix and lower the pH [50]. Postbiotics in fruits and vegetables, however, provide a number of benefits. Bacteriocins found in some postbiotics can help preserve fruits and vegetables. Exopolysaccharide-rich postbiotics can improve the flavor and texture of fruits and vegetables. Additionally, postbiotic solutions can be used to wash and sterilize fresh products [51-53]. Postbiotics for fruit and vegetable applications have frequently been made with the help of *Lactobacillus* and *Pediococcus* species. *L. plantarum* is a popular strain among them. Contrary to other species, this particular strain is usually isolated from fermented vegetables, making it very accepting with agricultural products. Additionally, *L. plantarum* produces a wide range of antimicrobial substances, including fatty acids, phenolic compounds, carbon dioxide, diacetyl, bacteriocins (plantaricin), organic acids (vanillic acid, gallic acid, and phenyllactic acid), and phenolic compounds (vanillin) [54]. Moreover *L. plantarum*, *L. lactis*, and *P. acidilactici* were among the most researched LAB for producing postbiotics in the case of meat, meat products, and seafood, while several LAB strains have been utilized in poultry. *L. plantarum* generate plantaricin, which is a class of bacteriocins that is highly effective against germs that cause foodborne illness and spoilage. Even at extremely high temperatures, like 121°C, this chemical maintains its stability and activity. It also displays a wide variety of activities. The postbiotics produced by *L. paracasei*, a popular strain utilized in fermented meat products like cooked sausages, chicken, fish, lambs, and fresh meat, have a strong negative effect on meat pathogens [55]. Additionally, beef can be effectively protected from contamination by *E. coli* ATCC 25922 or *L. monocytogenes* Scott A by being wrapped in whey protein films supplemented with *L. sakei* NRRL B-1917 cell-free bacteriostatic supernatant. This not only increases shelf life but also improves safety [19, 56]. Epsilon-polylysine, a novel extracellular antimicrobial made by *Streptomyces albulus*, has also been added to anti-microbial packaging or made into a bacteriostatic agent that was used to preserve longan fruit, sausage, pork, and vacuum-packed large yellow croaker by inhibiting Gram-positive and Gram-negative bacteria, fungi, and yeast [57].

Challenges and Future Perspective in the Application of Postbiotics in Foods

Despite the postbiotics' potential advantages in food preservation and packing, there are still a few issues that need to be researched further. For instance, there are still gaps in the authorization and law governing postbiotic foods, and there are no defined guidelines for their use. It's also unknown how often and at what dosage postbiotics are used in food [23]. Furthermore, certain possible postbiotic-derived strains' safety is still up for debate. Since some postbiotic combinations may have a high moisture content, a brownish or yellow color, or specific sensory properties, the use of postbiotics in food raises questions about the potential physical and chemical changes that could take place following their inclusion [58, 59]. Additionally, it is still uncertain how much postbiotics should be used to package and preserve food [19]. It is critical to take into account the quantity and quality of enzymes in postbiotic solutions made from advantageous microbial strains when employing postbiotics in foods. Proteolytic and lipolytic enzymes at high concentrations are present in some postbiotics, which could be problematic [24].

The precise postbiotic components are still challenging to determine and categorize under the available technical conditions. There are numerous technological challenges to be resolved in order to get and identify the individual postbiotics in order to explore the potential function of postbiotics systematically and thoroughly. In order to prepare postbiotics after the inactivation and lysis of microbial cells, effective extraction and purification processes, such as centrifugation, dialysis, freeze-drying, and column purification, must also be developed [60]. The precise mechanism by which postbiotics prevent specific diseases, the dose-effect relationship of postbiotics added to the food matrix, the qualitative and quantitative characterization of foods containing postbiotics, and new technologies for large-scale industrial production of postbiotic elements are all significant topics that require further research.

Conclusion

Postbiotics are projected to be used more frequently in the food industry, especially in food bio-preservation and the creation of functional meals that offer health advantages beyond basic nutrition. This chapter makes the case that postbiotics can act as nutritional and functional elements of food packaging and bio-preservation. The majority of current research focuses on creating postbiotics utilizing well-known probiotics and incorporating them into food products, while scientists are also looking into novel species that may have useful functions. LAB, in particular Lactobacillus, are widely used in the synthesis of postbiotics. Considering the antimicrobial properties of the majority of investigated postbiotics, using combined methods and compounds would likely yield improved functionalities. Although the direct incorporation of postbiotics into food products is a popular method, other approaches, such as spraying and incorporation into packaging materials, have gained significant attention. Postbiotics have been most studied, but it's important to see how postbiotics and paraprobiotics are absorbed in different foods. Based on the research exploring new uses for postbiotics, it is possible to increase their efficacy in food bio-preservation and packaging by using postbiotics within nanotechnology creating new nanomaterials from them. The main focus of the use of postbiotics for food biopreservation and packaging should be to conduct a comprehensive research aimed at addressing these problems.

Disclaimer

None.

References

[1] Guimarães J. T., Balthazar C. F., Silva R., Rocha R. S., Graça J. S., Esmerino E. A., Silva M. C., Sant'Ana A. S., Duarte M. C. K., Freitas M. Q. Impact of probiotics and prebiotics on food texture. *Current Opinion in Food Science*. 2020;33:38-44.

[2] O'Connor P. M., Kuniyoshi T. M., Oliveira R. P., Hill C., Ross R. P., Cotter P. D. Antimicrobials for food and feed; a bacteriocin perspective. *Current opinion in biotechnology*. 2020;61:160-7.

[3] Sheykhsaran E., Abbasi A., Baghi H. B., Ghotaslou R., Sharifi Y., Sefidan F. Y., Laghousi D., Hosainzadegan H., Hasani A., Sadeghi J. Staphylococcus aureus: A bacterial candidate for multiple sclerosis incidence and progression. *Reviews and Research in Medical Microbiology* 2022, *33*, 212-220.

[4] Abbasi A., Sabahi S., Bazzaz S., Tajani A. G., Lahouty M., Aslani R., Hosseini H. An edible coating utilizing Malva sylvestris seed polysaccharide mucilage and postbiotic from Saccharomyces cerevisiae var. boulardii for the preservation of lamb meat. *International Journal of Biological Macromolecules* 2023, *246*, 125660.

[5] Pujato S. A., del L. Quiberoni A., Candioti M. C., Reinheimer J. A., Guglielmotti D. M. Leuconostoc citreum MB1 as biocontrol agent of Listeria monocytogenes in milk. *Journal of Dairy Research.* 2014;81[2]:137-45.

[6] Sabahi S., Abbasi A., Mortazavi S. A. Characterization of cinnamon essential oil and its application in Malva sylvestris seed mucilage edible coating to the enhancement of the microbiological, physicochemical and sensory properties of lamb meat during storage. *Journal of Applied Microbiology.* 2022;133[2]:488-502.

[7] de Arauz L. J., Jozala A. F., Mazzola P. G., Penna T. C. V. Nisin biotechnological production and application: a review. *Trends in Food Science & Technology.* 2009;20[3-4]:146-54.

[8] Abbasi A., Rad A. H., Ghasempour Z., Sabahi S., Kafil H. S., Hasannezhad P., Rahbar Saadat Y., Shahbazi N. The biological activities of postbiotics in gastrointestinal disorders. *Critical Reviews in Food Science and Nutrition* 2022, *62*, 5983-6004.

[9] Abbasi A., Sanej K. D., Moradi S., Bazzaz S., Esmaeili A., Ghafourian K., Sabahi S., Lahouty M., Akrami S., Aslani R. Bioactive Compounds and Biological Activities of Allium sativum L. *Bioactive Compounds in the Storage Organs of Plants*: Springer; 2023. p. 1-40.

[10] Abbasi A., Bazzaz S., Da Cruz A. G., Khorshidian N., Saadat Y. R., Sabahi S., Ozma M. A., Lahouty M., Aslani R., Mortazavian A. M. A Critical Review on Akkermansia muciniphila: Functional Mechanisms, Technological Challenges, and Safety Issues. *Probiotics and Antimicrobial Proteins.* 2023:1-23.

[11] Singh V. P. Recent approaches in food bio-preservation-a review. *Open veterinary journal.* 2018;8[1]:104-11.

[12] Muthuvelu K. S., Ethiraj B., Pramnik S., Raj N. K., Venkataraman S., Rajendran D. S., Bharathi P., Palanisamy E., Narayanan A. S., Vaidyanathan V. K. Biopreservative technologies of food: an alternative to chemical preservation and recent developments. *Food Science and Biotechnology.* 2023:1-14.

[13] Ozma M. A., Abbasi A., Ahangarzadeh Rezaee M., Hosseini H., Hosseinzadeh N., Sabahi S., Noori S. M. A., Sepordeh S., Khodadadi E., Lahouty M. A critical review on the nutritional and medicinal profiles of garlic's (Allium sativum L.) bioactive compounds. *Food Reviews International.* 2022:1-38.

[14] Ghorbani-Tajani A., Mohammadi R., Shahrooz R. Effect of Local Transplantation of Bone Marrow Derived Mast Cells (BMMCs) Combined with Chitosan Biofilm on Excisional and Incisional Wound Healing: A Novel Preliminary Animal Study on Lamb. *Iranian Journal of Veterinary Surgery.* 2019;14(1):34-43.

[15] Lücke F. K. *Overview of Biopreservation*. 2023.

[16] Xu C., Ban Q., Wang W., Hou J., Jiang Z. Novel nano-encapsulated probiotic agents: Encapsulate materials, delivery, and encapsulation systems. *Journal of Controlled Release.* 2022;349:184-205.

[17] Hosseini H., Abbasi A., Sabahi S., Akrami S., Yousefi-Avarvand A. Assessing the Potential Biological Activities of Postbiotics Derived from Saccharomyces cerevisiae: An *In Vitro* Study. *Probiotics and Antimicrobial Proteins.* 2023:1-17.

[18] Siciliano R. A., Reale A., Mazzeo M. F., Morandi S., Silvetti T., Brasca M. Paraprobiotics: A new perspective for functional foods and nutraceuticals. *Nutrients*. 2021;13[4]:1225.

[19] Zhong Y., Wang T., Luo R., Liu J., Jin R., Peng X. Recent advances and potentiality of postbiotics in the food industry: Composition, inactivation methods, current applications in metabolic syndrome, and future trends. *Critical Reviews in Food Science and Nutrition*. 2022:1-25.

[20] Leylabadlo H. E., Heravi F. S., Soltani E., Abbasi A., Kafil H. S., Parsaei M., Sanaie S., Ahmadian Z., Ghotaslou R. The role of gut microbiota in the treatment of irritable bowel syndrome. *Reviews and Research in Medical Microbiology*. 2022;33[1]:e89-e104.

[21] Abbasi A., Hajipour N., Hasannezhad P., Baghbanzadeh A., Aghebati-Maleki L. Potential *in vivo* delivery routes of postbiotics. *Critical Reviews in Food Science and Nutrition*. 2022;62[12]:3345-69.

[22] de Almada C. N., Almada C. N., Martinez R. C., Sant'Ana A. S. Paraprobiotics: Evidences on their ability to modify biological responses, inactivation methods and perspectives on their application in foods. *Trends in food science & technology*. 2016;58:96-114.

[23] Sabahi S., Homayouni Rad A., Aghebati-Maleki L., Sangtarash N., Ozma M. A., Karimi A., Hosseini H., Abbasi A. Postbiotics as the new frontier in food and pharmaceutical research. *Critical Reviews in Food Science and Nutrition*. 2022:1-28.

[24] Ozma M. A., Abbasi A., Sabahi S. Characterization of postbiotics derived from Lactobacillus paracasei ATCC 55544 and its application in Malva sylvestris seed mucilage edible coating to the improvement of the microbiological, and sensory properties of lamb meat during storage. *Biointerface Res Appl Chem*. 2022;13.

[25] Pimentel T. C., Cruz A. G., Pereira E., da Costa W. K. A., da Silva Rocha R., de Souza Pedrosa G. T., dos Santos Rocha C., Alves J. M., Alvarenga V. O., Sant'Ana A. S. Postbiotics: An overview of concepts, inactivation technologies, health effects, and driver trends. *Trends in Food Science & Technology*. 2023.

[26] Barros C. P., Guimaraes J. T., Esmerino E. A., Duarte M. C. K., Silva M. C., Silva R., Ferreira B. M., Sant'Ana A. S., Freitas M. Q., Cruz A. G. Paraprobiotics and postbiotics: Concepts and potential applications in dairy products. *Current opinion in food science*. 2020;32:1-8.

[27] Ozma M. A., Nabizadeh E., Valiollahzadeh M. R., Rashedi J., Poor B. M., Asgharzadeh V., Kafil H. S., Khodadadi E., Taghinejad Z., Abbasi A. *Different Dimensions of the Effects of SARS-CoV-2 in Causing Fluctuations in the Blood Pressure of Patients*. 2022.

[28] Ozma M. A., Moaddab S. R., Hosseini H., Khodadadi E., Ghotaslou R., Asgharzadeh M., Abbasi A., Kamounah F. S., Aghebati Maleki L., Ganbarov K. A critical review of novel antibiotic resistance prevention approaches with a focus on postbiotics. *Critical Reviews in Food Science and Nutrition*. 2023:1-19.

[29] Abbasi A., Rad A. H., Maleki L. A., Kafil H. S., Baghbanzadeh A. Antigenotoxicity and Cytotoxic Potentials of Cell-Free Supernatants Derived from Saccharomyces

cerevisiae var. boulardii on HT-29 Human Colon Cancer Cell Lines. *Probiotics and Antimicrobial Proteins.* 2023:1-13.

[30] Abbasi A., Rad A. H., Maleki L. A., Kafil H. S., Baghbanzadeh A. Cytotoxic Potentials of Cell-Free Supernatant Derived from Lactobacillus casei CRL431 on HCT-116 and HT-29 *Human Colon Cancer Cell Lines.* 2022.

[31] Hossain M. I., Mizan M. F. R., Roy P. K., Nahar S., Toushik S. H., Ashrafudoulla M., Jahid I. K., Lee J., Ha S. D. Listeria monocytogenes biofilm inhibition on food contact surfaces by application of postbiotics from Lactobacillus curvatus B. 67 and Lactobacillus plantarum M. 2. *Food Research International.* 2021; 148:110595.

[32] Sheykhsaran E., Abbasi A., Ebrahimzadeh Leylabadlo H., Sadeghi J., Mehri S., Naeimi Mazraeh F., Feizi H., Bannazadeh Baghi H. Gut microbiota and obesity: an overview of microbiota to microbial-based therapies. *Postgraduate medical journal.* 2023;99[1171]:384-402.

[33] Ozma M. A., Abbasi A., Akrami S., Lahouty M., Shahbazi N., Ganbarov K., Pagliano P., Sabahi S, Köse Ş., Yousefi M. Postbiotics as the key mediators of the gut microbiota-host interactions. *Le infezioni in medicina.* 2022;30[2]:180.

[34] İncili G. K., Karatepe P., Akgöl M., Tekin A., Kanmaz H., Kaya B., Çalıcıoğlu M., Hayaloğlu A. A. Impact of chitosan embedded with postbiotics from Pediococcus acidilactici against emerging foodborne pathogens in vacuum-packaged frankfurters during refrigerated storage. *Meat Science.* 2022;188:108786.

[35] Homayouni-rad A., Aghebati-Maleki L., Samadi-Kafil H., Abbasi A., Khani N. Postbiotics as a safe alternative to live probiotic bacteria in the food and pharmaceutical industries. *HBI_Journals.* 2021;26:132-57.

[36] Rad A. H., Aghebati-Maleki L., Kafil H. S., Abbasi A. Molecular mechanisms of postbiotics in colorectal cancer prevention and treatment. *Critical reviews in food science and nutrition*. 2021;61[11]:1787-803.

[37] Abbasi A., Sheykhsaran E., Kafil H. S. *Postbiotics: science, technology and applications:* Bentham Science Publishers; 2021.

[38] Laursen M. F., Sakanaka M., von Burg N., Mörbe U., Andersen D., Moll J. M., Pekmez C. T., Rivollier A., Michaelsen K. F., Mølgaard C. Bifidobacterium species associated with breastfeeding produce aromatic lactic acids in the infant gut. *Nature microbiology.* 2021;6[11]:1367-82.

[39] Homayouni Rad A., Aghebati Maleki L., Samadi Kafil H., Abbasi A. Postbiotics: A novel strategy in food allergy treatment. *Critical reviews in food science and nutrition.* 2021;61[3]:492-9.

[40] Abbasi A., Aghebati-Maleki A., Yousefi M., Aghebati-Maleki L. Probiotic intervention as a potential therapeutic for managing gestational disorders and improving pregnancy outcomes. *Journal of reproductive immunology.* 2021;143:103244.

[41] Abbasi A., Aghebati-Maleki L., Homayouni-Rad A. The promising biological role of postbiotics derived from probiotic Lactobacillus species in reproductive health. *Critical Reviews in Food Science and Nutrition.* 2022;62[32]:8829-41.

[42] Rad A. H., Maleki L. A., Kafil H. S., Zavoshti H. F., Abbasi A. Postbiotics as promising tools for cancer adjuvant therapy. *Advanced Pharmaceutical Bulletin.* 2021;11[1]:1.

[43] Ramazanidoroh F., Hosseininezhad M., Shahrampour D., Wu X. Edible Packaging as a Functional Carrier of Prebiotics, Probiotics, and Postbiotics to Boost Food Safety, Quality, and Shelf Life. *Probiotics and Antimicrobial Proteins.* 2023:1-21.

[44] Rad A. H., Abbasi A., Kafil H. S., Ganbarov K. Potential pharmaceutical and food applications of postbiotics: a review. *Current pharmaceutical biotechnology.* 2020;21[15]:1576-87.

[45] Hosseini S. A., Abbasi A., Sabahi S., Khani N. Application of postbiotics produced by lactic acid bacteria in the development of active food packaging. *Biointerface Research in Applied Chemistry.* 2021;12:6164-83.

[46] Kudupoje M. B., Malathi V., Yiannikouris A. Impact of a Natural Fusarial Multi-Mycotoxin Challenge on Broiler Chickens and Mitigation Properties Provided by a Yeast Cell Wall Extract and a Postbiotic Yeast Cell Wall-Based Blend. *Toxins.* 2022;14[5]:315.

[47] Rajanikar R., Nataraj B. H., Naithani H., Ali S. A., Panjagari N. R., Behare P. V. Phenyllactic acid: A green compound for food biopreservation. *Food Control.* 2021;128:108184.

[48] Rad A. H., Maleki L. A., Kafil H. S., Zavoshti H. F., Abbasi A. Postbiotics as novel health-promoting ingredients in functional foods. *Health promotion perspectives.* 2020;10[1]:3-4.

[49] Homayouni-Rad A., Fathi-Zavoshti H., Douroud N., Shahbazi N., Abbasi A. Evaluating the role of postbiotics as a new generation of probiotics in health and diseases. *Journal of Ardabil University of Medical Sciences.* 2020;19[4]:381-99.

[50] Abbasi A., Saadat T. R., Saadat Y. R. Microbial exopolysaccharides–β-glucans–as promising postbiotic candidates in vaccine adjuvants. *International Journal of Biological Macromolecules.* 2022.

[51] Saadat Y. R., Khosroushahi A. Y., Movassaghpour A. A., Talebi M., Gargari B. P. Modulatory role of exopolysaccharides of Kluyveromyces marxianus and Pichia kudriavzevii as probiotic yeasts from dairy products in human colon cancer cells. *Journal of Functional Foods.* 2020;64:103675.

[52] Korcz E., Varga L. Exopolysaccharides from lactic acid bacteria: Techno-functional application in the food industry. *Trends in Food Science & Technology.* 2021;110:375-84.

[53] Abbasi A., Sanej K. D., Mohammadi A., Moradi S., Nayeri B. D., Bazzaz S., Hosseini H. *The Role of Postbiotics in Food Safety Promotion.*

[54] Abouloifa H., Gaamouche S., Rokni Y., Hasnaoui I., Bellaouchi R., Ghabbour N., Karboune S., Brasca M., D'Hallewin G., Salah R. B. Antifungal activity of probiotic Lactobacillus strains isolated from natural fermented green olives and their application as food bio-preservative. *Biological Control.* 2021;152:104450.

[55] Sharafi H., Divsalar E., Rezaei Z., Liu S. Q., Moradi M. The potential of postbiotics as a novel approach in food packaging and biopreservation: a systematic review of the latest developments. *Critical Reviews in Food Science and Nutrition.* 2023:1-31.

[56] Ghorbani Tajani A., Bisha B. Effect of Food Matrix and Treatment Time on the Effectiveness of Grape Seed Extract as an Antilisterial Treatment in Fresh Produce. *Microorganisms.* 2023;11[4]:1029.

[57] Lan W., Sun Y., Zhang N., Xie J. Effects of ε-polylysine and rosemary extract on quality attributes and microbial communities in vacuum-packaged large yellow croaker (Pseudosciaena crocea) during ice storage. *Food Science and Biotechnology*. 2021;30:465-74.

[58] Gervasoni L. F., Gervasoni K., de Oliveira Silva K., Mendes M. E. F., Maddela N. R., Prasad R., Winkelstroter L. K. Postbiotics in active food packaging: The contribution of cellulose nanocomposites. *Sustainable Chemistry and Pharmacy*. 2023;36:101280.

[59] Alesaeidi S., Kahrizi M. S., Ghorbani Tajani A., Hajipour H., Ghorbani M. Soy protein isolate/sodium alginate hybrid hydrogel embedded with hydroxyapatite for tissue engineering. *Journal of Polymers and the Environment*. 2023;31[1]:396-405.

[60] Tajani A. G., Carr J., Elbakush A., Bisha B., Gomelsky M. Evaluation of an Enzymatic Treatment to Control Listerial Biofilm on Produce. *IAFP* 2021. 2021.

Index

A

B

C

D

E

F

G

O

P

R

S

T

V